DVD contents

Video editor:

Kristin A. Boehm

- Local anesthesia for breast implants
  A. Aldo Mottura
- Correction of tuberous breast deformity
  Liacyr Ribeiro, Affonso J. Accorsi, Jr
- Mastopexy augmentation
  Mark A. Codner
- Primary augmentation mastopexy
  G. Patrick Maxwell, Allen Gabriel
- Circumvertical reduction mammaplasty
  A. Aldo Mottura
- Vertical reduction mammaplasty
  Elizabeth J. Hall-Findlay
- Vertical reduction mammaplasty with superior pedicle
  Foad Nahai
- No vertical scar mastopexy or breast reduction
  © *Donald H. Lalonde*
- Spiral flap breast reshaping in the massive weight loss patient
  Dennis J. Hurwitz
- Capsule dissection
  © *Bradley P. Bengtson*
- Short scar mastopexy and reduction mammaplasty
  Thomas Biggs, Ruth Graf

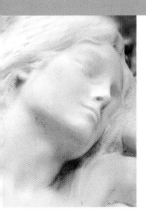

Aesthetic Breast Surgery

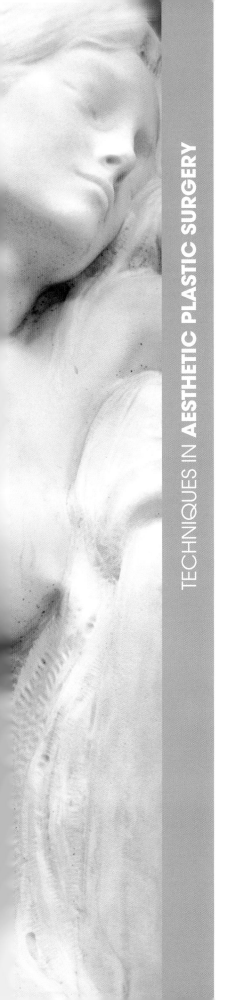

TECHNIQUES IN **AESTHETIC PLASTIC SURGERY**

Aesthetic Breast Surgery

Edited by

Louis P. Bucky MD, FACS

Associate Professor of Surgery, Department of Surgery,
University of Pennsylvania School of Medicine,
Philadelphia, PA, USA

A. Aldo Mottura MD, PhD

Plastic Surgeon, Private Practice, Córdoba, Argentina

Series Editor

Mark A. Codner MD

Plastic Surgeon, Private Practice, Paces Plastic Surgery,
Atlanta, GA
Clinical Assistant Professor, Division of Plastic and
Reconstructive Surgery, Emory University, Atlanta, GA,
USA

SAUNDERS

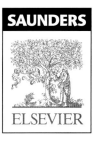

ELSEVIER

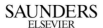

SAUNDERS
ELSEVIER

An imprint of Elsevier Limited

© 2009, Elsevier Limited. All rights reserved.

First published 2009

The right of Louis P. Bucky and A. Aldo Mottura to be identified as editors of this work has been asserted by them in accordance with the Copyright, Designs and Patents Act 1988.

ISBN 978-0-7020-3091-8

British Library Cataloguing in Publication Data
A catalogue record for this book is available from the British Library

Library of Congress Cataloging in Publication Data
A catalog record for this book is available from the Library of Congress

Notice
Medical knowledge is constantly changing. Standard safety precautions must be followed, but as new research and clinical experience broaden our knowledge, changes in treatment and drug therapy may become necessary or appropriate. Readers are advised to check the most current product information provided by the manufacturer of each drug to be administered to verify the recommended dose, the method and duration of administration, and contraindications. It is the responsibility of the practitioner, relying on experience and knowledge of the patient, to determine dosages and the best treatment for each individual patient. Neither the Publisher nor the authors assume any liability for any injury and/or damage to persons or property arising from this publication.

The Publisher

Printed in Spain
Last digit is the print number: 9   8   7   6   5   4   3   2   1

your source for books,
journals and multimedia
in the health sciences

www.elsevierhealth.com

The
publisher's
policy is to use
**paper manufactured
from sustainable forests**

Working together to grow
libraries in developing countries

www.elsevier.com | www.bookaid.org | www.sabre.org

ELSEVIER   BOOK AID
              International   Sabre Foundation

Commissioning Editor: Sue Hodgson
Development Editor: Martin Mellor
Project Manager: Camilla Cudjoe
Design: Charles Gray
Illustration Manager: Gillian Richards
Illustrator: Electronic Publishing Services Inc, NYC
Marketing Manager(s) (UK/USA): John Canelon/Brenna Christensen

Contents

Contents

Series Foreword

As editor of the *Techniques in Aesthetic Plastic Surgery* series, I would like to take this opportunity to foremost thank the reader and hope that you find this five-volume series as interesting and informative as I. As physicians, we have a number of responsibilities, including responsibilities to care for our patients and responsibilities to educate each other. In fact these two commitments intersect at the crossroads of publishing as sharing information allows us to cumulatively take better care of our patients. The goal of the *Techniques in Aesthetic Plastic Surgery* series is to blend a variety of techniques used internationally in synergistic subspecialties such as facial plastic surgery, oculoplastic surgery, dermatologic plastic surgery, and others. With that end in mind, I am delighted that the accomplished and internationally-esteemed colleagues who have contributed to this series have freely shared their thoughts, experiences, and techniques with the reader.

The *Techniques in Aesthetic Plastic Surgery* series is a unique compilation of chapters by authors who were personally invited by the editors. We sought out the best surgeons covering a variety of subject matter in an attempt to create five unique, comprehensive volumes in an easy-to-read format. While the field of plastic surgery has grown exponentially in breadth over the past ten years, the fundamental strength of our specialty revolves around maintenance of excellence across its breadth. Unification of the diverse aspects should be emphasized rather than allowing fragmentation of our specialty to develop.

I would like to thank the hard work and contributions made by the volume editors who have created an excellent educational resource, which includes some of the most recent technological breakthroughs in plastic surgery. The short time to publication allows the information in this series to be current, quick and nimble rather than obsolete by the time of publication.

The volume on *Aesthetic breast surgery* edited by Drs Bucky and Mottura is a fine overview of breast surgery which covers a number of very important topics, ranging from incision choices and preoperative evaluation to some of the most refined techniques in augmentation mastopexy and breast reduction. The international perspective is outstanding, and I would like to thank each of the individual authors for their superb chapters and enviable results. The book on *Facial rejuvenation with fillers* is going to be one of the most popular in the series since there has been an exponential surge in the use of non-surgical treatments, particularly with fillers for facial rejuvenation. I would like to congratulate Drs Cohen and Born who have done a terrific job organizing this volume. This text outlines commonly and less commonly used fillers as well as updated information on future fillers that are otherwise difficult to find.

Similarly, the volume on *Lasers and non-surgical rejuvenation* by Drs DiBernardo and Pozner is an absolute gem of a resource for the most effective and current lasers and non-invasive therapies for improving both the face and the body. These procedures are all very popular in the lay press and are among the most common inquiries we receive from patients. This volume is a good source of information as patients often seem to be ahead of the curve when it comes to some of these new non-surgical treatments. I would like to thank my practice associates Drs Farzad Nahai and Foad Nahai for helping put together the volume on *Minimally invasive facial rejuvenation*. The surgical techniques and non-surgical approaches provide a quick and easy review of the most current and popular techniques in this area. Many of the techniques have yet to be published and therefore provide the reader with new concepts that can be used to improve results and minimize complications. Lastly, I hope you will review with interest the volume on *Midface surgery* edited by myself and Drs de Castro and Boehm. I have long felt that surgery of the eyelid and peri-orbital area is the keystone to surgical rejuvenation of the face due to the challenges associated with surgery in this area. This volume is unique in that it provides a number of oculoplastic procedures in addition to some of the standard plastic-surgical procedures. It also presents a blend of oculoplastic surgery and plastic surgery, both in content and in the international spectrum of authors.

Another feature of these volumes is that the reader is able to obtain one or two of the individual books or the entire series. While this series is not meant to be an exhaustive comprehensive encyclopedia on the topics, it is designed to give an overview and description of the most useful and novel techniques. The individual volume editors are experts in their respective fields and have made sure that all of the cherry-picked chapters combine to create a complete review of the topic.

Lastly, I would like to take this time to thank the DVD editor, Dr Kristin Boehm, who is also an associate of mine from Atlanta. She has obtained, edited, and organized high quality videos to compliment each individual volume and demonstrate the techniques that are discussed in the chapters. While the video clips can be viewed without direct reference to the text, the purpose of the DVDs is to complement the text rather than act as a substitute. Since we are able to only show limited surgical techniques, the inclusion of the DVDs is to provide superior demonstration of surgical technique compared to the conventional figures included in the text. I hope you find the *Techniques in Aesthetic Surgery* series useful, whether you are a medical student, resident, fellow, or a seasoned veteran, and that the practical tools of wisdom and knowledge will serve to benefit not only you as a surgeon, but in addition your patients.

Mark A. Codner MD

Preface

It has been a pleasure to work together in the development of this very interesting and timely book on aesthetic breast surgery. Breast surgery is one of the most challenging areas of aesthetic surgery because it requires expertise in management of volume, shape, asymmetries, scars, and tissue/prosthesis interaction. Patients require an uneventful, quick recovery with high satisfaction and low revision rates. In recent years, aesthetic breast surgery has developed new short scars techniques, incorporated new anatomical planes, new implants, fat injections for breast augmentation and surgery on patients after massive weight loss.

These changes are widely publicized in the media and on the internet. Therefore, our patients are more rapidly introduced to the latest advancements. This book provides physicians with a clear, comprehensive opportunity to learn many of these new techniques and provide patients with a very thorough consultation, and advanced management.

The authors of this book are leaders in the field and provide an international experience describing a wide range of problems and techniques. The reader will find a practical view of contemporary breast augmentation, mastopexy, and breast reduction techniques. The chapters include sections on avoiding and managing their problems and complications. Each chapter was written to introduce the reader to key points, to the summary of the operative steps, to pitfalls and how to correct them. The book has nice illustrations artistically drawn and a DVD where some of the described techniques can be viewed. Although plastic surgery is another science of temporary truths, the readers will find here a 'state-of-the-art' book on breast surgery.

We would like to thank Dr Mark Codner for inviting us to participate in this book, which we accepted with enthusiasm. We extend our gratitude to the authors for the thorough preparation of each of the chapters and to the staff at Elsevier, especially to Devika Ponnambalam and Martin Mellor. We have learned a large amount of breast surgery from the contributors of this book and continue to be inspired by their commitment and expertise.

Louis P. Bucky MD, FACS, A. Aldo Mottura MD, PhD

Contributors

Affonso J. Accorsi Jr MD
Plastic Surgeon, Private Practice, Niterói, RJ, Brasil

Bradley P. Bengtson MD, FACS
Plastic Surgeon, Grand Valley Surgical Center Associate Professor, Plastic Surgery, Medical Education Research Center, Michigan State University, Grand Rapids, MI, USA

Giorgio Bronz MD
Private Practice, Clinica Dr. Bronz, Lugano, Switzerland

Daniel A. Del Vecchio MD, MBA
Consultant, Department of Surgery, Massachusetts General Hospital, Harvard Medical School, Boston, MA, USA

L. Franklyn Elliott MD
Plastic Surgeon, Private Practice, Atlanta Plastic Surgery; Clinical Professor, Section of Plastic Surgery, Emory University, Atlanta, GA, USA

Allen Gabriel MD
Director of Clinical Research, Department of Plastic Surgery, Loma Linda University, Loma Linda, CA, USA

Ruth M. Graf MD, PhD
Professor of Plastic Surgery, Hospital de Clínicas, Federal University of Paraná (UFPR), Paraná, Brazil

James C. Grotting MD, FACS
Clinical Professor of Surgery, Division of Plastic Surgery, University of Alabama School of Medicine and The University of Wisconsin-Madison; Private Practice, Grotting Plastic Surgery, Birmingham, AL, USA

Elizabeth J. Hall-Findlay MD, FRCSC
Private Practice, Banff, Alberta, Canada

Dennis J. Hurwitz MD, FACS
Clinical Professor of Surgery (Plastic), University of Pittsburgh Medical Center; Attending Plastic Surgeon, University of Pittsburgh Medical Center at Magee Women's Hospital and South Side Hospital, Pittsburgh, PA, USA

Roger K. Khouri MD, FACS
Private Practice, PlasticandReconstructive Surgery.com, Miami, FL, USA

Phillip L. Lackey MD
Aesthetics and Breast Reconstruction Fellow, Grotting Plastic Surgery, Birmingham, AL, USA

Donald H. Lalonde MD
Professor Plastic Surgery, Dalhousie University, Saint John, NB; Atlantic Health Sciences Corporation Breast Health Program, Saint John, NB, Canada

Janice F. Lalonde RN, CPSN, CPN(C)
Plastic Surgery Nurse, Private Plastic Surgery Practice, Saint John, NB, Canada

G. Patrick Maxwell MD, FACS
Assistant Clinical Professor, Department of Plastic Surgery, Vanderbilt University; Private Practice, Maxwell Aesthetics, Nashville, TN, USA

A. Aldo Mottura MD, PhD
Plastic Surgeon, Private Practice, Córdoba, Argentina

Maria Cecília C. Ono MD
Resident in Plastic Surgery and Post-graduate in Surgery, Hospital de Clínicas, Federal University of Paraná (UFPR), Curitiba, Brazil

Contributors

Mark A. Pinsky MD, PA
Chief, Division of Plastic Surgery, St Mary's Medical Center, West Palm Beach, FL, USA

Liacyr Ribeiro MD
Plastic Surgeon, Private Practice, Rio de Janeiro, Brazil

Roberto B. Rocha MD
Plastic Surgeon, Private Practice, Rio de Janeiro, Brazil

Michael Scheflan MD
Private Practice, Atidim Medical Center, Tel Aviv, Israel

Kenneth C. Shestak MD
Chief of Plastic Surgery, Magee Women's Hospital, Pitttsburgh; Professor of Plastic Surgery, University of Pittsburgh School of Medicine, Pittsburgh, PA, USA

Constantin Stan MD, RASS, ACPR
Plastic and Aesthetic Surgeon, Director of Medical Service Clinic, Bacău, Romania

Steve Teitelbaum MD, FACS
Assistant Clinical Professor of Surgery, David Geffen School of Medicine at UCLA, Los Angeles, CA, USA

André R.D. Tolazzi MD, MSc
Plastic Surgeon, Hospital de Clínicas, Federal University of Paraná (UFPR), Curitiba, Brazil

Dedication

Before I dedicate this book, I would like to thank all of the volume editors and individual authors for their dedication of time, talent, and thought which has created a series of texts most exemplary of the evolution of technique culminating in the current state of the art in plastic surgery. I would also like to thank key individuals at Elsevier who captured this international synergy and brought it from vision to production in a timely fashion: Sue Hodgson, Devika Ponnambalam, and Martin Mellor.

I would like to take this honor to dedicate this five-volume series to my teachers in plastic surgery Drs Jurkiewicz, McCord, Bostwick, Nahai, Hester, Baker, Gordon, and Stuzin, to my friends who have been my teachers in life, and my family who have been my teachers in love including my parents, my wife Jane and our children Molly and Blake. I am grateful for all I have learned from each of you.

MAC

This book is dedicated to my patients who make the practice of plastic surgery interesting, challenging and – ultimately – satisfying. They provide the impetus to improve as a surgeon. I would like to thank my office staff who help care for our patients and allow me the time to continue my education. Lastly, I want to thank my family – Elizabeth, Alexandra and Caroline – who continue to support my professional and educational pursuits with love and encouragement that only a family can offer.

LPB

This book is dedicated to my staff, secretaries and residents for their help supporting my daily activities. It is also dedicated to my son Julian, to my daughters Elisa and Celina – who co-work in my clinic – and to my wife Rosa.

AAM

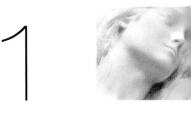

Pre-operative evaluation, preparation and education of the breast augmentation patient

Kenneth C. Shestak

Key points

- Understand what the patient wants and perform a careful pre-operative evaluation.
- Breast and torso dimensions and amount and thickness of breast tissue.
- Breast ptosis.

- Inframammary fold anatomy.
- Asymmetry (IES).
- Transmission of information to patient.
- Pre-operative management of patient expectations and informed consent.

Introduction

Consistently systematic and precise pre-operative patient evaluation, combined with informative patient teaching and pre-operative management of patient expectations is essential for the successful practice of aesthetic plastic surgery. This is especially true in breast augmentation surgery. The following pages outline an approach that has worked for me in minimizing complications and re-operation rates while producing a high level of patient satisfaction following breast augmentation. It is a methodical approach in the evaluation of the prospective patient seeking breast augmentation which includes a careful history with an emphasis on size concerns and a thorough physical examination entailing both an anatomic and aesthetic analysis resulting in an individualized surgical plan (Bostwick 2000, Shestak 2006, Spear 2006b).

As is true in all fields of medicine, the interaction with the patient begins with a careful history and physical examination. This also applies when approaching the prospective breast augmentation patient. Careful attention must be paid to the patient's breast development, whether or not the breast development has been symmetric, the patient's age at menarche and whether there is an appreciable change in breast size or sensitivity during the course of the menstrual cycle. A history of pregnancy is elicited from every patient and if they have been pregnant it is important to inquire about the changes in the breast following such pregnancies. Many patients are concerned by the loss of volume and the change in shape which may have occurred with pregnancy or breast feeding. If a patient has been pregnant I find it helpful to ask how the large the breasts became during pregnancy and whether the patient was comfortable with or liked the size of her breasts during her pregnancy.

Carefully noting the patient's opinion regarding breast settling or ptosis is important. When appropriate, suggestions regarding breast ptosis correction in conjunction with breast augmentation can be made by the plastic surgeon. It is important for the plastic surgeon to inquire about any lumps or masses that the patient may have had in either breast during the course of her lifetime and what treatment was given for this problem. Specifically, it is important to determine exactly what the diagnosis was and how it was resolved. In patients who are older than 35 years of age, the physician must inquire whether the patient has had a mammogram, and if so, the results of the study must be known. I ask the patient whether the mammograms have been normal and will often request that the report be sent to my office for inclusion in the patient's chart. If there is any question about a previous mammogram I will request that the films be sent to my office. I find it helpful to personally review these mammograms with the help of a radiologist. If a patient has not had a mammogram by the time they have reached 35, one should be ordered and the results verified prior to a planned surgical procedure (The American Cancer Society).

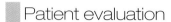

Patient evaluation

Important aspects of the pre-operative physical examination

The plastic surgeon performing breast augmentation must perform a systematic examination of the breasts on each patient. The visual, tactile and artistic senses as well as communication skills of the plastic surgeon all come into play during this essential part of the pre-operative evaluation process (Bostwick 2000, Shestak 2006, Spear 2006b). The surgeon must note the general appearance of the breasts, scanning them for symmetry in terms of contour, fullness, nipple areola position, position of the areola complex relative to the infra-mammary fold and the amount of 'skin show' peripheral to the nipple in all directions (Figure 1.1). The relationship of the breast to the mid-sternal area (cleavage) and the position of the breast relative to chest wall structures is also noted. Examine the anterior and posterior aspect of the patient's torso looking for musculoskeletal abnormalities such as scoliosis and soft tissue abnormalities that can produce asymmetry(ies). Both obvious and subtle asymmetries are noted.

As alluded to previously, I find it helpful to measure the dimensions of the breast including the base width (Tebbetts 2002), height (i.e., the extent of upper pole fullness when the breast is gently compressed against the chest wall) and various distances of the breast architectural features from a fixed point on the torso (Figure 1.2). Most frequently, I measure the distance from the nipple to the supra-sternal notch on each side followed by the distance of nipple to the IM fold

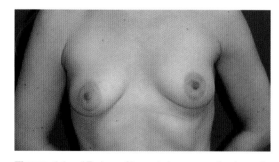

Figure 1.1   AP view of breasts in prospective breast augmentation patient. Note differences in nipple position, lateral contours and skin show peripheral to the nipple–areola complex.

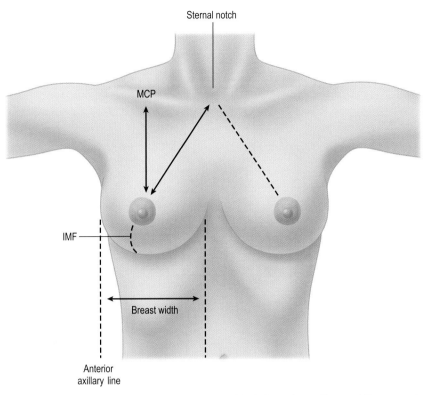

Figure 1.2 Diagram of breasts illustrating important topographical dimensions of base width, supra-sternal notch to nipple (SSN-nipple), nipple to infra-mammary fold (IMF) distances which are important in planning.

in the mid-meridian of the breast and also the distance from the inferior aspect of the areola complex to the IM fold. I record all these measurements on a breast diagram (Figure 1.2) and incorporate the information on a worksheet (Shestak 2006) compiled for use in breast augmentation and kept in the patient's chart (Figure 1.3).

The inframammary fold (IMF) is perhaps THE critical structure in determining breast shape and lower breast pole aesthetics. It is also a key indicator of breast abnormalities, developmental problems and asymmetries. The inframammary fold is formed by a condensation of connective tissue arising as a coalecence of anterior and posterior leaves of the superficial fascia which is an extension of Scarpa's fascia in the abdomen which inserts into the dermis at the lowest aspect of the inferior pole of the breast. There have been many anatomic studies on the anatomy of this structure and I believe the most informative is that published by Muntan et al (2000). The inframammary fold outlines an arc beginning near midline and continuing laterally

where it extends to the lateral aspect of the breast and its juncture with the lateral chest wall at the anterior axillary line (Bostwick 2000, Shestak 2006, Spear 2006b).

The surgeon should evaluate the fold for its degree of tightness, position on one side of the chest relative to the opposite breast and for any degree of asymmetry. Normally the fold is roughly symmetric when comparing both breasts. Asymmetries in the fold are not uncommon (Figure 1.4) and must be noted by the surgeon and pointed out to the patient pre-operatively. Any flattening or straightness in the curve at any point of this arc may indicate a form of a constricted breast (Figure 1.4A). It may be unilateral or bilateral. When it occurs unilaterally it may not be possible for the breast plastic surgeon to correct this and thus the asymmetry noted pre-operatively will be present post-operatively. A fold that is high and 'tight' (Figure 1.4C) presents potential difficulties when the operative plan entails lowering the fold to accommodate a large implant and in my experience is a

Breast Augmentation Worksheet

Chief complaint: _____

Breast history
Age breast development:_____ Age at menarche: _____
Menses:_____ Change in breasts w/ menses:_____

Height:_____ Weight:_____
Changes in weight:_____

Bra size:_____

Pregnancy history:_____
Size of breasts w/ pregnancy:_____
Did patient like size: _____
Changes after pregnancy:_____

Surgeries on breast:_____
Pathology report:_____

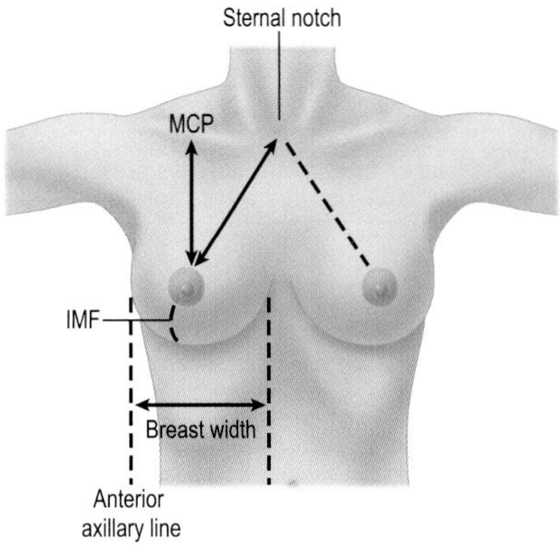

Nipple sensation:_____
Chest wall
Scoliosis:_____
Pectus excavatum:_____
Breasts
Scars:_____
Striae:_____
Constriction:_____
Ptosis/clamifuatim:_____

Breast Dimensions

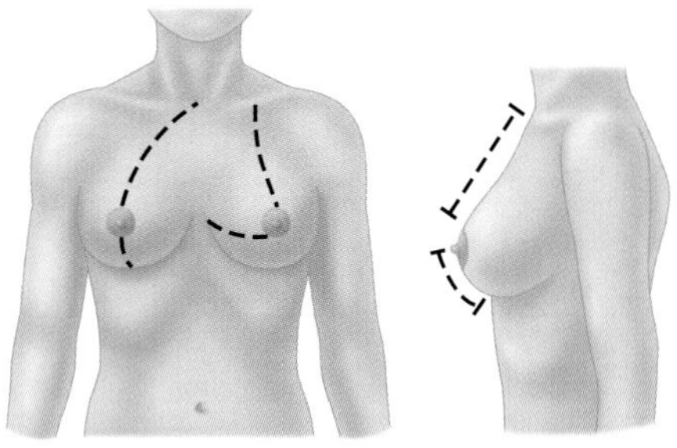

Mammogram reports: _____

Medications: _____

Allergies: _____

Smoking history: _____

Information: Packets:_____ Consent: _____
Silicone information:_____
Questions: Answered:_____
Consent: Signed:_____

Analysis:_____

Recommendations:_____
_____
_____

Plan
Incision:_____
Implant position:_____
Implant characteristics:_____

Figure 1.3 Breast augmentation worksheet containing important pre-operative information and diagrams used for planning the procedure.

predictor of an increased chance for re-operation following breast augmentation (Shestak 2006).

The surgeon should note the thickness, distribution and elasticity of the breast parenchyma (Tebbetts & Adams 2006). The upper pole breast thickness can be determined by grasping the parenchyma 4 cm above the areola in a maneuver described by Tebbets as the 'pinch test' (Figure 1.5) (Tebbetts & Adams 2006). A thickness of at least 2 cm is necessary for the draping the implant if sub-glandular placement of the implant is contemplated. Distances from the nipple to IMF are measured (Figure 1.6A). Other maneuvers to stretch

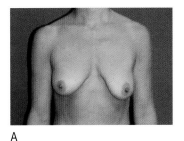
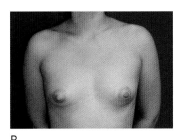
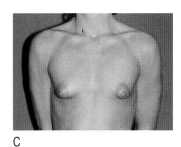

A   B   C

Figure 1.4   Variations in Infra-mammary fold (IMF) morphology. (A) Patient illustrating a flatness of the medial aspect of the IMF medially on the right side indicating a mild focal constriction. This asymmetry of the IM folds may be hard to eliminate at surgery and it should be mentioned to the patient pre-operatively. (B) IM fold asymmetry with higher fold on right than left and bilateral mild constricted breast deformity. (C) Bilateral significant constricted breast deformity with 'high, tight folds'.

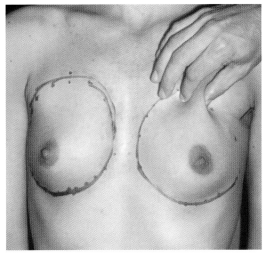

Figure 1.5   Assessing thickness of the soft tissue padding in the upper pole of the breast using the 'pinch test'. A minimum of 2 cm of breast tissue is necessary to minimize implant visibility if a sub-glandular placement of a breast implant is contemplated.

the breast tissue in a superior and anterior direction are helpful in evaluating the potential effects of the implant on the breast tissue (Figure 1.6B,C). Similarly evaluation of skin condition of the breasts is noted with the surgeon keying into the elasticity, the presence of striae and existence of previous scars on the breast skin. Pre-existing striae may become worse following breast augmentation, and a lax skin envelope indicates that the skin will play no role in helping to support a breast implant.

Implant position is determined by tissue factors, degree of ptosis and patient desires. Partial sub-pectoral positioning is the most common site of implant placement in my practice. It provides the maximum thickness of soft tissue padding and thus concealment for the implant, is associated with a lower chance of capsular contracture as reflected in every study in the literature, and it provides the best possible mammograms. This latter benefit of facilitating mammographic evaluation of the breasts cannot be understated. Minimal degrees of breast ptosis are better treated with sub-glandular implant placement. Sub-glandular placement allows a minimally ptotic breast to be re-distributed over the entire implant. The dual plane approach allows redistribution of the lower pole tissue over the implant and is helpful in cases of mammary pseudo-ptosis (Spear 2006b).

It is true that almost no woman's breasts are perfectly symmetric (Bostwick 2000, Shestak 2006). That is to say a careful physical examination will almost always reveal some element of breast asymmetry (Rohrich et al 2006, Spear 2006a). It is essential that the plastic surgeon point out asymmetries to the patient pre-operatively (Shestak 2006, Rohrich et al 2006, Spear 2006a) as these will remain after surgery. Following augmentation of the asymmetric breasts, the overall breast appearance is usually markedly enhanced and the patient will look right past them. Essentially, this is always true if the patient is made aware of the asymmetries prior to surgery. The adage that 'an explanation prior to surgery is an explanation, an explanation after surgery is an excuse' is true in most areas of aesthetic surgery.

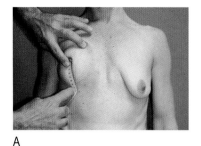 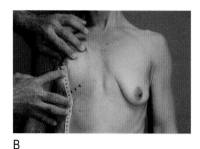 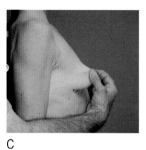

A   B   C

Figure 1.6   Measurement of breast dimensions in repose and with the breast tissue on stretch. These are done to obtain an estimate of potential tissue drape over an implant. (A) Nipple to IM fold without the tissues on stretch. (B) Nipple to IM fold with tissues on stretch. (C) Anterior stretch of the breast tissue.

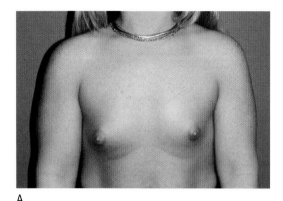 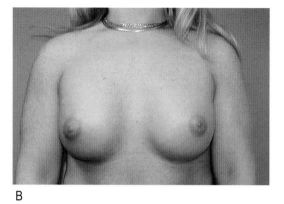

A   B

Figure 1.7   Patient with multiple breast asymmetries including contour, volume, IM fold level, nipple position, nipple inclination and areola size. (A) Pre-operative AP view. (B) One year post-operative view following placement of 12.3 cm base diameter smooth walled saline implants with 360 mL volume, into partial retro-pectoral position. Note that all of the pre-operative asymmetries persist following surgery.

Many elements of asymmetry are illustrated by the patient seen in Figure 1.7. Her pre-operative evaluation revealed multiple breast asymmetries including breast volume, infra-mammary fold level, breast contour with definite difference in the infero-lateral contour, nipple position, nipple inclination, and areola size (Figure 1.7A). The patient underwent the partial retro-pectoral placement of 12.3 cm diameter 360 mL smooth walled moderate profile implants. Note that all of the pre-operative asymmetries are present post-operatively but the breasts show more fullness and overall aesthetic enhancement (Figure 1.7B). Wide set breasts have a wide cleavage (Figure 1.8). This anatomic condition cannot be changed by implants and the cleavage will remain wide after surgery.

Discussion about breast size and implant selection

It is interesting to note that patients have different ideas concerning what is most aesthetic in a breast augmentation and many are interested in obtaining a certain look which they individually feel is most aesthetic. This is illustrated by the fact that many patients bring in pictures pre-operatively indicating how they want their breasts to appear post-operatively. This can be helpful to the surgeon. However, the surgeon must decide if the patient's desires can or should be realized.

Concepts about breast attractiveness relative to size are different in different cultures with women in Europe and South America generally desiring less

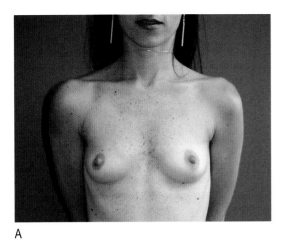
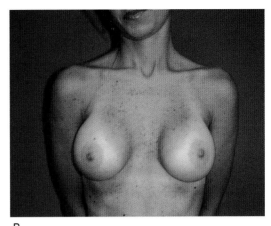

A   B

Figure 1.8 Appearance of a patient with wide cleavage due to lateral displacement of the right breast. (A) Pre-operative AP view. (B) Post-operative AP view following the placement of 11.7 cm base diameter smooth walled saline implants with volume of 300 mL into partial retro-pectoral position.

breast volume enhancement from a breast augmentation. I try to listen very intently to every idea and intention a particular patient has about her perceived post-operative size. As previously mentioned, I have come to understand that what patients want and find desirable is often very different than what the plastic surgeon considers to be an aesthetically desirable result. After my breast analysis which focuses on an analysis of breast dimensions and tissue characteristics and speaking with the patient I can usually narrow the implant choice to either one or two implants.

I perform a final cross-check of the probable implant selection by reviewing photographs brought in by the patient at my request (Shestak 2006). These are images which can be downloaded from a variety of websites containing pre- and post-operative images of actual breast augmentation patients (not models) (Figure 1.9). These provide an important insight into a particular patient's desires and expectations for both volume and shape following breast augmentation. Most often it coincides with my choice of an implant but occasionally there are surprises when a patient wants to be either larger or occasionally smaller than my analysis and communication with the patient has led me to believe. I find, however, that the process of a patient's bringing in photos is helpful to me and more so than having patients place implants in a bra over the surface of their breasts. I do not subscribe to this practice but would suggest it is known for sur-

geons to 'go up one size in the implant' to compensate for the compression effect of the breast and muscle tissue on the implant.

Although the topic of implant selection is covered in other chapters of this volume suffice it to say the pre-operative planning and implant selection depend to a significant degree on patient anatomic factors including breast dimensions, torso dimension, degree of ptosis, tissue elasticity, and pre-existing asymmetry. In my practice, implant selection is governed mostly by anatomic surface relationships, as well as breast and torso dimensions. The 'paradigm shift' of emphasizing correlating implant dimensions (Tebbetts 2001) to important anatomic dimensions of the breast and torso was a positive benefit of using saline implants almost exclusively for breast augmentation from 1992 until 2006 in the United States.

The most important dimension is the base width of the breast (Figure 1.2) or the distance from the area immediately lateral to the lateral edge of the sternum to the mid-axillary line. This distance determines the largest implant which can be placed especially if a round implant is selected. The center of a round implant should be positioned beneath the nipple. If the implant has too great a diameter (i.e., is too large) then the breast will elongate vertically or produce an abnormal horizontal contour. A helpful rule of thumb is that when using a round implant the largest radius which should be used is equal to the distance from the

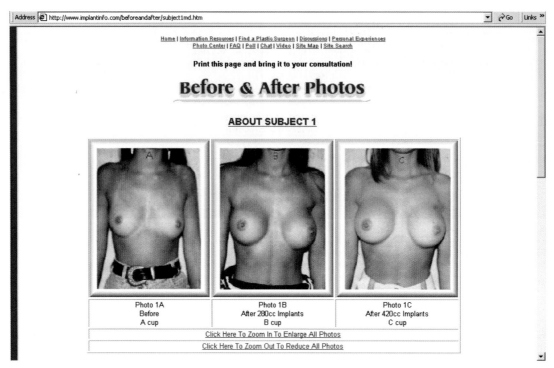

Figure 1.9 Pre- and post-operative images of patient who underwent a bilateral breast augmentation downloaded from the internet from a website called implantinfo.com.

nipple to the immediate parasternal area. This is because the tissues between the nipple and the parasternal area are fixed, i.e., the distensibility of the breast tissue there is less than it is laterally in the area between the nipple and lateral breast. The height of the implant is also important but since the IM fold is often lowered the accomodatable height can vary. The distance from the nipple to the lateral silhouette of the breast on AP is also variable due to the distensibility of those tissues as mentioned above. Therefore, the horizontal distance from the nipple to the parasternal region represents the greatest implant radius that should be used. I will generally choose an implant which is smaller in dimension than this distance.

After carefully recording these dimensions I will consult various implant charts provided by the manufacturers to select an implant which will best satisfy the patient's desires and 'fit' her anatomy. If there are other anatomic considerations such as petite or small stature, or narrow torso, it is often desirable to select an implant with more volume for a given base dimension. In such a patient, a high profile implant (one with greater projection and volume for a given base diameter) may be helpful. Such implants are very helpful in patients who place a premium on a large volume in the face of smaller breast and torso dimensions. Alternatively, a shaped textured implant can be used. These implants are designed with variable heights and volumes for a given base width and they give the illusion of greater projection and volume for a given base diameter dimension (Figure 1.10). I will use a shaped implant with a relatively short vertical dimension in patients of small stature who desire a very full breast. Conversely, I have found that shaped implants which have a long vertical dimension are helpful in the very tall patient (more than 6 feet in height) who requires upper pole fullness as part of their augmentation.

Important information transfer

Information about the options previously discussed is presented to the patient in an interactive format. This is done to encourage active patient participation

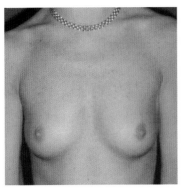
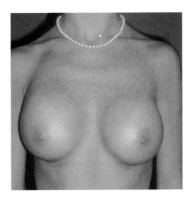

Figure 1.10   Pre- and post-operative views of patient with petite stature who desires large breast volume with minimum upper pole fullness and is an ideal candidate for a shaped implant. The augmentation was performed with a shape textured implant with a base dimension of 12.3 cm and saline fill volume of 370 cc.

in the decision-making process prior to breast augmentation. There is a substantial amount of information which must be presented to the patient who is considering breast augmentation. It is an opportunity for important patient learning and for developing a doctor–patient relationship with the idea of building communication and the trust which is important in helping the patient through the operative experience. This is especially important in helping the patient through post-operative complications. During this time instructions regarding important perioperative and post-operative care are also given to the patient.

Informed consent

Informed consent is an active process during which time the physician (plastic surgeon) presents important information to the patient about a proposed procedure (Gorney 1999, Gorney & Martelo 1999, Gorney 2001, Shestak 2006). Treatment options including no treatment are discussed along with the potential risks and complications associated with each treatment option. These should be presented to the patient in understandable terms and the patient should be allowed to process this information and to ask whatever questions she may have. It is an opportunity for the physician to communicate to the patient that they are entering into the surgical experience together and for the patient to understand that there are no absolute guarantees as to outcome. This allows the patient to see the surgeon not as someone who is omnipotent

but rather as a person with the patient's best intentions as his/her priority in undertaking the procedure.

Plastic surgeons virtually always explain both surgical risks and cosmetic risks of a given procedure. The operation of breast augmentation entails complications that can potentially come into play when an implant is placed. I have defined these as inherent risks of the procedure (Shestak 2006). I will often use the American Society of Plastic Surgeons specially compiled consent form for breast augmentation as a patient resource for learning and as the informed consent document that the patient signs in the office (Figure 1.11). Alternatively, there are check list documents that the patient can initial, such as the one compiled by Mark Gorney of the Doctors Company (Figure 1.12), which details the important aspects of the procedure that the patient needs to understand as a means of consistently explaining and cataloguing the risks of breast augmentation to the patient.

I explain the potential complications of breast augmentation to each patient in terms of surgical, cosmetic and inherent risks. The surgical risks or potential complications with breast augmentation encompass specific risks related to wound healing including issues such as bleeding, hematoma formation, seroma, infection, wound healing imperfections such as wound separation, scar tissue abnormalities, loss of sensation in the skin or nipple–areola complex, and breast pain (a rare but recognized complication following breast augmentation). Infection and wound separation are particularly worrisome complications in that they may result in implant loss. Placing a breast implant in

CONSENT FOR SURGERY / PROCEDURE or TREATMENT

1.   I hereby authorize Dr. _____**Kenneth C. Shestak**_____ and such assistants as may be selected to perform the following procedure or treatment:

     _____ .

     I have received the following information sheet:

INFORMED-CONSENT FOR AUGMENTATION MAMMAPLASTY

     _____ .

2.   I recognize that during the course of the operation and medical treatment or anesthesia, unforeseen conditions may necessitate different procedures than those above. I therefore authorize the above physician and assistants or designees to perform such other procedures that are in the exercise of his or her professional judgment necessary and desirable. The authority granted under this paragraph shall include all conditions that require treatment and are not known to my physician at the time the procedure is begun.

3.   I consent to the administration of such anesthetics considered necessary or advisable. I understand that all forms of anesthesia involves risk and the possibility of complications, injury, and sometimes death.

4.   I acknowledge that no guarantee has been given by anyone as to the results that may be obtained.

5.   I consent to the photographing or televising of the operation(s) or procedure(s) to be performed, including appropriate portons of my body, for medical, scientific or educational purposes, provided my identity is not revealed by the pictures.

6.   For purposes of advancing medical education, I consent to the admittance of observers to the operating room.

7.   I consent to the disposal of any tissue, medical devices or body parts which may be removed.

8.   I authorize the release of my Social Security number to appropriate agencies for legal reporting and medical-device registration if applicable.

9.   IT HAS BEEN EXPLAINED TO ME IN A WAY THAT I UNDERSTAND:
     a.   THE ABOVE TREATMENT OR PROCEDURE TO BE UNDERTAKEN
     b.   THERE MAY BE ALTERNATIVE PROCEDURES OR METHODS OF TREATMENT
     c.   THERE ARE RISKS TO THE PROCEDURE OR TREATMENT PROPOSED
                         SIGN A OR B

A.   I CONSENT TO THE TREATMENT OR PROCEDURE AND THE ABOVE LISTED ITEMS (1-9). I HAVE BEEN ASKED IF I WANT A MORE DETAILED EXPLANATION, BUT I AM SATISFIED WITH THE EXPLANATION, AND DO NOT WANT MORE INFORMATION.

     _____

     Patient or Person Authorized to Sign for Patient

     Date _____   Witness _____

B.   I CONSENT TO THE TREATMENT OR PROCEDURE AND ABOVE LISTED ITEMS (1-9). I REQUESTED AND RECEIVED, IN SUBSTANTIAL DETAIL, FURTHER EXPLANATION OF THE PROCEDURE OR TREATMENT, OTHER ALTERNATIVE PROCEDURES OR METHODS OF TREATMENT AND INFORMATION ABOUT THE MATERIAL RISKS OF THE PROCEDURE OR TREATMENT.

     _____

     Patient or Person Authorized to Sign for Patient

Figure 1.11   Two pages of ASPS informed consent document for breast augmentation.

Breast augmentation is the implantation of artificial material inside the female breasts to enlarge them or give them a different shape for: 1) restoration of normal breast appearance after a mastectomy, 2) enlargement of the breasts in patients who have less breast tissue than they desire, or 3) correction of asymmetry of the breasts.

I authorize and direct _____, M.D., with associates or assistants of his or her choice, to perform the following procedure of Breast Augmentation on _____.

(patient name)

Patient's Initials

_____   The details of the procedure have been explained to me in terms I understand including but not limited to:

subglandular vs. submuscular　　*anticipated size and shape*
preferred technique and why　　*constraints of individual anatomy*
available methods of anesthesia　　*if asymmetry exists, complete correction unlikely*
type of implant to be used

_____   Alternative methods and their benefits and disadvantages have been explained to me.

_____   I understand and accept the most likely risks and complications but are not limited to:

bleeding　　*uncertain life span of implant*
hematoma　　*compromised detection of early breast cancer*
change in nipple sensation　　*possible effects on nursing*
chronic pain　　*capsular contracture*
asymmetry　　*possibility of late calcification*
scarring　　*general disappointment*

_____   I understand and accept the less common complications, including the remote risk of death or serious disability that exists with any surgical procedure.

_____   I am aware that smoking during the pre- and postoperative periods could increase chances of complications.

_____   I have informed the doctor of all my known allergies.

_____   I have informed the doctor of all medications I am currently taking, including prescriptions, over-the-counter remedies, herbal therapies, and any other.

_____   I have been advised whether I should avoid take any or all of these medications on the days surrounding the procedure.

_____   I am aware and accept that no guarantees about the results of the procedure have been made.

_____   I accept financial responsibility for revisions or complications.

_____   I have been informed of what to expect post-operatively, including but not limited to: estimated recovery time, anticipated activity level, and the possibility of additional procedures.

_____   Pre- and post-operative photos and/or videos will be taken of the treatment for record purposes. I understand that these photos and/or videos will be the property of the attending physician.

_____   The doctor has answered all of my questions regarding this procedure.

continued

A

Figure 1.12　Checklist consent document for breast augmentation assembled for use by the Doctors Company. (A) Breast augmentation form.

Pre-operative evaluation of the breast augmentation patient

I authorize and direct _____, M.D., with associates or assistants of his or her choice, to perform the following procedure of breast implant removal on _____.

(patient name)

Patient's
Initials

_____   The details of the procedure have been explained to me in terms I understand.

_____   Alternative methods and their benefits and disadvantages have been explained to me.

_____   I understand and accept the most likely risks and complications of breast implant removal include but are not limited to:
  - *Strong, negative impact on my physical appearance, including distortion, wrinkling, and significant loss of volume, and/or an appearance worse than prior to the initial augmentation*
  - *Severe psychological disturbance, including depression*
  - *Loss of interest in sexual relations by either myself or my partner*
  - *Scar contractures precluding reconstruction later*
  - *Infection, hematoma (swelling or blood mass), or scarring*
  - *Loss of breast tissue resulting in loss of breast sensation*
  - *Inability to breast-feed*
  - *Implant rupture and inability to remove 100% of the residual silicone from the breast cavity*

_____   I understand and accept the less common complications, including the remote risk of death or serious disability that exists with any surgical procedure.

_____   I am aware that smoking during the pre- and post-operative periods could increase chances of complications.

_____   I have informed the doctor of all my known allergies.

_____   I have informed the doctor of all medications I am currently taking, including prescription, over-the-counter, herbal, and any other.

_____   I have been advised whether I should take any or all of these medications on the days surrounding the procedure.

_____   I am aware and accept that no guarantees about the results of the procedure have been made.

_____   I have been informed of what to expect post-operatively, including but not limited to: estimated recovery time, anticipated activity level, and the possibility of additional procedures.

_____   Pre- and post-operative photos and/or videos will be taken of the treatment for record purposes. I understand that these photos and/or videos will be the property of the attending physician.

_____   I understand that the removed implant will be examined and sent to pathology, if necessary.

_____   I understand that if the implant is intact I may take it with me, or it will be destroyed.

_____   The doctor has answered all of my questions regarding this procedure.

I certify that I have read and understand this treatment agreement and that all blanks were filled in prior to my signature.

_____   _____
Patient or Legal Representative Signature / Date   Relationship (self, parent, etc.)

_____   _____
Print Patient or Legal Representative Name   Witness Signature / Date

I certify that I have explained the nature, purpose, benefits, risks, complications, and alternatives to the proposed procedure to the patient or the patient's legal representative. I have answered all questions fully, and I believe that the *patient / legal representative* fully understands what I have explained.   *(circle one)*

_____
Physician Signature / Date

_____ copy given to patient   _____ original placed in chart
initial   initial

B

Figure 1.12 *Continued* (B) Breast implant removal form.

either the sub-glandular or sub-muscular location will decrease the amount of breast tissue which can be imaged on a mammogram.

Cosmetic risks of breast augmentation relate mainly to asymmetries (Rohrich et al 2006) of the breast or implant position following surgery. These include differences in size or volume of the breast, shape, contour, or level of the IM folds or lower part of the breasts. As noted above (Rohrich et al 2006, Spear 2006a), in many cases these asymmetries are very frequently present prior to surgery, again underscoring the importance of allowing the patient and the surgeon to anticipate their persistence after the procedure is completed. In this way, they will not be viewed from the perspective of patient disappointment. The findings of implant edge palpability or visibility as well as the potential for palpable or visible ripples, ridges or folds is also important to mention, especially in patients who have thin chest tissues. Post-operative implant malposition which may be present in the immediate post-operative period or that which occurs down the road from the original surgical procedure should also be explained.

A category of risks which is not entailed in the informed consent for other procedures but one which plays a prominent role in the discussion with the patient who is considering breast augmentation is that of inherent risks. Inherent risks are those risks which are 'inherent' for patients who will have a breast implant placed as a part of their procedure. This includes both prospective breast augmentation patients and those who are considering implant-based breast reconstruction. They relate to anticipated events such as implant firmness or 'capsular contracture' (Burkhardt 1998), implant failure (Cunningham et al 2000), and the likely event of re-operation to address a problem with the breast most often due to a problem with the implant.

I present capsular contracture to the patient not as a complication but as a potential side-effect of implant placement. I explain this as a form of their own biologic incorporation of the breast implant during which the scar tissue deposited around the implant produces an undesirable amount of firmness in the overlying breast tissue. I also explain that there is no known cure or consistently effective treatment strategy for it. I inform the patient that additional surgery to modify the scar tissue can be performed and that this frequently may be helpful (Spear et al 2003) but I emphasize that there is not definite cure for firmness around

the implant. It is important to explain that unplanned additional surgery on the breast following breast augmentation is not uncommon. I will mention a re-operation rate of approximately 20% at 5 years following the original surgery.

Finally, we talk about implant failure. I mention that saline implants have a deflation rate of 2% per year per implant which has been established by several studies (Cunningham et al 2000). I also let the patient know that the exact failure rate of silicone gel implants is not known with much certainty at the present time but data is accruing to illustrate that the failure rate of gel implants is similar to that of the saline filled devices. At this point I give the patient the opportunity to ask questions and provide the best answers that I can.

Revision policy

From the standpoint of pre-operative disclosure, it is important that the plastic surgeon makes his or her revision policy very clearly understood by the patient. In other words, fees for operative re-intervention in either the immediate or long-term phases of the post-operative period must be explained. This includes facility fees and fees for additional implants should removal and replacement become necessary. This is another way of showing the patient that we care about them and are willing to follow them indefinitely and provide long-term surveillance of their breast health and implant condition.

Summary

Breast augmentation continues to be an operation with extremely high patient and plastic surgeon satisfaction. As with every cosmetic procedure that we perform 'an informed patient is your best ally'. By its very nature (placing a biomedical implantation device), breast augmentation requires an extensive amount of interaction and information transfer between the patient and the plastic surgeon. Adequate preparation and understanding of the procedure on the part of both the plastic surgeon and the patient is essential for consistently satisfactory outcomes. The approach I have overviewed has been effective for me in more than two decades of breast augmentation practice.

. . . .

Further reading

Bostwick J III Plastic and reconstructive breast surgery. Quality Medical Publishing, St Louis. 2000.

Burkhardt BR. Capsular contracture: hard breasts, soft data. Clin Plast Surg 1998;15:521.

Cunningham BL, Lokeh A, Gutowski KA. Saline-filled breast implant safety and efficacy: a multicenter retrospective review. Plast Reconstr Surg 2000;105:2143–2149, discussion.

Gorney M. The wheel of misfortune, Clin Plast Surg 1999;26:15.

Gorney M. Preventing litigation in breast augmentation. Clin Plast Surg 2001;28:607.

Gorney M, Martelo J. The genesis of plastic surgery claims – a review of recurring problems. Clin Plast Surg 1999;26:123.

Muntan CD, Sundine MJ, Rink RD, Acland RD. Inframammary fold: a histologic reappraisal. Plast Reconstr Surg 2000;105:549–556, discussion.

Rohrich RJ, Hartley W, Brown S. Incidence of breast and chest wall asymmetry in breast augmentation: a retrospective analysis of 100 patients. Plast Reconstr Surg 2006;118(7 Suppl):7S–13S; Plastic & Reconstructive Surgery 2006;111:1513–1519.

Shestak KC. Re-operative plastic surgery of the breast. Lippincott Williams & Wilkins, Philadelphia, PA 2006.

Spear SL. Discussion of incidence of breast and chest wall asymmetry in breast augmentation: a retrospective analysis of 100 patients. Plast Reconstr Surg 2006a;118(Suppl):15S–17S.

Spear SL. Surgery of the breast: principles and art. Lippincott Williams & Wilkins. Philadelphia, PA 2006b.

Spear SL, Carter ME, Ganz JC. The correction of capsular contracture by conversion to 'dual plane' positioning: technique and outcomes. Plast Reconstr Surg 2003;112:456–466.

Tebbetts JB. Patient evaluation, operative planning, and surgical techniques to increase control and reduce morbidity and reoperations in breast augmentation. Clinics in Plastic Surgery 2001;28:501–521.

Tebbetts JB. A system for breast implant selection based on patient tissue characteristics and implant-soft tissue dynamics. Plast Reconstr Surg 2002;109:1396–1409

Tebbetts JB, Adams WP. Five critical decisions in breast augmentation using five measurements in 5 minutes: the high five decision support process. Plast Reconstr Surg 2006;118(7 Suppl):35S–45S.

The American Cancer Society. Mammography Guidelines.

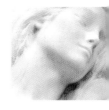

2

Breast augmentation: incision selection

Mark A. Pinsky

Key points

- Inconspicuous incision location.
- Adequate incision length for accurate and meticulous pocket dissection.
- Large enough incision so as not to damage the breast implant.

- Accurate anatomic realignment of the tissues.
- Tension free skin closure.

Introduction

The chosen incision technique should be based upon the type of breast surgery to be performed, the patient's anatomy, the type and size of the breast implant and the preferences of the patient and surgeon. If a mastopexy is planned as a part of the procedure then, ideally, one of the mastopexy incisions should be utilized so as to avoid additional unnecessary scarring on a woman's breast. The same is true if a scar already exists on a breast and the procedure is not otherwise compromised. Patients often choose an incision based upon it leaving the least conspicuous scar. The surgeon should share this goal, leaving as little surgical evidence as possible.

Basic principles should include placing incisions inconspicuously and along relaxed skin tension lines regardless of location. The incisions should be as short

as possible, but as long as necessary so as not to compromise accurate and meticulous pocket dissection and insertion of the breast implant without damage. Even though some implants can be placed through an incision as short as 2 cm, the quality of the scar is more dependent upon minimizing tissue trauma from retraction injury than upon the length of the scar. In general, it is important that tissues disrupted by surgery be accurately and anatomically realigned. Reapproximating the fascia, when available, provides a strong closure and minimizes tension on the edges of the wound. Deeper layers should be sutured to eliminate any dead space. Closure of the deep dermis should create eversion of the wound edges so the skin suture can perfectly align the skin edges without any tension.

Suture selection should be based upon utilizing the least amount of suture material necessary to effectively close the wound. It should resorb as quickly as possible after adequate tissue strength in the healing wound has been accomplished. Typically, deeper layers of tissue require larger absorbable sutures. The scar is minimized if the skin suture is placed below the skin as a permanent running or pullout subcuticular suture.

Incision selection

Inframammary incision

Historically, the inframammary incision has been the most commonly used incision since the inception of breast implantation surgery (Cronin 1964). Women who have a well-defined inframammary fold and slight glandular breast ptosis are the best candidates for this incision. Incisions that are planned correctly and lie precisely in the new inframammary fold heal very well and are difficult to see not only from a standing position, but also while lying down (Figure 2.1). An incision in this location (a relaxed skin tension line) has very little tension on it from the stretch of the new implant, but it must be placed accurately (Figure 2.2). A scar misplaced superiorly on the breast mound becomes apparent when the patient lies down whereas a scar placed too low is evident in any posi-tion. Sometimes even a well planned incision becomes too high as an implant descends, a phenomenon less likely with the tissue adhesion from aggressively textured implants. Some surgeons shy away from the inframammary incision because of this inherent unpredictability. Discussions will follow as to how to more precisely predict the location of the inframammary scar.

The inframammary incision is perhaps the simplest and quickest of all breast augmentation incisions. It allows immediate and direct access to any desired dissection plane with very little disruption of breast tissue. This incision is often necessary in patients who receive larger implants or those requiring textured implants where longer length incisions are frequently necessary. It is an ideal incision for anatomic shaped implants where the orientation of the implant is crucial to the overall success of the surgery. This is also the incision of choice for secondary or revision breast implant surgery. The inframammary incision is not a good choice in patients with a non-existent inframammary fold or a high inframammary fold which is to be lowered as a part of the surgical plan (Hidalgo 2000). Usually a 4 cm incision provides sufficient exposure to facilitate accurate pocket dissection for most saline breast implants and smaller silicone breast implants. Textured surface implants, larger smooth surface silicone implants and cohesive gel implants may require incisions up to 6 cm in length for proper insertion while avoiding damage to the implant.

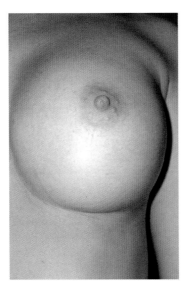

Figure 2.1 An inframammary incision perfectly positioned in the inframammary fold making detection virtually impossible.

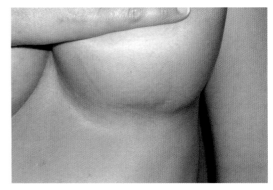

Figure 2.2 The breast is lifted up to reveal the inframammary scar. The scar is very thin as a result of accurate placement (relaxed skin tension line).

Operative technique

The most important consideration in the placement of the inframammary incision is predicting the final position of the inframammary fold. There are two methods for determining the post-operative inframammary fold location, one simple and the other more complex. Keep in mind that regardless of the method chosen, other variables must be accounted for such as the type of breast implant selected for the patient, the pocket location and the fibrous connections from the deeper tissues to the skin.

The type of implant selected makes a significant difference in the final location of the inframammary fold. Smooth implants are known to 'drop' in the early post-operative course. How far they drop is dependent upon the volume (weight) of the implant and how tight the attachments are from the superficial tissues to the deeper tissues; stronger in young nulliparous women and weaker in older patients especially if they have had children. Placement is another consideration. Subpectoral implants in a dual plane pocket tend to drop more than implants placed in a submammary position or complete submuscular position. Lastly, breast implants with a more aggressive textured surface tend to be more predictable in terms of their final position because of adherence from the implant to the surrounding tissues. Thus, the ultimate inframammary location becomes more predictable since these implants are less likely to drop.

The simplest method for determining the post-operative inframammary fold location is by marking the patient's existing inframammary fold while the patient is in the standing position (Figure 2.3). Markings for the new inframammary fold are made with the patient on the operating room table in the supine position. The covered nipple is held with the thumb and index finger pulling it away from the chest wall. The remaining fingers are used to push the breast gland inferiorly (Figure 2.4). The new curvilinear inframammary fold is marked along the crease created by this maneuver (Figure 2.5).

A more comprehensive method for determining the inframammary fold location utilizes the tissue based planning principles in the High Five System (Tebbetts & Adams 2005). This method analyzes variables such as breast implant volume, implant base width; the patient's measured breast width, anterior pull skin stretch, nipple

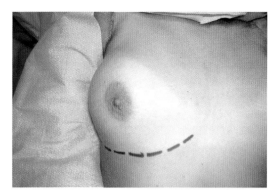

Figure 2.3 The patient's original inframammary fold is marked.

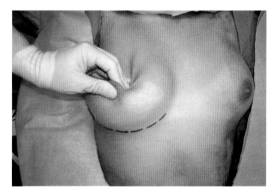

Figure 2.4 The nipple is held in the surgeon's index finger and thumb pulling the breast away from the chest wall while the other fingers are used to push the breast gland caudad.

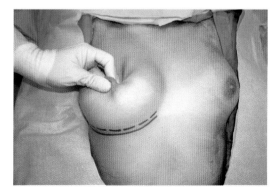

Figure 2.5 The new inframammary fold is marked.

17

to IMF distance on stretch and breast parenchyma to stretched breast envelope fill. Once an implant has been selected based upon these variables, a reference chart is used to determine the recommended new IMF fold location. This selection is based in part upon the base width and volume of the breast implant, the recommended nipple to inframammary distance based upon the author's experience and the patient's preoperative nipple to inframammary fold distance under maximal stretch. The inframammary fold location is then determined based upon the difference in the recommended and measured IMF fold position. This new fold position is calculated prior to surgery, noted in the patient's chart and physically marked in the preoperative holding area or in the operating room.

Ultimately, the goal in planning the location of the inframammary fold is to have the inferior border of the implant lay at the fold with the point of maximum projection of the implant located directly behind the nipple. Therefore, the radius of a round implant or the distance from the point of maximum projection to the lower edge of an anatomic implant should equal the distance from the nipple to inframammary fold. Once the inframammary fold position has been determined, a vertically oriented paramedian line is drawn from the medial aspect of the areola inferiorly to bisect the newly drawn inframammary fold (Figure 2.6). This marks the medial extent of the planned inframammary incision. The marking is then carried laterally along the new inframammary fold for 4–6 cm depending upon the procedure to be performed and the implant type and size (Figure 2.7).

The incision is performed with a 10 or 15 blade down through skin into the mid dermis. Further dissection is carried out while holding the breast between the fingers and thumb lifting it away from the chest wall. Dissection proceeds superiorly at about a 20 degree angle down to the chest wall with an electrocautery device (Figure 2.8). The electrocautery device should be set on the lowest possible setting to avoid collateral thermal damage to the tissues. The dissection passes through the subcutaneous tissue and Scarpa's fascia to the retroglandular fatty tissue. From this point, the lateral diagonal border of the pectoralis major muscle and its fascia as well as the breast gland are visible making it easy to proceed with the desired pocket dissection.

Closure of the inframammary fold should include Scarpa's fascia with simple interrupted 3-0 or 4-0 absorbable sutures placed approximately 1 cm apart

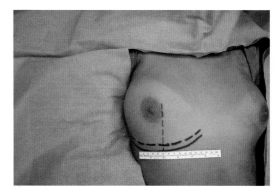

Figure 2.7   The length of the incision is dependent upon the type of implant to be used.

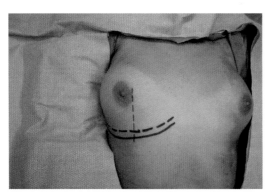

Figure 2.6   A vertical paramedian line is drawn from the medial border of the nipple areolar complex to the newly marked inframammary fold.

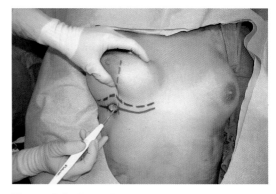

Figure 2.8   Dissection proceeds at a 20 degree angle from the chest wall while lifting the breast away from the chest wall.

(Figure 2.9). There should be closure of the subcutaneous tissue and deep dermis with simple interrupted 4-0 absorbable suture with eversion of the wound edges so the skin edges are touching one another without tension. Finally, there should be perfect alignment of the epidermis with a permanent running or pullout subcuticular suture or skin glue (Figure 2.10). Depending upon the thickness of the tissues, Scarpa's fascia, the subcutaneous tissue and the deep dermis may all be included in a single suture.

Periareolar incision

The periareolar incision was first described by Jenny in 1972. Because the scar is usually very difficult to detect, breast augmentation patients often present to the plastic surgeon requesting the periareolar incision (Figure 2.11). This is particularly true in patients where there is a marked color contrast between the areola and the surrounding breast skin and when the areola has a discrete sharp edge to it. This approach is less ideal for patients who have lightly colored areola or patients in which the edge of the areola is irregular and appears to diffuse into the surrounding breast skin. This incision should not be recommended in patients with a history of poor scars as the incision is placed near the center of the breast where it would be readily visible. Though unpredictable, some scars in this area may become hypopigmented and therefore more apparent if the incision is made within the pigmented areola. Hypopigmentation is less noticeable in lighter skinned patients when the incision is placed appropriately (Figure 2.12).

Patients should have an areola diameter large enough to accommodate accurate pocket dissection and place the implant without damage. An areola of 3 cm should provide a curvilinear distance on the inferior half of the areola of approximately 4 cm, just large enough to place an unfilled saline breast implant. There is limited exposure for areolas smaller than 3 cm. In those patients the periareolar approach

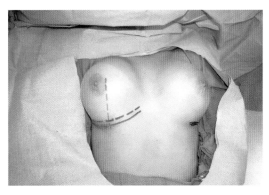

Figure 2.10   Final closure of the inframammary incision.

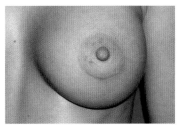

Figure 2.11   An example of a well placed periareolar incision. The patient has a discrete areolar border and marked color contrast between the areola and breast skin.

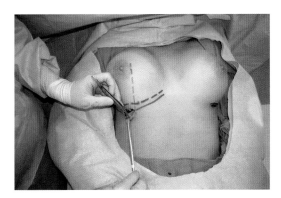

Figure 2.9   Closure should include the fascia of the breast located above and below the incision.

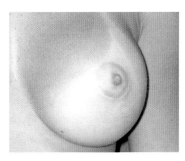

Figure 2.12   A hypopigmented periareolar scar.

incision should be avoided. Patients with limited areola dimensions should also avoid a periareolar incision if they require larger breast implants, larger textured breast implants and possibly cohesive gel implants, all of which typically require longer incisions to avoid damage to the implant. This is particularly true in patients with larger breasts, especially when the breast tissue is dense because the tunnel to pass the implant is longer and the breast tissue is less compliant. Operative procedures with incisions around the areola or through the areola involve more time because there is more tissue to dissect through and the closure takes longer. Dissection through the breast tissue may result in scarring or cyst formation necessitating future breast biopsies.

The periareolar incision is ideal for patients with tuberous breast deformities or constricted breasts where division of the radial bands is a part of the operative plan. In patients with slight glandular ptosis, the periareolar incision is an excellent choice as a small amount of breast tissue can be strategically resected from the lower pole of the breast (Pinsky 2005). It is also a good incision in patients with mild ptosis when the decision to commit to a mastopexy is deferred until the time of surgery. In this situation the periareolar incision can be incorporated into the mastopexy without the need for an additional incision on the breast. The most common placement of the periareolar incision is along the inferior edge of the areola. Exceptions are those designed on the superior edge and others oriented more medially, i.e., from one to seven o'clock on the left breast, to preserve sensory innervation (Karabulut et al 2002). There have been many transareolar incisions described in an effort to conceal the scar. Those include incisions directly across the diameter of the areola through the nipple (Kompatscher et al 2004), across the areola but under the nipple (Atiyeh et al 2002), 'W' plasty incisions through the areola (Fernandez et al 1999) and incisions isolated around the nipple (Becker 1999) as well as others.

Incisions through the nipple are particularly problematic as the glands of the breast harbor bacteria increasing the incidence of capsular contracture. It has recently been reported that the difference in capsular contracture rate in breast augmentation with the periareolar incision versus the inframammary incision is 9.5% and 0.59% respectively (Weiner 2008). There is a higher risk of infection and colonization of the breast pocket with *Staphylococcus epidermidis* with all areolar incisions due to the abundance of this bacterium in ductal secretions. The periareolar incision has been implicated in lactation insufficiency which is defined as inadequate volume of expressed milk and/or infant growth (Michalopoulos 2007). The intricate process of lactation may be influenced by one or more consequences of breast augmentation surgery and the periareolar incision. The NAC is innervated by the lateral and medial branches of the third through sixth intercostal nerves. Damage to these nerves can occur during pocket dissection with any of the incision techniques, but is at greater risk for injury when using the periareolar incision. Damage to this nerve may result in decreased nipple sensitivity which may affect the suckling reflex.

When performing a periareolar incision the surgeon can reach the desired plane of pocket dissection either by dissecting through the breast tissue or a path between the breast tissue and the subcutaneous tissue. The latter tends to be more difficult in thin women and may result in temporary or permanent contour abnormalities on the skin. More often the breast tissue is divided in order to arrive at the desired tissue plane for pocket dissection. Transecting mammary ducts may interrupt the drainage system to the nipple and thereby lead to lactation insufficiency (Michalopoulos 2007). In addition, transecting the mammary ducts may prevent decompression of those portions of the gland when the breasts are engorged during breastfeeding. This pressure may cause atrophy of those portions of the breast gland and also contribute to lactation insufficiency.

It is important to discuss these issues with patients of child bearing age requesting the periareolar approach to breast augmentation. The immediate desire for breast enhancement may eclipse her ability to make the best decision with regard to her ability to breastfeed at a future date. Recently, the dogma of decreased nipple areola complex sensitivity with the periareolar incision has been challenged. Two studies utilizing advanced computerized testing devices have found no difference in nipple areolar complex sensitivity with either the inframammary or periareolar incision (Mofid et al 2006, Okwueze et al 2006). It appears as though nipple areolar complex sensitivity may actually have a more inversely proportional relationship to the size of the breast implant rather than the type of incision utilized (Mofid et al 2006). All patients undergoing breast augmentation with either the inframammary or periareolar incision had decreased nipple areolar complex sensitivity compared to nonoperated controls. On the other hand, the periareolar incision may produce less sensory loss in the lower pole of the breast compared to the inframammary incision (Okwueze et al 2006).

Operative technique

The inferior periareolar incision is marked with the patient asleep on the operating room table in the supine position. Markings are made as a series of dots along the interface between the pigmented areola and the lighter color of the native breast skin (Figure 2.13). Dots are used instead of a line so that the surgeon can better visualize the different colors of the areola and the breast skin for a more accurate incision. Poor scars may occur as the result of incisions extending onto the breast skin. The incision does not have to be a smooth arching curve, but rather needs to be placed precisely at the junction of the areola and the breast skin even if the incision is irregular in its path. The incision is placed equidistant, medial and lateral from the meridian of the areola the length of which is determined by the procedure to be performed and the implant to be utilized. The length is usually no longer than 50% of the perimeter so as to not undermine the nipple areolar complex.

With the assistant stretching out the areola with both hands, an incision is made with the 15 scalpel through the skin to the mid dermis. Further dissection is carried out with the electrocautery device on the lowest possible setting so as to avoid collateral thermal injury to the tissues. The dissection proceeds inferiorly through the breast tissue with either a vertical or horizontal orientation, or between the interface of the breast tissue and the subcutaneous tissue not traversing the breast tissue (Figure 2.14). With both approaches, dissection proceeds inferiorly so not to undermine and compromise the blood supply to the nipple areolar complex (Figure 2.15). Dissection continues until the retroglandular fat is encountered where the lateral border of the pectoralis major muscle and fascia are clearly visible and the desired plane of pocket dissection can begin (Figure 2.16).

It is important during wound closure to approximate the tissues of the breast gland as they existed prior to the surgery with one or two layers of simple interrupted 3-0 absorbable sutures (Figure 2.17). The deep dermis and subcutaneous tissue should be closed with simple interrupted 4-0 absorbable sutures evert-

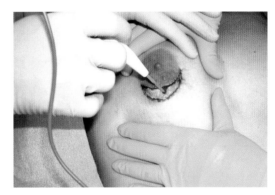

Figure 2.14 Inferiorly oriented dissection through the breast tissue.

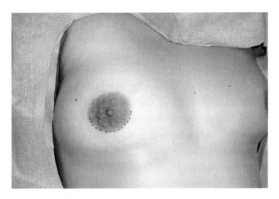

Figure 2.13 Dot markings for the planned periareolar incision.

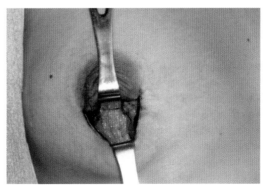

Figure 2.15 Deeper dissection through the breast tissue.

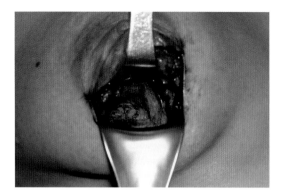

Figure 2.16 The pectoralis muscle at the base of the dissection.

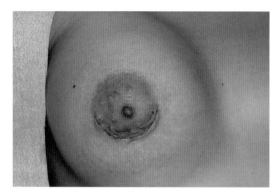

Figure 2.18 Final closure of the periareolar incision.

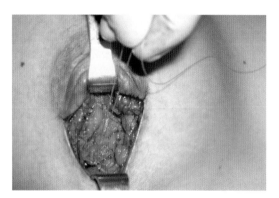

Figure 2.17 Closing the first of two layers of breast tissue.

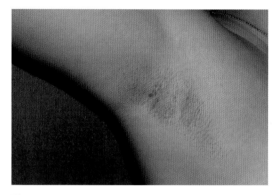

Figure 2.19 Post-operative appearance of a transaxillary incision.

ing the skin edges. Finally, there should be perfect alignment of the skin edges with a running subcuticular permanent or pullout suture or tissue glue (Figure 2.18).

Transaxillary incision

Transaxillary breast augmentation was first described by Hoehler in 1973. The advantage of this method is that it avoids placement of an incision on the breast gland (Figure 2.19). It is indicated in women who do not want to have a scar on their breast or in those having a small nipple areolar complex or indiscreet inframammary fold. The best surgical candidates for this incision are patients with little or no ptosis and a breast positioned high on the chest wall. Conversely, patients with breasts positioned low on a long chest wall will pose a greater challenge (Hidalgo 2000).

The disadvantage to the transaxillary incision is two-fold; the difficulty obtaining adequate exposure and achieving satisfactory hemostasis without endoscopic assistance. Originally described with a blind, blunt dissection technique, it is now often performed with endoscopic assistance as direct visualization of the plane of dissection is virtually impossible. More instrumentation and time is required when using the endoscope although the latter becomes less significant with greater endoscopic experience by the surgeon (Tebbetts 2006). This incision may not be the incision of choice for textured implants, large silicone implants or in the case of anatomical implants where correct implant orientation is critical to the success of the procedure. It is also not the incision of choice in more complex breast surgery such as a tuberous breast deformity. Revision surgery often requires an inframammary fold incision or periareolar incision.

Operative technique

The patient is marked in the standing position with her hands placed on her hips. A single dot is placed at the apex of the axillary fossa (Figure 2.20). A line is then drawn within or parallel to the relaxed skin tension lines of the axilla, perpendicular to the long axis of a hair bearing axilla (Figure 2.21). The markings begin just inside the anterior edge of the hair bearing axilla and extend posteriorly for 4–6 cm depending upon the procedure to be performed and the implant selected. Care should be taken not to extend the incision beyond the posterior aspect of the hair bearing axilla as it may be seen from behind. The markings should be checked by viewing the patient from the front and back to make sure the incisions are not visible.

An alternative transaxillary incision design is one that places the incision just inside the anterior inferior aspect of the hair bearing axilla almost parallel to the anterior axillary fold. Although this incision is perpendicular to the relaxed skin tension lines of the axilla, it is camouflaged by the hair of the axilla and is behind the anterior axillary fold. Access to the lateral border of the pectoralis major muscle is easy. Patients best suited for this incision design are those with a low breast position and long chest wall or in the event that

larger prefilled breast implants are being used. As described above, the highest point within the axillary fossa should be marked and a line should be drawn from this point to the anterior border of the hair bearing axilla along the relaxed skin tension lines. This identifies the superior limit of the planned incision. The marking is then carried inferiorly inside the anterior hairline almost parallel to the anterior axillary fold (Figure 2.22). It is important to be sure this line is hidden behind the anterior axillary fold with the patient's arms at her side.

Unlike the more common inframammary fold incision and the periareolar incision, there are many important neurovascular structures in the axilla. Care must be taken to avoid the sensory nerve branches including the intercostobrachial nerve that course through the axillary fat pad and the deeper brachial plexus as well as subclavian artery and vein. In order to do this, it is important to keep the dissection plane in the subcutaneous tissue and not enter the axillary fat pad. The patient is positioned on the operating room table in the supine position with the arms abducted 90 degrees. An incision is made in the skin down to mid dermis with either a 10 or 15 blade. Further dissection is carried out with the electrocautery device at the lowest possible setting so as to avoid collateral thermal damage to the tissues. Once through

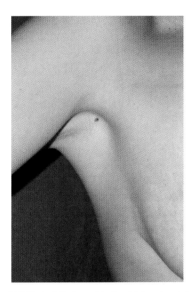

Figure 2.20 A dot placed in the highest point of the axillary fossa.

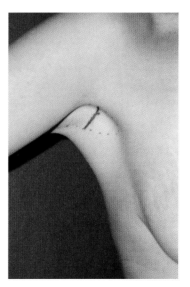

Figure 2.21 The planned incision line is drawn within the relaxed skin tension line across the hair bearing axilla.

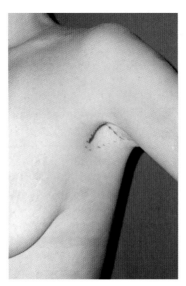

Figure 2.22 The planned incision line is drawn within the hair bearing axilla behind the anterior axillary fold.

the deeper dermis and into the subcutaneous tissue skin retractors are held by the assistant. The heel of the assistant's hands can be utilized to retract the breast gland into a more medial position thereby displacing the incision closer to the lateral border of the pectoralis major. Dissection should proceed to the lateral border of the pectoralis major muscle. It is easy to visualize the pectoralis major and minor as well as the pre-pectoral plane for either subpectoral or prepectoral pocket dissection.

When closing the wound it is important to realign the anatomic structures as they were prior to surgery. The pectoralis major fascia should be realigned with 3-0 absorbable sutures. This will realign the axillary fat pad which falls away and superior from its pre surgical position. The skin is then closed with simple interrupted 4-0 absorbable sutures in the deep dermis and subcutaneous tissue to create mild eversion of the skin edges. The skin is now poised for perfect alignment using either a permanent or pullout running subcuticular suture or skin glue.

Abdominoplasty incision

The abdominoplasty incision, originally described by Planas in 1972, can be utilized as the access incision to place either submammary or subpectoral breast implants. The advantage of this incision is the absence of scars on the patient's breast. The primary disadvantage of this incision is poor visibility during pocket dissection which requires both a blind and blunt dissection. Once the abdominoplasty dissection is complete and prior to rectus abdominus fascia plication, tunnels are created above the rectus abdominus fascia under each breast (Wallach 2004). The medial inframammary fold is disrupted in order to gain access to the appropriate plane of pocket dissection. Each pocket should be kept separate to avoid synmastia but large enough for atraumatic insertion of the implants. Once the breast augmentation procedure is completed the tunnels can be closed with simple interrupted 2-0 absorbable sutures to recreate the inframammary fold. This is particularly necessary in heavier women and in cases of subpectoral implant placement. In lieu of closing the tunnels in thinner patients a bra can be worn to apply gentle compression over the costal margin for several weeks. The abdominoplasty incision is closed in the typical fashion.

Transumbilical incision

Transumbilical breast augmentation (TUBA) was originally described by Johnson and Crist in 1993 where an unfilled saline breast implant is inserted through a tunnel from the umbilicus to the breast. This procedure has not been readily adopted by plastic surgeons for a variety of reasons which will be discussed below. With the approval of silicone breast implants the popularity of this procedure may further wane. While originally described as a blind procedure, it has been performed by some surgeons with endoscopic assistance. As in the case of the axillary incision, patients frequently ask about the procedure because this technique avoids placement of an incision on the breast gland.

The concept of the procedure was borne out of performing breast augmentation through an abdominoplasty incision without a breast incision, wherein tunnels are created near the sternum at the top of the abdominoplasty dissection to each breast. A breast pocket could then be created using blunt technique either above or below the pectoralis major muscle. The TUBA procedure was the natural progression from this approach in patients not undergoing abdominoplasty, but distinctly averse to scarring (Pound & Pound 2001). The shortcoming of this approach is poor access to the implant pocket for accurate and meticulous pocket dissection. In addition, this procedure does not lend itself to prefilled implants or shaped saline implants as it is very difficult to assess proper orientation of these types of implants. As in the case of the transaxillary incision, this is not the incision of choice in more complex breast problems such as a tuberous breast deformity or revisions that are better served by an inframammary incision or periareolar incision.

The incision is very straight forward in that a 15 blade is used to make an incision on the upper half of the umbilicus under the umbilical hood. Dissection proceeds subcutaneously above the rectus abdominus fascia with a blunt dissector to the breast. The path of dissection is from the umbilicus to the nipple wherein the plane of pocket dissection is performed. Closure is simple with simple interrupted 4-0 absorbable suture placed in the dermis followed by a 5-0 permanent or pull out suture or tissue glue for the skin. Occasionally the deeper tissues can be included with the deep dermal suture triangulating the closure to recreate the occasional depression above the navel.

Conclusion

The overall success of breast augmentation surgery is directly related to choosing the proper incision location. Incision choice should be predicated on the type of breast surgery to be performed, the patient's anatomy, the type and size of the breast implant, the patient's preference and surgeon's preference and skill set. It is best if the surgeon is familiar with several of the more common incision techniques (inframammary, periareolar, and endoscopic transaxillary incisions) in order to accommodate the multitude of variables associated with each patient and surgery.

The incision should not leave pronounced evidence of plastic surgery invasion of the breast. Incisions should be placed in locations as inconspicuous as possible and along relaxed skin tension lines. Tell-tale scars can become the patient's focal point and ultimately skew their perception of an otherwise successful surgical result. In order to obtain the best scars incisions need to be positioned precisely. There should be minimal tissue trauma when making the incision. The incisions should be large enough to perform uncompromised pocket dissection without tissue trauma from retractors and also large enough to accommodate placement of the implant without damage.

Closure of the incision should realign all the anatomic structures as they existed prior to surgical invasion; including fascia when available, closing all dead space, everting the superficial tissues and perfect realignment of the skin. If despite proper precautions, a less than desirable scar occurs, patients may benefit from silicone sheeting/ tape or pharmaceutical scar products. Patients who eventually develop poor scars may benefit from tattooing the scar. In prioritizing incision techniques, the surgeon should marry the patient's goals and anatomy with the benefits and consequences of each incision technique. Adopting the associated techniques discussed above will lead to more consistently exceptional results for you and your patients.

Further reading

Atiyeh BS, Al-Amm CA, El-Musa KA. The transverse intra-areolar infra-nipple incision for augmentation mammaplasty. Aesth Plast Surg 2002;26:151–155.

Becker H. The intra-areolar incision for breast augmentation. Ann Plast Surg 1999;42:103–106.

Fernandez CP, Lopez FM, Burrieza PI. Our experience with the triple-v transareolar incision for augmentation mammaplasty. Aesth Plast Surg 1999;23:428–432.

Hidalgo DA. Breast augmentation: choosing the optimal incision, implant, and pocket plane. Plast Reconstr Surg 2000;105:2202–2216.

Karabulut AB, Aydin H, Sirin, F, Tumerdem B. Augmentation mammaplasty by medial periareolar incision. Aesth Plast Surg 2002;26:291–294.

Kompatscher P, Schuler C, Beer GM. The transareolar incision for breast augmentation revisited. Aesth Plast Surg 2004;28:70–74.

Michalopoulos K. The effects of breast augmentation surgery on future ability to lactate. Breast J 2007;13:62–67.

Mofid MM, Klatsky SA, Singh NK, Nahabedian MY. Nipple-areola complex sensitivity after primary breast augmentation: a comparison of periareolar and inframammary incision approaches. Plast Reconstr Surg 2006;117:1694–1698.

Okwueze MI, Spear ME, Zwyghuizen AM, et al. Effect of augmentation mammaplasty on breast sensation. Plast Reconstr Surg 2006;117:73–83.

Pinsky MA. Radial plication in concentric mastopexy. Aesth Plast Surg 2005;29:391–399.

Pound III, EC. Pound Jr, EC. Transumbilical breast augmentation (TUBA). Clin Plast Surg 2001;28: 597–605.

Tebbetts JB. Axillary endoscopic breast augmentation: processes derived from a 28-year experience to optimize outcomes. Plast Reconstr Surg 2006;118(7 Suppl):53S–80S.

Tebbetts JB, Adams WP. Five critical decisions in breast augmentation using five measurements in 5 minutes: the high five decision support process. Plast Reconstr Surg 2005;116:2005–2016.

Wallach SG. Maximizing the use of the abdominoplasty incision. Plast Reconstr Surg 2004;113:411–417.

Weiner TC. Relationship of incision choice to capsular contracture. Aesth Plast Surg 2008;32:303–306.

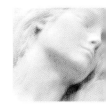

Subpectoral approach for primary breast augmentation

A. Aldo Mottura

Key points

- The subpectoral pocket can be dissected through the submammary, areolar or axillary incisions and each of these approaches is different.
- The submuscular dissection includes the pectoralis major and the serratus anterior muscles.
- The muscles are transected at the submammary area to avoid implant displacement.
- Textured silicone implants have now been used routinely for 15 years.

- The superior breast mound is not visible with subpectoral breast implants.
- The implant is more protected when it is covered by the muscles and rippling is not visible with the subpectoral implants.
- Breast lumps diagnostics and treatment are facilitated when the implant is placed subpectorally and capsular contracture is less frequent.

Introduction

The subglandular technique described in numerous papers and books has been widely used worldwide for the last 45 years. The subpectoral approach is only used by some surgeons and has received less attention in the international literature. This paper will, therefore, expand mainly on the subpectoral technique.

Patient selection

There are three usual pockets used for breast implants and the election depends on several factors:

- The surgeon studies the thickness of the skin and muscles and the size of the implant the patient wishes to have in relation to her thoracic width.
- The patient's opinion as to whether she would like a visible superior breast mound is explored during

interrogation. If she does, then I consider placing the implant subglandularly but if she refuses, then the submuscular technique is chosen.

● It is also important to educate young patients regarding the future possibility of having parenchyma pathology like fibroadenomas, cysts or breast cancer.

In cases where the subglandular approach is chosen, the implant will attach to the parenchyma. In future mammograms, the parenchyma will be more difficult to study and in case of a tumor or a cyst, biopsies or puntions into the breast will be dangerous. In cases where the implant is submuscular, the parenchyma is more visible in mammograms and biopsies and puntions can be done in a safer way. If the implant is retropectoral, in cases of a quadrantectomy or mastectomy, the parenchyma can be removed while the implant is kept safely under the muscle. My personal preference is to use the subpectoral and the subglandular approaches. There are surgeons who prefer the subfascial approach rather than the submuscular one and this is a third possibility.

Indications

Submuscular implants are indicated when:

● patients have small breasts, thin skin and subcutaneous tissue where the implant will be covered in its superior part, by the thin skin.
● the patient has a history of multiple fibroadenomas or family history of breast cancer.
● the patient has submammary breast implants with capsular contracture.

Submuscular implants are not indicated:

● when the patient has a thick subcutaneous layer or a flat breast parenchyma.
● in competitive sport players.
● where bigger implants than the submuscular dimensions have to be used.

Pre-operative preparation

At home, the patient has to scrub the pectoral and axillary areas with iodopovidone and before the markings are made, the skin is defatted with alcohol. With the patient in a standing position, breast symmetry, submammary crease and areola positions are studied in relation to the size of the implant. The new sub-

mammary position, 2 cm beyond the implant limits and the extension of the pocket are penciled onto the skin.

Technique

With the patient under deep sedation, I prepare an anesthetic solution with 25 mL lidocaine 2%, 25 mL bupivacaine 0.5%, 1 mL epinephrine 1 : 1000 and 450–550 mL saline solution. The infiltration is performed touching the external aspect of the sixth rib and injecting the anesthesia in an radial way in order to facilitate the subpectoral and serratus anterior dissection. The infiltration continues at the medial part of the breast, at the border with the sternum where the cutaneous branch of the intercostal nerves emerges and at the lateral emergence of the lateral cutaneous nerves. I also introduce the needle into the inferior border of each rib, blocking the third, fourth, fifth and sixth intercostal nerves, adding extra anesthesia and also producing vasoconstriction at the intercostal arteries and veins. In cases where the approach is axillary, the anesthesia is complemented with an infiltration under the incision lines, at the subcutaneous tissue, all the area to be dissected and in the path to the subpectoral space. In the peri-areolar approach, under the incision line, I infiltrate the parenchyma and the submammary space. With the submammary technique, I also infiltrate under the incision line, at the submammary space and at the submuscular plane.

In the axillary approach, the incision is marked in one of the axillary creases. Then 5 cm subcutaneous is dissected downwards and, with the index finger, I try to determine the pectoralis major muscle and to enter through its posterior aspect (Figure 3.1). In the submammary technique, the incision is made 1 cm above the new submammary fold and at the lateral half of the gland. The pectoralis major muscle is divided obliquely along and separating 5–7 cm of its fibers all along their course first touching and dissecting over the external aspect of a rib, this way avoiding dissecting the intercostal muscles (Figure 3.2). If the areolar approach is used, the incision of preference is at the inferior half of the areola but in cases where there is a small areola, a round periareolar incision brings a wide tunnel for the dissection and introduction of the implant. The parenchyma is divided and the submammary space is dissected obliquely making only a small space for the dissection of the pectoralis major muscle

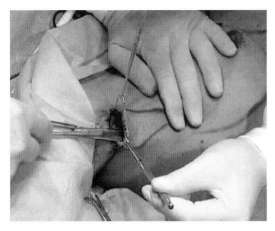

Figure 3.1   From the axilla, the subcutaneous tissue is undermined.

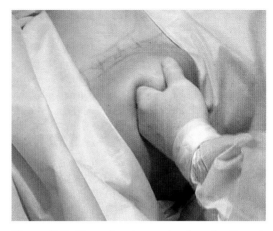

Figure 3.3   Finger tip submuscular dissection through a subareolar incision.

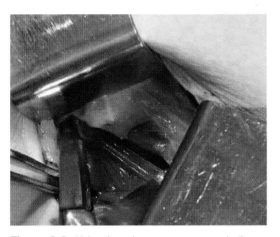

Figure 3.2   Using the submammary approach, the pectoralis muscle is divided along the direction of its fibers.

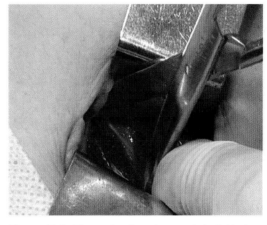

Figure 3.4   The pectoralis major muscle is divided along the muscle direction.

which is carried out in the same way as in the submammary approach (Figure 3.3).

The submuscular pocket dissection differs according to the approach selected. In the axillary approach, the finger tip dissects the pocket beginning from the superior part where the muscle is detached from the thoracic wall. The index finger releases the insertion of the muscle at the costal surfaces then separates the serratus anterior insertion from the ribs using the finger tip with the nail detaching the muscle from the external aspect of the ribs making tunnels and then connecting these two to three tunnels. This dissection continues laterally until the finger tip feels strings emerging perpendicularly from the thoracic wall.

These are the lateral intercostal perforator nerves. Finally, I disrupt the long muscle fibers that are usually present more medially by trespassing the SMF. In the dissection of the pocket from the axilla, sometimes the length of my finger is shorter than the extent of the planned pocket so it is necessary to use a dissector as a prolongation of my finger tip (Figures 3.4–3.6).

In the areolar approach, I make a 5 cm incision at the fascia, and with scissors, I separate the muscle fibres along the oblique direction of the fibers above the external surface of a rib. Once I have introduced my index finger, I dissect the pocket in the same way. In the submammary approach, I make the same oblique fascia incision and dissection but the inferior fiber detachment of the pectoralis major muscle is not easy to perform at the inferior IMF area from this lateral approach so sometimes the scissors are helpful. The disruption of the pectoral fibres from the ribs is different in the three approaches because from the axilla, the direction of the index finger is from the superior part of the breast, from the areolar approach it is from the medial part of the breast and from the infra-mammary approach it is from the inferior and lateral part.

As soon as the pocket is completed on one side, I insert three big compresses into the pocket and move to the other side. While I am working on the second breast; the compresses stop the bleeding and distend the cavity. Once I have inserted the three compresses in the second breast I come back to the first one and I remove all the compresses one by one watching which of them has a significant blood spot. In this way, I can observe where bleeding has occurred (Figures 3.7–3.9). The coagulator is very seldom used because after the profuse local anesthesia with vasoconstrictors and 15 min compression, almost all the vessels are coagulated. Frequently, I use two compresses when the implant is small (less than 220 mL) and four compresses when the implant is over 360 mL.

I wash all the operated surfaces, the cavity, the implants and the gloves with antibiotic solution before the introduction of the implants. Once the textured

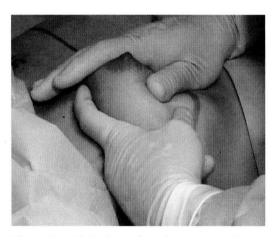

Figure 3.5 Using finger dissection, the pectoralis major muscle is detached.

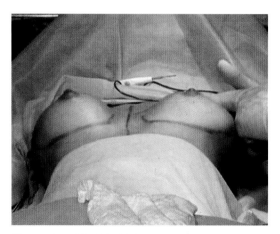

Figure 3.7 The left side has three compresses already in place.

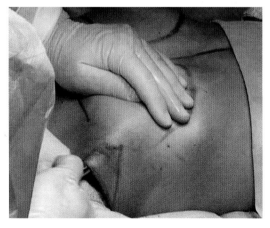

Figure 3.6 Using the metal dissector the pectoralis major dissection is completed.

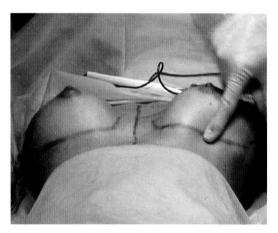

Figure 3.8 On the right side, an insufficient submammary muscle detachment in the submammary area is observed.

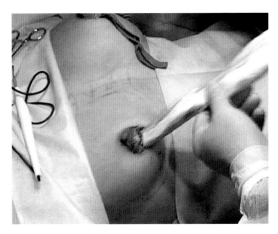

Figure 3.9 Removing the third clean compress, without any blood spot.

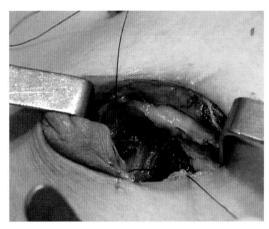

Figure 3.11 Once the textured implant is placed, the muscle is sutured.

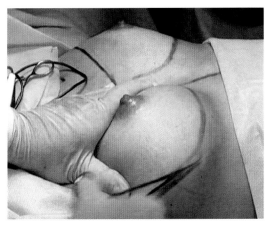

Figure 3.10 The implant was observed filling the infra-mammary space.

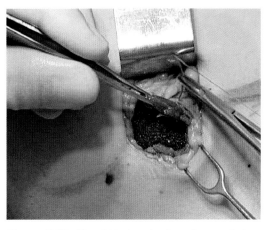

Figure 3.12 The divided pectoralis major muscle is sutured.

implant is introduced, it should reach and fill all the inferior edge of the dissection. With the patient in a supine position with the arms away from the table, the implant is placed in the inferior half of the breast (Figure 3.10).

Closure

In the areolar and submammary approaches, both edges of the divided muscle are mobilized separating each side from the implant surface with the fingertip to approxi-

mate each other for suturing using two to three separated 3/0 vicryl stitches (Figures 3.11, 3.12). The skin is closed with a subdermal vicryl suture and epidermal 5/0 suture. In my procedure, no drains are used.

Operative steps

- Lidocaine, bupivacaine and epinephrine anesthetic solutions are used.
- Skin incisions and subcutaneous dissection without cautery.

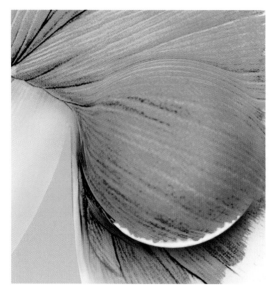

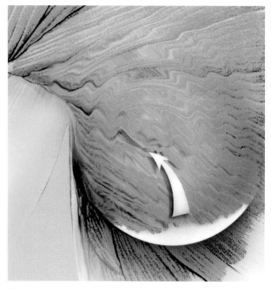

Figure 3.13 The implant is covered by the pectoralis major and the serratus anterior muscles. The inferior part of the pectoralis major muscle is transected.

Figure 3.14 When the pectoralis major muscle is in motion, the muscle slides over the implant as its inferior part is free.

- In the axillary and submammary approach direct submuscular dissection.
- In the areolar approaches, first the parenchyma has to be divided.
- The submuscular pocket includes the pectoralis major and the serratus anterior muscles (Figures 3.13, 3.14).
- The implant and the pocket are washed with a cefuroxone solution.
- Textured silicone implants are used.
- In the submammary and areolar approaches, the divided pectoralis is sutured.
- No drains are used.

Results

I usually use round, high profile implants and seldom use anatomical or low profile implants. By using textured cohesive silicone implants in the subpectoral approach I do not see any rippling or visible superior implants edges. The capsule contracture Baker II is less than 2%, implant extrusions are not observed, seromas are less than 1%, perioperative infections is less than 0.5% and implant displacement when there is muscle contraction is very rarely observed. The only problem is the implant malposition, having a rate of around 5% for early re-operation.

Case **1**

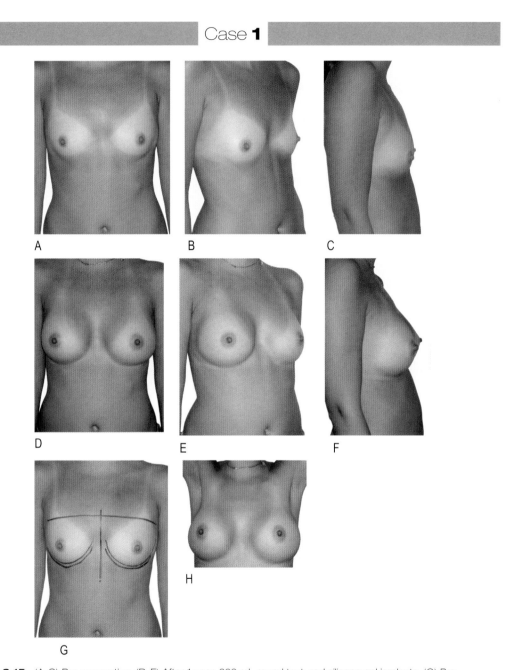

A

B

C

D

E

F

G

H

Figure 3.15 (A–C) Pre-opperative. (D–F) After 1 year, 300 mL round textured silicone gel implants. (G) Pre-operative axillary marks. (H) Axillary scars.

Subpectoral approach for breast augmentation

Case **2**

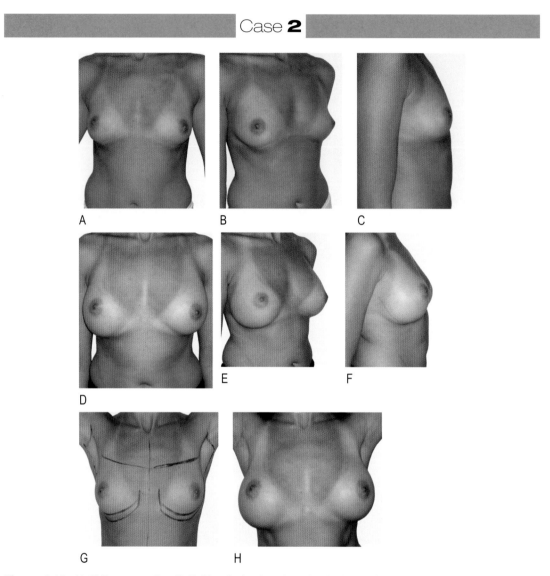

A   B   C

D   E   F

G   H

Figure 3.16 (A–C) Pre-opperative. (D–F) After the implantation of 320 mL round textured silicone gel implants. (G) Pre-op, submammary fold markings 2 cm below it. ••

Case **3**

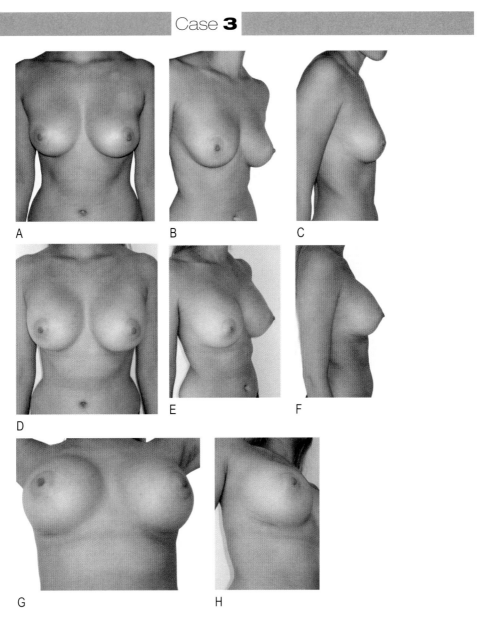

Figure 3.17   (A–C) Pre-op. (D–F) Thirteen months post-op.; 340 mL textured silicone implants were used. (G) From a frontal view the submammary scar is not visible. (H) From the inferior-lateral view, the scar is hardly visible.

Case **4**

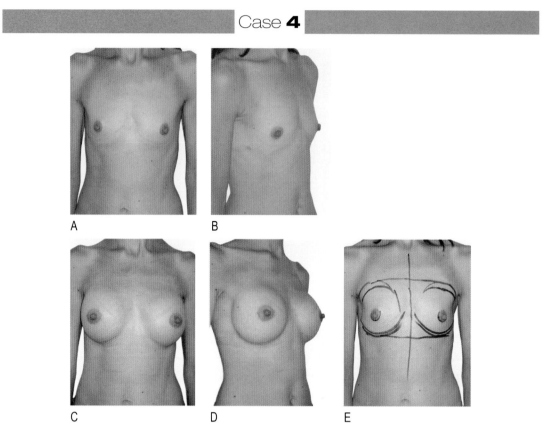

Figure 3.18   (A, B) Pre-op. (C, D) Two months after periareolar breast augmentation with 340 mL round texture silicone gel implants. (E) Pre-operative markings.

Case **5**

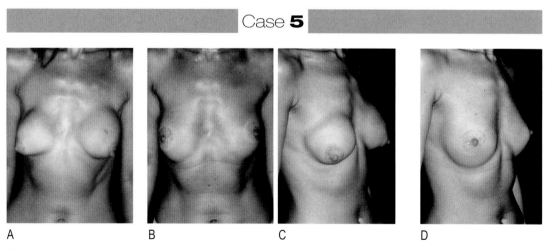

Figure 3.19   (A, C) Submammary breast implants. Capsule contracture and visible implant edges. (B, D) One year post-op. subpectoral approach using new round 300 mL textured silicone implants. Ptosis was corrected.

Case **6**

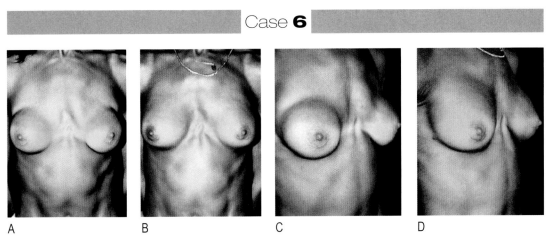

A   B   C   D

Figure 3.20 (A, C) Submammary breast implants. Capsule contracture Baker III. (B, D) Subpectoral approach using new 280 mL round textured silicone implants. No capsulectomy. The superior breast mound is no longer visible.

Pitfalls and how to prevent them

For minimal bleeding during surgery, profuse local anesthesia with vasoconstrictors should be used. To facilitate the submuscular pocket dissection, profuse infiltration is suggested. If post-operative pain relief is sought, then Bupivacaine should be added to the anesthetic solution. To detach the pectoralis major and the serratus muscles from the costal surfaces, the use of the finger tip is advised. To avoid implant displacement, highly textured implants are used and the muscles are transected at the new submammary fold area. To stop bleeding and to elongate the pocket, three compresses are placed in each of them. To avoid herniation of the implants, the pectoral muscle is sutured. In cases where malposition of the implant is detected, it should be reviewed and corrected as soon as possible. If this is done in 2–3 days re-operation will be easier to perform. To avoid visible implant edges, submuscular implants are used (Figures 3.15, 3.19).

Post-operative care

Patients may begin mobilization of their implants on the post-operative seventh day for 10 mins three to four times daily. The patient is advised not to practice any sport for 4 weeks.

Conclusion

The submuscular implant technique has several advantages when compared to the submammary approach. This technique is not widely adopted because it is more demanding than the submammary technique. I am hereby reporting my experience with the submammary, areolar and axilar approaches placing the implants submuscularly. Profuse local anesthesia is infiltrated to avoid bleeding, to facilitate the surgery and to bring some post-operative pain relief. The pocket is dissected detaching the pectoral major and anterior serratus muscles. Both muscles are disrupted at the new submammary fold projection to avoid the implant displacement. Textured silicone implants are used. Drains are not routinely used.

· ·

Further reading

Aldo MA. Breast augmentation: particular pears (?)for the subpectoral technique. Innovations in Plastic Surgery. Springer Verlag, Berlin. 2007. Ch 48, p. 389–396.

Hendricks H. Complete submuscular breast augmentation. 650 cases managed using an alternative surgical technique. Aesth Plast Surg 2007;31:147–153.

Rohrich R. Silicone breast implants: outcomes and safety update. Plast Reconstr Surg 2007;120:1s–3s.

Takanayagi S, Nakagawa C, Sugimoto Y. Augmentation mammaplasty: where should the implant be placed? Aesth Plast Surg 2004;28:83–88.

Tebbets J. Does fascia provide additional meaningful coverage over a breast implant? Plast Reconstr Surg 2004;113:777–779.

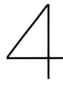
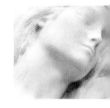

4

Saline implants: indications, techniques and precautions

L. Franklyn Elliott

Key points

- Understanding of the continued need and success of saline implants in aesthetic breast surgery.

- Acquiring an appreciation for when not to use saline breast implants.

- A simplified method for choosing the proper saline breast implant without extensive pre-operative measuring.

- A straightforward technique for saline implant primary augmentation.

- Understanding of possible complications that can ensue with saline implants and how to correct these complications.

Patient selection

Saline implants continue to have an important place in aesthetic breast surgery. In fact, the most commonly used breast implants in the United States for aesthetic breast surgery are saline. In my opinion, however, there remain certain patients who are better candidates for gel breast implants over saline breast implants. Certainly, since gel implants have become more available, many of us consider gel breast implants more broadly than was possible before January 2008. Nonetheless, despite the 'opening up' of the possible uses for gel breast implants, there are certain groups of patients in whom I continue to use saline breast implants.

One of the most frequent indications for the use of breast implants in aesthetic breast surgery is primary breast augmentation. In this group, patient selection is important. The primary quality which differentiates my general recommendation for a patient to have saline or gel implants is the pre-operative amount of the patient's breast tissue. Akin to the amount of breast tissue is the amount of subcutaneous fat, particularly in the chest area. Usually these two qualities are closely related such that a patient with very small amounts of breast tissue is a fairly thin patient as well. This patient, who would properly be termed an A cup and a very thin patient with low body fat (less than 10%) is probably a better candidate for gel implants for primary breast augmentation. In these patients, the borders of any implant are felt, particularly inferiorly and laterally. In these locations, the less resilient or 'thin' feel of a saline implant may be more apparent as opposed to the thicker, more natural feel of the gel implant when in situ. Thus, the thin patient with scant breast tissue is a better candidate for the gel implant than the saline implant for primary breast augmentation.

All other patients, i.e. those with A–B cup breasts or larger and whose body fat would not place the patient in the 'thin' category, are probably better candidates for saline implants. First of all, the implant becomes less palpable peripherally as the patient gains body fat and breast tissue. The palpable nature of the breast implant remains the gel implant's best advantage over the saline. As this becomes less of an advantage, the advantages of the saline implant take prominence. Significant advantages of the saline implant include less contamination upon insertion of the uninflated implant, a smaller incision with easier insertion of the implant, the adjustability of the saline breast implant, the fact that if they leak they only leak saline, and that the patient knows when the implant leaks. All of these are significant advantages of saline over gel implants.

While a whole host of causes have been suggested for capsular contracture, two of the primary causes for capsular contracture that are on everyone's list are microorganism contamination of the pocket and silicone gel stimulation of the capsule itself. The fact that the saline implant is inserted uninflated markedly reduces the opportunity for contamination of the implant itself or the internal space for the breast implant. This is in marked contrast to the force that is necessary to insert a gel implant and is a striking advantage of the saline breast implant. Certainly, skin protection can be used, which does help with insertion of the gel implant, but clearly there is less opportunity for contamination with the saline implant insertion techniques as opposed to the gel implant insertion techniques. Alternately, when considering silicone gel

stimulation of the capsule and its relation to capsular contracture, it is obvious that the saline implant contains no silicone gel and, thus, that causative factor is not present when saline implants are used. These advantages of the saline implant remain significant when advising patients upon their choice of saline or gel implants for primary breast augmentation.

At the time of the initial conversion from gel to saline in the United States in 1992, textured implants were in common use and were felt to be a significant improvement over smooth implants in terms of incidence of capsular contracture and naturalness of final result. The capsular contracture decrease was felt to be due to the texturing which 'broke up' the otherwise spherical smooth capsule around a smooth implant. The naturalness with a textured implant was felt to be due to the adherence of the implant to the capsule which stabilized its position on the chest wall giving a more natural relationship to the overlying breast as opposed to the smooth implant which could, and would, relatively slide around on the chest wall. This thinking accompanied the switch from gel to saline implants and thus most surgeons continued using textured implants. Over time it was noticed that capsular contracture, both incidence and intensity, was less with saline versus gel implants and it became increasingly clear that this was due to less contamination when inserting the saline implant and no occurrence of gel bleed as the implants did not contain gel.

As data was accumulated from both textured and smooth saline use, it became increasingly apparent that textured saline implants leaked more often and more quickly after implantation than smooth saline implants. Since capsular contracture was less of a problem with saline implants, it became obvious that the smooth saline implant was decidedly better than the textured saline implant and that is what we use today. Ultimately, though, it is the patient's choice. Patients are encouraged to educate themselves through any legitimate means possible. This would include information and literature from the implant companies themselves, which can be found in hard copy or on the internet. Any strong desire to use one or the other type of breast implant is honored. On the other hand, it is important for the surgeon to discuss the pros and cons of each implant type as listed above. It is not appropriate, in my opinion, to push a patient into the use of either implant against their wishes. Indeed, either the gel or saline implant is quite successful in essentially any clinical setting for breast augmentation, even in the thin patient using the saline implant. If the patient expresses a strong antipathy to the use of gel implants it is probably not a good idea to force this issue even if one feels the gel implant would be better. Patients with strong antipathy one way or the other will continue to worry post-operatively.

In secondary aesthetic breast surgery, it is generally a good idea to use the same type of implant on the second operation as was used on the first one. This is because the patient has become used to the feel of the saline or gel implant over time. Thus, keeping the same type implant is almost always better accepted by the patient. A caveat to that is that almost every patient who has had previous breast implants is characterized by the compression of the overlying breast tissue and a thinning of the overlying coverage of the breast implant. This should be thoroughly discussed with the patient, as the gel implant may be the better choice, depending on the degree of thinning of the overlying coverage.

There is generally no need for the use of shaped saline implants in aesthetic breast surgery. With overlying breast tissue the round saline implant achieves, on the upright chest wall, a more contoured confirmation and, thus, a contoured or shaped implant is not needed. This is also true for gel implants, where the round implant achieves a more contoured position on the upright chest. The literature is filled with declamations of the round implant due to superior pole fullness, allegedly due to the round breast implant. This is not the case, however, as almost all this superior pole fullness is due to inadequate inferior dissection or the formation of capsular contracture, which shifts the implant superiorly and leads to superior pole fullness no matter what type implant is used. In addition, the round implant has no polarity and, thus, its position in the pocket is unimportant as it rotates naturally in the pocket postoperatively. This, of course, is not true for the contoured or shaped implants.

For reconstruction, the saline implant use is limited to that of tissue expanders. Obviously, tissue expanders must be saline so they can be adjusted appropriately post-operatively. A tissue expander is a device used to achieve a specific purpose, that of expansion of the overlying skin and coverage in particular areas of the breast, usually inferior. This device is not appropriate for the reconstruction of the final breast.

Exchange of the tissue expander is almost always performed using a subsequent gel implant. Tissue coverage over implants after mastectomy is predictably thin, even when a muscle flap has been used. While the flap thickens the coverage over the anterior surface of the implant, at the periphery coverage is always thin. Thus, the gel implant is the best choice for the final implant in breast reconstruction.

Indications

Saline breast implants are indicated for primary augmentation in the patient who is not excessively thin and has at least an A–B cup of breast tissue preoperatively. This, of course, is a judgement call and there are certainly patients who fall in a gray zone. On the other hand, results with either the saline or gel implant are so good that the use of a saline or gel implants in these gray zone patients is generally successful. Secondary aesthetic breast surgery usually follows the rule that whatever the patient had preoperatively is usually used for the second procedure. Exceptions to this are patients who have a desire to change from one filler to the other. Often these patients are significantly influenced by previous leak of the breast implant. This can be the case with a saline implant that has leaked, causing the patient to want to use gel or the patient who has had a gel leak and now wants to use saline. In these cases, a patient's desires are almost always followed.

On secondary aesthetic breast surgery if the patient's tissues have thinned to a significant degree due to the longstanding breast implant, a gel implant is probably the best choice. There are a few indications for the use of the saline implant as the final implant in reconstructive breast surgery. There may be the very rare patient who has a very strong antipathy to the use of gel breast implants, but those patients are uncommon.

Operative technique

Pre-operative preparation

For the primary breast augmentation patient, preoperative markings are kept to a relative minimum. The round, smooth saline breast implant is the primary choice, thus size remains the main quality for discussion with the patient. We each have our own method of reaching a conclusion as to the proper size. There are many methods that work. Focusing on cup size seems to be an excellent way to communicate with the patient in a manner that both doctor and patient understand and generally agree upon. In general, it is suggested that the patient choose between a B–C cup, a full C cup or larger than a C cup. This usually enables the patient to communicate to the surgeon the general size they wish to be. One can also examine the types of bra the patient uses pre-operatively to give an idea of what size they are comfortable with and would like to be. Coupling these two methods generally directs the surgeon to the appropriate size. For instance, for a B–C cup the patient would generally get a 275–300 mL implant. For a full C the patient would receive a 325–375 ml implant. A person who wanted to be larger than a C would generally get a 400–475 ml implant. We rarely go over 475 ml in primary breast augmentation. Indeed, most patients fit into the first two categories.

The other quality of the implant to be decided upon is projection – normal, normal–plus and high. The typical patient gets normal projection implants for primary breast augmentation. Secondary cases may get normal plus or high projection implants depending on the chest dimension, the skin envelope and patient desires. As projection increases for any given size implant, the base narrows. This relationship can be utilized for a desired effect. However, these features rarely are necessary in primary augmentation. Once the appropriate implant size and projection have been chosen, the patient is marked by marking the inframammary line bilaterally. We are careful to be sure that those lines are symmetrical. In addition, it is extremely important to note any differences in amounts of breast tissue on each side, as the saline implants can be adjusted mL for mL. This is often not easy to do once the implants are in place. If one has evaluated the patient preoperatively and finds that one breast is larger than the other, this should be noted and preparations made.

The best incision for saline implant insertion is the periareolar incision. This incision fades rapidly and is barely noticeable post-operatively. One of the drawbacks to this incision is that one must dissect around the breast tissue inferiorly and not through the breast tissue. This is slightly more difficult than if the inframammary incision is used, but the periareolar incision has the strong advantage of being less visible than the inframammary incision. However, if one is uncomfortable about dissecting around the breast

tissue through the periareolar incision, the inframammary incision is a better choice. With a small amount of breast tissue, it is quite easy to dissect caudal around the breast tissue to achieve the postmammary plane. Positioning is supine with the arms extended laterally. Infiltration of both the proposed incision site as well as fourth and fifth intercostal blocks is done with bupivacaine with epinephrine.

Technique

The periareolar incision is made transversely as far as the areolar dimensions allow, from approximately the 4 to 8 or 9 o'clock position. Since the incision site has already been injected, the dissection caudal subcutaneously, superficial to the breast tissue, proceeds with little or no bleeding. The inferior breast tissue is then elevated over the pectoralis major muscle for 2–3 cm. The anterior surface of the pectoralis muscle can then be seen and the pectoralis entered, splitting the fibers not cutting them. The submuscular plane is reached by visualizing the underlying ribs, which can be palpated through the muscle prior to dissection.

The subpectoral pocket is preferred for the following reasons. The pectoralis muscle gives an additional layer of coverage to the breast implant, particularly superiorly. The pectoralis muscle provides a layer of separation between the breast tissue and the subpectoral breast implant, helpful for possible subsequent mammographic visualization. The subpectoral pocket has been shown in some studies to lead to less capsular contracture than the pre-pectoral placement. For these reasons, the subpectoral placement of the saline implant is preferred. It is true though that if the subpectoral placement of the implant seems to lead to a constriction of the pocket inferiorly, there is no hesitation in dividing the muscle inferiorly to allow for an appropriate, rounded shape of the inferior pole of the augmented breast.

The subpectoral pocket is dissected to the dimensions of the breast. It is particularly important to divide digitally the insertion of the pectoralis fibers medially from the 8 to the 10 o'clock position (if looking at the left breast). It is not necessary to divide all of these fibers, but digital disruption of these fibers to an extent that is equal bilaterally and adequately frees up the tension in that portion of the pocket is most important. It is important not to dissect too far laterally prior to placement of the implant, as this dissection can be completed once the implant is in place. Once the pocket has been dissected to essentially 95% of its planned dimensions, the pocket is irrigated with triple antibiotics. The saline implant, which has been soaked in antibiotics, is then inserted in an uninflated state with its injection tubing previously inserted into the implant. The implant is unfurled digitally in the pocket and inflation begins. We use a closed system for inflation from a sterile bag of intravenous fluid.

Once the implant has been inflated to within 20% of the desired size, the implant is carefully adjusted in the pocket to be sure that it is completely unfurled and oriented properly. Inflation of the implant is then completed. With the patient in a sitting, upright position, the position of the implant and the shape of the breast is assessed. As mentioned previously, if the inferior pole is not nicely rounded, there is no hesitation in division of the muscle inferiorly. This can be continued down to the inframammary line within the pocket. Normally this technique gives nice release of the inferior pole and rounds out the inferior pole. The injection tubing is left in place as attention is turned to the opposite breast.

A similar procedure is carried out on the opposite side, including the incision, the dissection, placement of the implant, and inflation of the implant. Division of the muscle inferiorly as well as medial dissection is performed, depending on the symmetry of the breasts. At this point, with the patient in a sitting, upright position, all quadrants of the breast are finally critiqued. Often, additional lateral dissection is indicated into order to achieve symmetry. In addition, a final assessment of size can be done and milliliters of saline added or removed to make the sizes as exact as possible. Once size, shape and symmetry are achieved, the injection tubings can be removed and the plugs palpably placed.

Closure

Closure is straightforward, with two layers of absorbable sutures. This is followed by sterile tape. No other dressings are used. Drains are never used for primary breast augmentation. No post-operative bandaging or bra used except as mentioned above. In fact, patients are advised to not wear a bra for at least 1 week after surgery, as it is felt that the bra can shift the breast implant up in the pocket, bringing it out of the space in which it was inserted intraoperatively. After a week, bras are allowed. Patients are not instructed to perform post-operative massage.

Operative steps

- Pre-operative assessment of asymmetry, shape and size.
- Periareolar and intercostal injections.
- Periareolar incision with dissection around, not through, breast tissue.
- Digital dissection of the subpectoral pocket with careful inspection for any bleeding.
- Insertion of the saline breast implant into one side, with inflation to the appropriate size.
- Division of inferior musculature if necessary.
- Completion of the opposite side and assessment of both breasts with the patient in a sitting position, followed by possible additional lateral dissection.
- No bra post-operatively.

Results

Case **1**

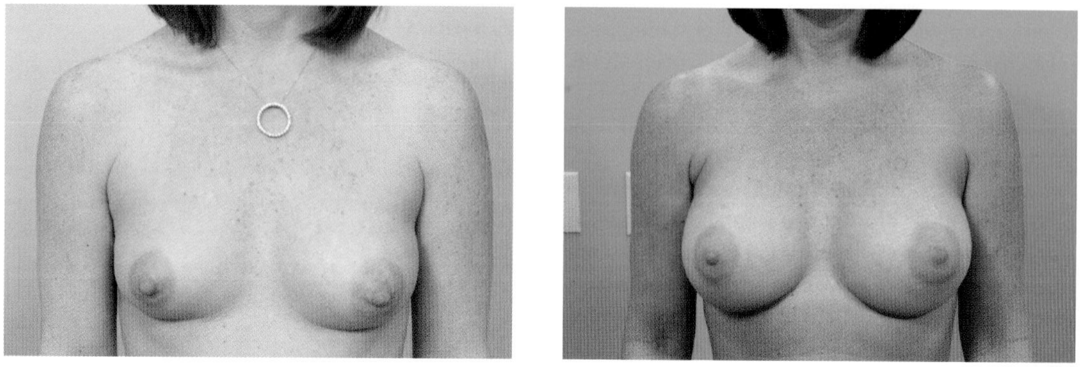

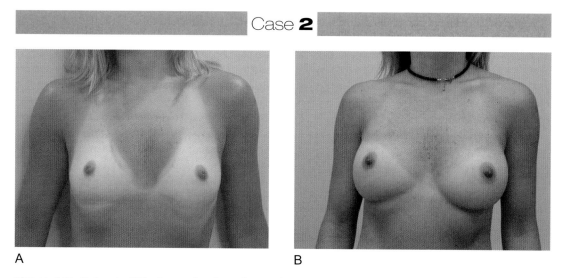

A   B

Figure 4.1   Periareolar submuscular saline implant breast augmentation. (A) Before. (B) Six months post-op. 350 mL left, 325 mL right.

Case **2**

A   B

Figure 4.2   Periareolar 275 mL smooth saline submuscular. (A) Before. (B) Ten months post-operative.

Case **3**

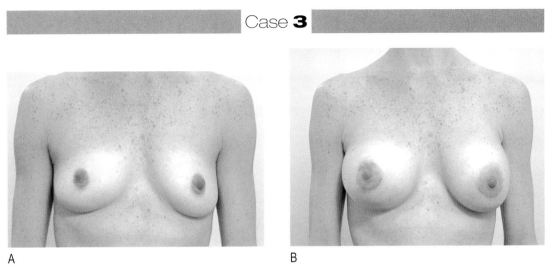

A   B

Figure 4.3 Periareolar submuscular smooth saline: 325 mL inflated to 350 mL (A) Before. (B) Eight months post-operative.

Case **4**

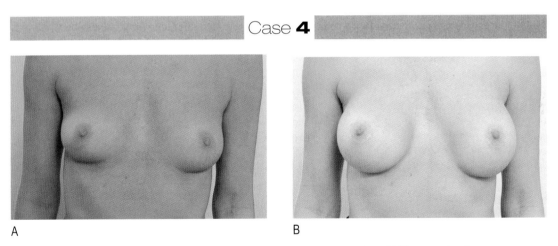

A   B

Figure 4.4 Smooth saline submuscular: 325 mL inflated to 350 mL (A) Before. (B) Nine months after.

Case **5**

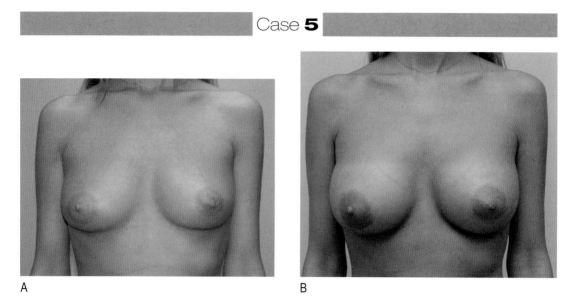

A   B

Figure 4.5 Submuscular saline smooth: periareolar 300 mL (A) Before. (B) Nine months post-operative.

Pitfalls and how to correct

With the above-described technique, one should achieve the appropriate shape and size in essentially all primary breast augmentation patients. However, it is certainly possible to over-dissect or under-dissect the pocket in any direction. In the first example this patient indicates an instance where the dissection has been carried too low inferiorly. If this is noted within the first couple of weeks after surgery, taping along with continuous bra wear might alleviate the problem. On the other hand, generally if the implant is too low, it remains too low. In this case an additional operation involving inferior capsulectomy and capsulorrhaphy with permanent suture was necessary to give the proper post-operative result (Figure 4.6).

There is the occasional instance wherein a patient has an appropriate result after saline implant augmentation but loses weight. This may shift the patient from an acceptable indication for placement of a saline implant to one in whom the borders of the implants can now be palpated more than they would like. The second patient began running multiple triathlons postoperatively. Her body fat dropped to less than 10% and she complained of being able to palpate the breast implants. Because of her thinness, there was a good bit of doubt that exchanging the implants from saline to gel would completely alleviate her concerns.

Thus, in this case we used fat injections in specific areas to actually add fat to remove the palpability of the breast implant borders (Figure 4.7).

Under-dissection inferiorly can also be a problem, resulting in the implant being shifted cephelad leading to unattractive superior pole fullness and a lack of natural lower pole roundness. As mentioned in the operative steps, the division of the pectoralis major muscle inferiorly along with its overlying fascia should be strongly considered if one detects lack of filling of the inferior pole. This certainly places the 'submuscular implant' in a 'dual plane' position. This terminology has made this part of the operation unduly complex. The simple fact is that the muscle must be divided if there is any constriction of the lower pole. Having the lower pole of the breast implant subcutaneous instead of submuscular may lead to some degree of increased palpability. However, in most cases an excellent postoperative result easily cancels minor palpability inferiorly.

Post-operative care

Post-operative care begins intraoperatively in that the exact position of the breast implant is paramount. Once the implants are placed in the exactly correct position intraoperatively they will remain in that position unless they are unduly manipulated postopera-

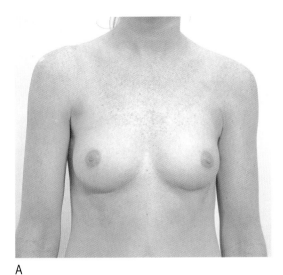

A

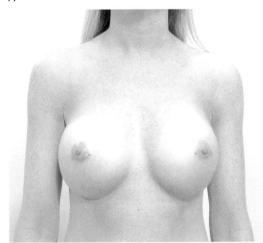

B

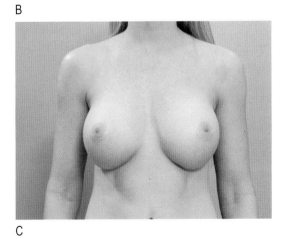

C

Figure 4.6 Submuscular implants. 300 mL textured saline. (A) Before. (B) Too low: needs capsulorrhaphy. (C) Six months status post-inferior capsulectomy/ capsulorrhaphy.

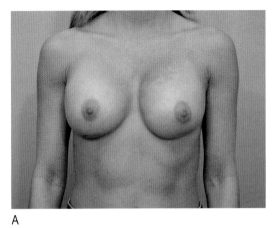

A

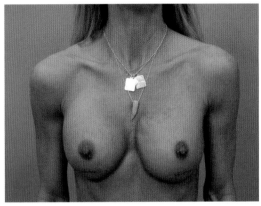

B

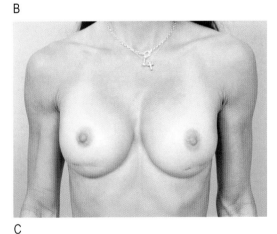

C

Figure 4.7 (A) One year after 325 mL gel augmentation (secondary). (b) Six years after. After fat loss due to training for triathlons: note rippling in upper inner quadrant left breast. (C) Six months after fat injections to upper inner pole left breast. Rippling has largely resolved.

47

tively. Thus, any kind of bras or dressings placed inferiorly on the primary augmentation patient are contraindicated. Patients can begin driving and doing normal daily activities 2–3 days post-operatively, depending on their discomfort. Pain relievers and muscle relaxants are also used during this time. Bras are contraindicated until at least one week post-op.

Conclusion

The saline breast implant remains an important tool in achieving successful primary breast augmentation. While there is the occasional very thin patient who is not a good candidate for the saline implant, most patients desiring breast augmentation are good candidates for the use of the saline breast implant. The technique is a relatively simple one but an exact one.

Ultimately, it is judged on the operating table with the patient in a sitting, upright position. Any variance in symmetry must be corrected at that time through implant filling or implant positioning. No bra or other inferior dressing should be used in the first post-op week.

Saline breast implants are also indicated for secondary aesthetic breast surgery, particularly if the patient has had saline breast implants prior to the secondary operation. On the other hand, patients who have had saline breast implant leak sometimes choose to use gel implants for their second or third operations and these desires should certainly be honored. Smooth saline implants are preferred over textured saline implants, as the textured saline implants have a higher incidence of leakage. Saline implants are rarely, if ever, used for the final implant in breast reconstruction.

Further reading

Araco A, Gravante G, Araco F, Delogu D, Cervelli V, Walgenbach K. A retrospective analysis of 3000 primary aesthetic breast augmentations: post-operative complications and associated factors. Aesth Plast Surg 2007;341:532.

Elliott LF. Breast augmentation with round, smooth, saline or gel implants: the pros and cons. Clin Plast Surg 2001;28:523.

Gancedo M, Ruiz-Corro L, Salazar-Montes AR, et al. Pirfenidone prevents capsular contracture after mammary implantation. Aesth Plast Surg 2008;32:32.

Henriksen TF, Fryzek JP, Hölmich LR, et al. Surgical intervention and capsular contracture after breast augmentation: a prospective study of risk factors. Ann Plast Surg 2005;54:343.

Kjöller K, Hölmich LR, Jacobson PH, et al. Epidemiological investigation of local complications after cosmetic breast surgery in Denmark. Ann Plast Surg 2002;48:229.

McCarthy CM, Pusic AL, Kerrigan CL. Silicone breast implants and MRI screening for rupture. Plast Reconstr Surg 2008;121:1127.

Nanigian BR, Wong GB, Khatri VP. Inframammary crease: positional relationship to the pectoralis major muscle origin. Aesth Surg J 2007;27:509.

Rohrich RJ, Reece EM. Breast augmentation today: saline vs silicone: what are the facts? Plast Reconstr Surg 2008;121:669.

Stokes RB. Breast augmentation in thin women: patient satisfaction with saline-filled implants. Aesth Plast Surg 2004;28:153.

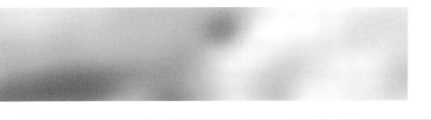

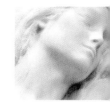

Silicone implants

Giorgio Bronz

Key points

- Atraumatic operation.
- Operation under vision.
- Textured implants.

- Subglandular position.
- Periareolar or inframammary approach.

Introduction

When I started performing breast augmentation surgery in the late 1970s, I was using round, smooth implants. The operation was done blind with the pocket dissected using the fingers rather than by sight. Complication rates were high with incidences of infection, hematomas and capsular contractures. To improve the quality of life of my patients I knew I had to do something to improve this technique and to reduce complications.

Patient selection

The evaluation of the quality, volume, dimensions of the breast parenchyma and soft tissue envelope is very important. The ideal patient is slim, has adequate soft tissue coverage over the implant and good skin quality. The major cause for re-operation is breast implants that are too large for the patient's tissue. To choose the correct implant, measurements of thorax width, the distance between sternal notch and areola, breast width, areola width, the distance from nipple to infra-mammary fold, and inter-mammary distance are necessary.

Indications

All the patients with the above mentioned qualities are good candidates for breast augmentation

Operative technique

Pre-operative preparation

At least 1 week before surgery and with the patient in the standing position, I visually analyze the body, the existing breasts and take measurements. Because I am a private surgeon I have to determine and order the implants that I use 1 week before surgery. For this reason, I cannot use sizers. On the day of surgery, I make the markings. According to the implant size, I mark the future inframammary fold and the medial, lateral and cranial pocket extent. Depending on patient preference, the incision is periareolar or infra-mammary. If a ptosis or asymmetry are to be corrected, the marking takes care of this problem.

The patient is placed in a supine position on the operating table with their arms out to the side at a 75 degree angle. The anesthetist begins the sedation and after careful disinfection, I start the infiltration first circumferentially with 0.5% mepivacaine and then infiltrate the medial and the lateral plane of dissection. I do not use more than 60 mL of 0.5% local anesthesia and keep the needle of infiltration horizontal so as not to provoke pneumothorax.

Technique

Depending on patient preference, the incision is made in the future inframammary line or the periareolar. The plane of dissection is retroglandular and supramuscular. The dissection is carried out under direct vision with the electrocautery. I dissect the pocket 2–4 cm wider than the implant; 2 cm wider if the skin is very loose and 4 cm if it is tight enough. If I use the periareolar approach, the incision is made to also transect the parenchyma. Caudally, the dissection is carried out to the desired inframammary line. Careful vessel coagulation is performed until the pocket is very dry. I never use drainage during the primary operation. The anesthetist administers a single injection of antibiotics.

The selected implants are placed accurately in the pocket. The implant is only exposed to the air for a few seconds. If the approach is inframammary, the superficial fascia is sutured to the profound one with interrupted 3-0 resorbable sutures. A second layer is sutured with 4-0 subcuticular sutures, and finally I use an intradermal 5-0 running suture. With the periareolar approach, the breast parenchyma is carefully closed with interrupted 3-0 resorbable sutures. If the periareolar approach is combined with a periareolar mastopexy, I first place a purse-string suture (round block suture) in the outer diameter with 2-0 nylon tightened to the chosen inner diameter. Then, 4-0 resorbable sutures are placed in the dermis. Finally, a 5-0 resorbable suture completes the closure and I tape with paper tape. In cases where I use drains (secondary cases only), these are removed after 24–48 h. A bra is worn after 24 h.

Operative steps

- Exact drawing.
- Pre-selected implants.
- Careful disinfection.
- Atraumatic pocket dissection under vision.
- Pocket dissection 2–4 cm larger than the implants.
- Closure in three layers with resorbable sutures (only round block suture in non resorbable nylon).

Post-operative care

- Pain pills for 24 h.
- Bed rest for 24 h.
- The paper tape bandage is changed after 24 h and replaced with a sports bra.
- The patient can resume driving after 1 week.
- No active sport allowed for 6 weeks.

Results

Case 1

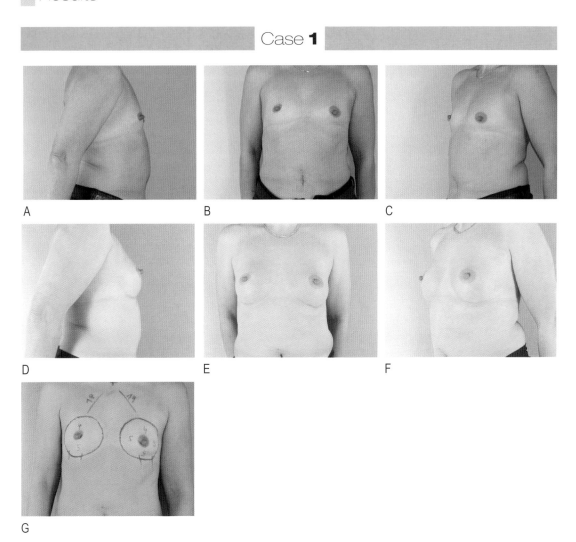

Figure 5.1 (A–C) Pre-operative view of a 49-year-old woman. (G) Exact measurements determine the pre-operative markings. Extent of the pocket dissection for a small implant. Lowering of the inframammary fold 5 cm below the inferior areolar border. Inframammary approach. Incision 5 cm. (D–F) Post-operative views 2 years following surgery. Sub-glandular augmentation with McGhan Style 410 MM185g implant via an inframammary approach. The inframammary fold was lowered 5 cm below the infra-areolar border.

Case **2**

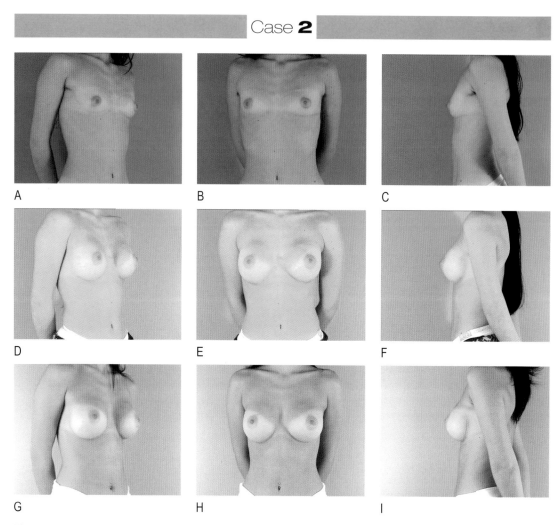

Figure 5.2 (A–C) Pre-operative view of a 20-year-old woman. (D–F) Post-operative view 1 year after sub-glandular augmentation via an inframammary approach 5.5 cm below the infra-areolar border with McGhan Style 410 270cc implant. (G–I) Post-operative view 9 years after surgery. In Part I the marks of a bra which was too small are visible.

Case **3**

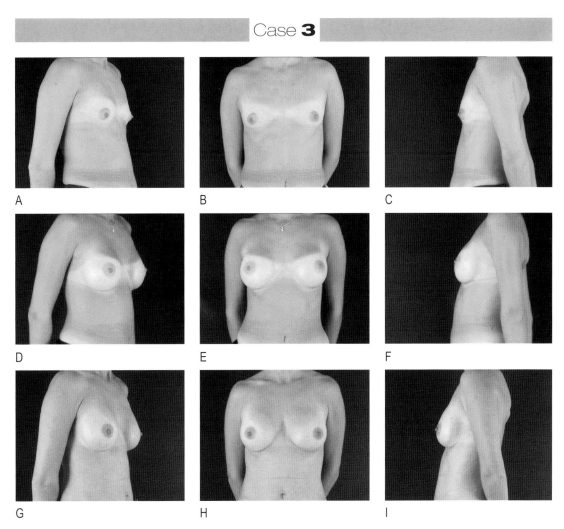

A   B   C

D   E   F

G   H   I

Figure 5.3 (A–C) Pre-operative view of a 23-year-old woman. (D–F) Postoperative view 1 year after sub-glandular augmentation via an inframammary approach 5.5 cm below the inferior areolar border with McGhan Style 410 240cc implant. (G–I) Post-operative views 10 years after surgery.

Case **4**

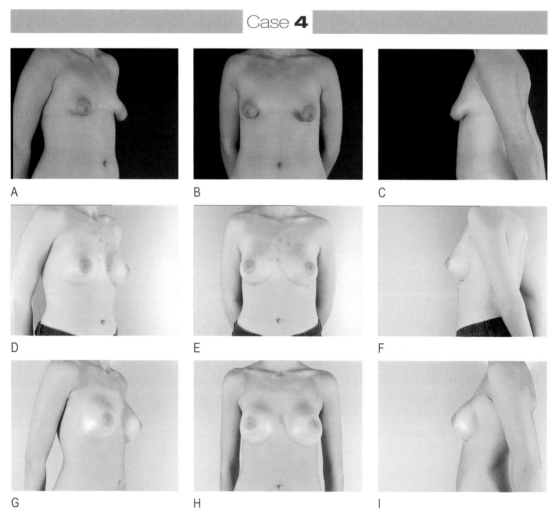

A B C
D E F
G H I

Figure 5.4 (A–C) Pre-operative view of a 19-year-old woman with tuberous breasts. (D–F) Post-operative view 1 year after sub-glandular augmentation via a periareolar approach. The areola is reduced to a 4.5 cm diameter. The inferior constricted parenchyma is released from deep to superficial with multiple horizontal and vertical cuts. After this procedure a McGhan Style 410 240g anatomical implant is placed in the pocket, dissected 5.5 cm below the areola. (G–I) Post-operative view 11 years after surgery. The round block permanent suture in 3-0 nylon is still in place.

Case 5

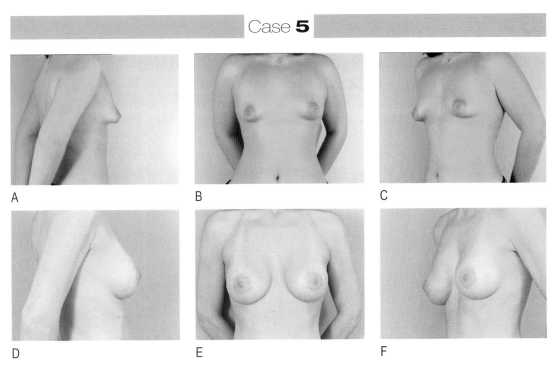

A B C

D E F

Figure 5.5 (A–C) Pre-operative view of a 22-year-old woman with tuberous breasts. (D–F) Post-operative view 9 years after periareolar, sub-glandular augmentation with a McGhan Style 410 FM 205g implant. The procedure is the same as in Case 4.

Silicone implants

Pitfalls and how to correct them

Case **6**

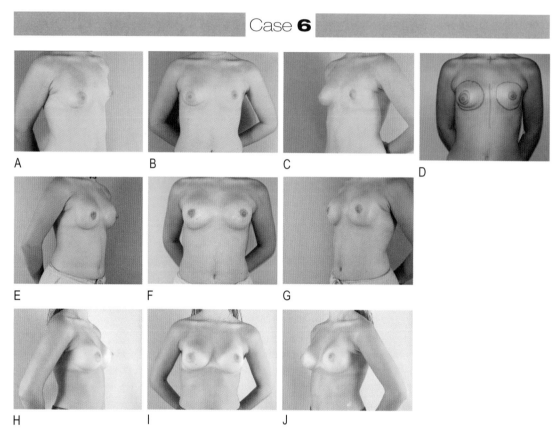

A

B

C

D

E

F

G

H

I

J

Figure 5.6 (A–C) Pre-operative view of a 18-year-old woman with asymmetric breasts. (D) Pre-operative marking: Left breast: periareolar approach 2 cm lowering of the inframammary fold. Right breast: periareolar mastopexy, 1 cm lowering of the inframammary fold. (E–G) Post-operative views 6 months after sub-glandular augmentation with a McGhan Style 410 MM 185g on the left smaller side and with a McGhan Style 110 90cc implant round block suture on the right side. (H–J) Post-operative view 3 years after surgery. Note the minimal enlargement and ptosis of the right breast.

Case 7

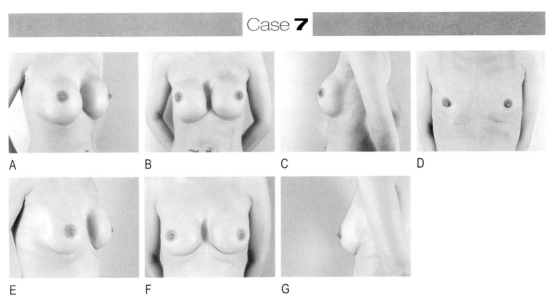

A   B   C   D

E   F   G

Figure 5.7 (A–C) A 42-year-old woman who underwent breast augmentation with too large implants (335 mL) with distortion of the areola. (D) Three months after capsulectomy and implant removal. (E–G) Post-operative view 6 months after secondary sub-glandular inframammary augmentation with McGhan Style 410 MF 255g.

Conclusion

Careful pre-operative evaluation of the volume, consistency and dimensions of the existing breast and careful operative planning with precise drawing and precise execution lead to desired surgical results for both the surgeon and the patient.

Further reading

Bronz G. How reliable are textured implants used in breast surgery? A Review of 510 Implants. Aesth Plast Surg 1999;23:424–427.

Bronz G. A comparison of naturally shaped and normal implants. Aesth Surg J 2002;23:238–246.

Bronz G. Mamma reconstruction with skin-expander and silicone protheses: 15 years experience. Aesth Plast Surg 2002;26:215–218.

Maxwell P. Breast asymmetry. Aesth Surg J 2001;21:552–561.

Tebbetts JB. Patient evaluation, operative planning, and surgical techniques to increase control and reduce morbidity and reoperations in breast augmentation. Clin Plast Surg 2001;28:501–521.

Tebbetts JB. The best breast. CosmetXpertise, Dallas, 1999.

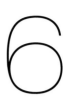
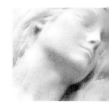

Semi-cohesive gel implants

Michael Scheflan, Constantin Stan

Key points

- Patients often ask for enhancement of breast shape, so the new breast must be controlled dimensionally. The extension must be controlled horizontally, vertically and anteriorly.

- Consideration of the new way of approaching a breast augmentation including patient education and information.

- Size is less important. Proportion, shape and acceptance of patient limits must be discussed and agreed upon.

- Introduction and consideration of a new generation of implants: implant shape, designed to reshape the final breast shape more closely to anatomical shape; and gel consistency to keep the implant shape and to control the soft tissue distribution.

- Introduction of a plan to evaluate the patient dimensions and characteristics, select an appropriate implant and plan the surgical technique.

- Introduction of new principles and surgical techniques to match the pocket limits and internal soft tissue modification to achieve the best results from the outset.

Introduction

For the past four decades we have primarily been using round, soft, 'responsive' silicone gel implants for breast augmentation. Our best attempts however, have often been unsuccessful in producing a long-term, predictable, stable and attractive enhancement of the breast. It is not surprising that in an organ subjected to monthly hormonal changes, pregnancies and fluctuation of body weight, it is difficult to achieve a lifelong attractive and stable result by placing an implant in it as while the implant itself does not change much over time, everything surrounding it does (Drever 2003).

During this era, with few implant options to choose from, the only decision that had to be made concerned the size of the implant. While some of our patients had good long-term results, others seemed to deteriorate with time. Silicone gel implants appeared to keep the breasts of some of our patients attractive and rejuvenated but accelerated breast aging in many others. If all patients and breasts were alike and the only change that occurred following insertion of the implant in a breast was making the breast bigger, then issues such as individual tissue and implant characteristics and the dynamics between the two would be irrelevant. The rationale behind the evolution of and the movement towards cohesive, form stable implants was driven by patients and surgeons who were looking for better long-term outcomes. A stable appearance of an augmented breast requires a shape stable device and a stable interaction between the implant and the soft tissue envelope surrounding it.

As we cannot prevent hormonal changes and aging from occurring in the breast, we need to establish a predictable relationship with an implant. This means that the implant should fit the breast like a 'hand in a glove', have an even, constant distribution of gel throughout the shell in any position and be perfectly filled with cohesive gel so that there are almost no wrinkles on its surface. Form stable implants maintain a constant shape in and outside the breast, and the cohesive gel used to fill them does not spread when broken (Spear et al 2001). The first introduction of anatomical, form stable implant (style 410 FM by McGhan) was in 1994 by Tebbetts. Originally these implants were conceptualized to produce a durable, longer-lasting, wrinkle free implant and to stabilize the shape of the implant and the breast over time. Soft gels (responsive) implants easily deform into a sphere by even a mild fibrous capsule while cohesive silicone gel implants retain their shape and form even when cut or compressed and hence breast shape remains stable (Figure 6.1). A form stable, cohesive gel implant retains its shape even in unfavorable parenchymal environment such as thin soft tissues.

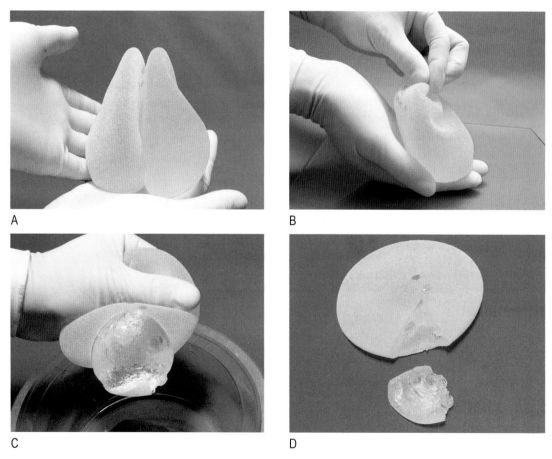

A

B

C

D

Figure 6.1   Cohesive gel breast implants – advantages. (A,B) Cohesive gel/stable shape implants do not collapse or fold and maintain their shape. (C,D) The whole implant or even a piece of it should maintain its shape when cut apart.

Advantages of form stable implants

Form stable implants cause fewer deformities such as rippling, traction folds, buckling, knuckling, vertical implant displacement and bottoming out (Tebbetts 2006). Our personal experience over the last decade has shown that the overall shape stays the same after a long period of implantation. Textured form stable implants move less during the capsular contracture compared with smooth, soft gel implants (Figures 6.2, 6.3). The wide variety of different implant shapes and

dimensions available today cater to more existing and desired breast types and makes customized fitting of an implant to a breast specific and individualized.

The high consistency of the filler gel influences the wear of the envelope. Improved device durability means less risk for implant rupture (0.3–1%). Hence, according to the same study, responsive gel implants have five to thirty times higher rupture risk and the removal of a ruptured, form stable implant is easy and more complete as the gel does not spread (Figure 6.4). A well planned and executed, dimensional pocket with snugly fitting, elastic soft tissues overlying the stable shape implant better controls the final breast shape.

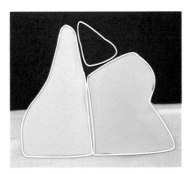

Figure 6.2 Round vs anatomical shaped implant, low responsive gel vs high cohesive gel. Allergan Matrix 410 high cohesive gel (maintenance of shape and free from folds) vs round, low responsive gel (relatively under-filled and the gel moves within the shell to the bottom, without knowing what the shape will be in the pocket).

Disadvantages of form stable implants

Cohesive gel implants result in a slightly firmer breast, similar to Baker II consistency. While acceptable for young, nuliparous women, it may feel less favorable in multiparous woman with more softness, laxity and thinning of their breasts. Rarely, however, patients complained about firmness and in no instance were we asked to exchange form stable, cohesive gel implants to softer ones. The process of implant selection and surgical technique is more technically demanding with a need for a change in concept and a steeper learning curve for the surgeon. Because of the risk of damaging the implant by forcing it through a short incision, the incision must be larger (5.5–6 cm incisions are often necessary). In more than 90% of

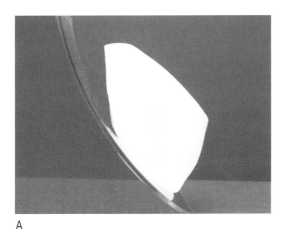

A

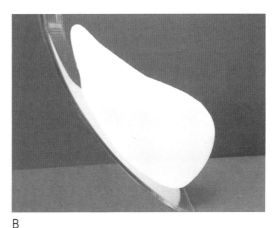

B

Figure 6.3 Cohesive gel implants – advantages. (A) Round, lower responsive gel implants do not maintain the shape and are subject to the forces of gravity (B) Cohesive gel implants with form stable shape do not collapse or fold and do maintain the shape even in upward position.

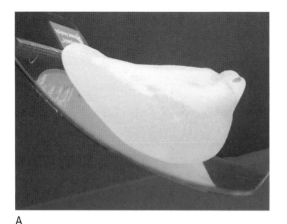
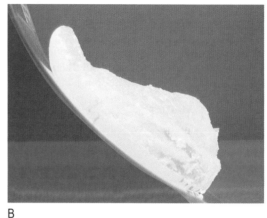

A   B

Figure 6.4   (A) Cohesive gel implants will not leak when the shell might break or (B) if the shell is peeled of the implant, the cohesive gel filler will maintain its shape.

patients, the inframammary approach is the recommended route. Axillary and periareolar approaches are possible but less desirable. Using cohesive shaped implants carries 0.7% risk of rotation with major impact on the breast shape. The more complex technology of implant manufacturing has resulted in higher implant costs.

The gel confusion

Since the introduction of the first high cohesive gel implant, it was obvious that cohesivity had no common denominator and that highly cohesive devices were different from each other in more than one way. Firmness depended on how much 'cross linking glue' was added to the original liquid formula. There is large variability related to the gel consistency amongst different manufacturers and in the way it is perceived by plastic surgeons. Consistency, degree of fill and shapes differ from one producer to another. Both major manufacturers, Allergan and Mentor, refer to their products as anatomical, high cohesive gel implants (Allergan: Matrix family, Style 410, 410 Soft Touch™ and Style 510 Dual Gel (Figure 6.5). Mentor: CPG™ MemoryGel™ (Figure 6.6). These two leading products differ not only in the fill but also in the feel and shape. It is impossible to compare both implant families in terms of gel consistency only by a subjective definition of examining and palpating the implants. The shape of anatomical and round implants produced by different companies is different. While it

is clear that the final shape and the gel consistency are important for breast shape control, it is difficult to compare or verify which shape controls and creates a better looking breast in the same setting for a longer period of time.

The Allergan (McGhan) Style 410 was the first shaped cohesive gel implant introduced. The expanded 410 product line includes 12 different shapes for any given width. Each implant is designated by width, and two letters. The first relates to the height (low, medium, full) and the second to the projection (low, medium, full). In 1997, the original high cohesive gel consistency was softened and the style 410 Soft Touch™ was added as an entire second matrix choice. An extra (X) projection implant was added 4 years ago forming a 12 '410 Matrix'. All original nine cells of the 410 series are available in the Soft Touch™ variety to cater to patients and surgeon's needs and desires. It is not clear and there is no consensus whether softening the gel somewhat causes the implant to lose its shape primarily in the upper pole. There is agreement however that the thinner the soft tissue envelope of the patient, the more form stability is needed. In other words, a firmer shaped implant helps produces a better looking breast in thin patients.

The contour profile gel (CPG™) high cohesive gel from Mentor was initially made in a single shape (medium height, medium projection), and filled with a gel slightly softer than their competitors. In a series of Mentor's gel consistencies from 1 (responsive gel), 2 (Lumera, similar to Soft Touch™), the new consistency

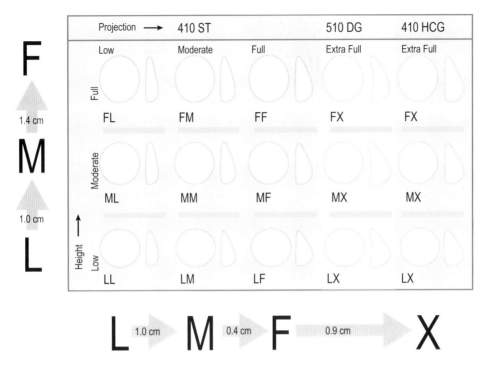

Figure 6.5 Allergan implants chart. Courtesy of Allergan.

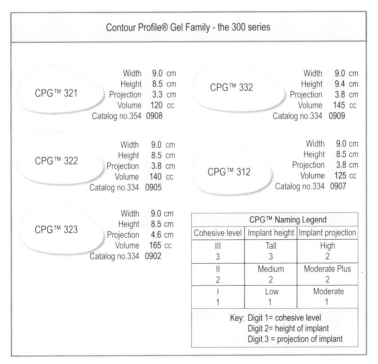

Figure 6.6 Mentor implants chart. Courtesy of Mentor.

was MemoryGel™ 3, the most highly cohesive gel in their series. The CPG line has later expanded to include three different projections and three additional heights. The huge choice of implant shapes and fillers further increases the 'gel confusion'.

Patient selection

Both authors have had extensive experience using cohesive, form stable implants with a long-term follow up primarily with style 410/510 matrix family from Allergan. Ten years experience using cohesive, form stable implants in Europe and Israel clearly demonstrates the lowest reported incidence of rupture, fibrous capsule formation and reoperations rates (Bengtson 2007). Some misconceptions associated with breast augmentation need to be clarified, discussed, sharpened and nuanced before embarking on the journey of using form stable implants. Among them are that the only change caused by implants is size increase, that the implant does not cause changes in the breast tissues and that the implant's fill, size or shape has no bearing on the long-term result. Implants firm up and lift the breast and therefore keep it looking young. Large implants permanently fill the upper pole and high profile implants correct breast ptosis. Round implants appear spherical and anatomical implants give a more natural but ptotic look.

Unsubstantiated working hypothesis like these are commonly verbalized by physicians and patients alike and require reeducation of both groups. Using the new cohesive, form stable implants requires a new way of thinking and a major paradigm shift from size to shape, from a fixed, steady state to a dynamic process, and from volume to dimensions. A recent large demographic study demonstrated that women are concerned about shape just about as or even more than about size (Palidwar 2007). Placing large implants under a limited and restricted soft tissue envelope weakens and displaces the fold and stretches the lower pole. This phenomenon ignores short- and long-term interaction between implant and soft tissues.

Thinning and atrophy of breast tissues due to heavy and extra-projecting implants make the final result unstable and less predictable. Soft tissue laxity and ptosis further complicates the task of breast enhancement and makes the process of implant selection even more crucial and more complex. The larger the implant, the greater the imbalance with the sur-

rounding soft tissues and the less predictable the final result. Any implant may become a powerful manipulator of soft tissue and act as a tissue expander even if we do not want it to do so. Therefore if we want to shift from soft 'responsive' to cohesive 'form stable' implants, we need to change more than just our way of thinking.

Patient education, consultation, physical examination and measurements, implant selection, surgical technique and post-operative management must all be dealt with in a new and different way. Other questions that should be discussed prior to undertaking a major shift in clinical practice towards breast enhancement surgeries are concerned with the shape of the implant. Round or anatomical? Does implant shape influence breast shape? (Friedman et al 2006, Hamas 1999). Is there an identifiable characteristic shape for each device? Do round implants appear spherical while anatomical appear more natural? What are the indications and contraindications to use one or the other?

For practical purposes let us first consider young nuliparous patients presenting for primary breast augmentation with no ptosis, laxity or other signs of breast aging. Implant shape is chosen in such patients according to the thickness of the soft tissue coverage. Patients with a thick upper pole pinch could choose either a round or an anatomical device as the ample padding obscures the implant's contours. On the other hand, patients with thin upper poles benefit more from an anatomical shaped device as round devices appear spherical even when placed underneath the muscle.

A well selected implant (dimension and size) that is in good equilibrium with the soft tissues of the patient will have a long-term rejuvenating effect on the breast whether it is round or anatomical, except that in our experience, shaped implants will better enhance the upper pole and therefore appear more natural (Tebbetts 1994). In the parous patient or any patient with an aging breast (including young women with weight loss), a well selected shaped anatomical implant will better correct a mild ptosis when combined with controlled lowering of the inframamary fold and internal tissue manipulations as will be described below. This is true only for patients with a mild degree of ptosis and a reasonably good skin quality. Trying to correct second degree ptosis with a large, high-profile implant and lowering the inframammary fold is destined to fail.

No correction of patients with poor quality skin, skin excess, laxity and ptosis should be attempted using implants only. It is tempting at first to mistakenly assume that the new generation of form stable implants with the wide variety of shapes and profiles may obviate the need for tightening the envelope and lifting the breast. The wishful thinking that the lower pole curvature of a high profile, form stable implant may support and redrape the excess tissues in the inferior hemisphere of the breast and raise the nipple areola complex is not supported by our experience. The preferred approach remains mastopexy/augmentation using moderate size cohesive implants, avoiding future stretching, thinning, atrophy and recurrent ptosis.

While shaped (anatomical implants) seem to offer a better and more balanced upper pole fill with good projection under the nipple and areola complex, their use in patients with aging breasts and skin is fraught with a higher incidence of implant rotation. This tradeoff must be carefully discussed when selecting the shape of the implant. A recent study demonstrated an incidence of rotation of 0.7% over an 8-year period (Bengtson 2007). Implant rotation was typically more frequent during the early experience and was due to poor patient selection, improper surgical technique, primarily large pockets, seroma and early mobilization of the breasts.

To minimize rotation, there should be a perfect 'hand in glove' fit between the implant and the surrounding soft tissue envelope, no massaging, restricted upper torso exercising and gentle breast handling during sexual activity for 3 months. Patient education and consultation on form stable/high cohesive gel implants requires a different approach when compared with the traditional way of selecting a round, responsive gel implant (Tebbetts 2002a,b, 2006). The first step is usually conducted by a patient educator and contains information about shapes, gel consistency and available widths, heights and projections correlated with the patient's desires and individual tissue characteristics. After viewing and feeling available consistencies and implants, patients are informed about the steps of selecting an appropriate implant. Often, a shaped implant is preferred to create shaped, natural and proportional results. Common and significant risks and complications are discussed, including the showing of photos of the most frequent complications to help create a realistic understanding of potential risks.

The second stage of the consultation process is done by the surgeon in front of a large mirror. The consultation process is more specific and directly oriented towards customized implant selection, related to and limited by the patient own tissues. Only through objective evaluation of the patient's current breast and thorax can we dimensionally select the specific implant aimed to achieve the desired result. Dimensional patient evaluation considers current breast parenchyma, soft tissue envelope and the thorax. Some of the measurements (direct measurements) help in final implant selection while others (indirect measurements) are used to demonstrate and explain current asymmetries and limiting individual factors which may influence outcomes. Measurements and their interpretation with the patient's active participation help create a realistic patient perspective about options, limitations, and outcomes.

To do this we are assisted with software (BioDynamic™ Breast Analysis System, distributed by Allergan) that guides the patient through a series of steps towards the final implant selection. First, we measure the patient's thorax characteristics then the soft tissues (Figure 6.7) Next, we enter into the software the patient desires regarding the size and shape of her future breasts (Figure 6.8A). This is followed by the actual implant selection where, within the limits of the patient's characteristics, the software suggests the most appropriate available implant to fulfill her desires (Figure 6.8B). The final step simulates the prospective result using a family of external sizers suggested by the software. The sizers are placed inside a bra and an elastic T-shirt is placed over it (Figure 6.9). Looking in a mirror, the patient provides her feedback to the physician. Based on this feedback, implant selection may be adjusted towards a smaller or larger implant (if possible).

The biodimensional process of measurement and implant selection

The most important measurements for selecting the implants are base width, soft tissue thickness (measured pinch) in the medial, lateral, lower and upper pole as well as the distance under maximum stretch from the nipple to the inframammary fold (Figure 6.10). As implants are designed by choosing a width, a proportional height and a balanced projection, the

Semi-cohesive gel implants

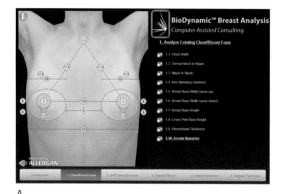
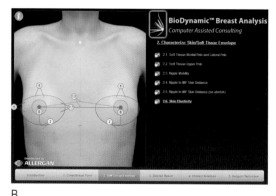

A

B

Figure 6.7 BioDynamic™ software: (A) Thorax dimensions and (B) soft tissue characteristics. Devised by Dr C. Stan; distributed by Allergan.

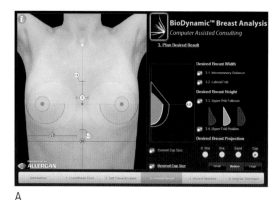
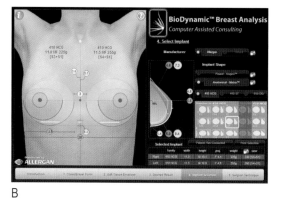

A

B

Figure 6.8 BioDynamic™ software: (A) Patient desires and (B) implant selection. Devised by Dr C. Stan; distributed by Allergan.

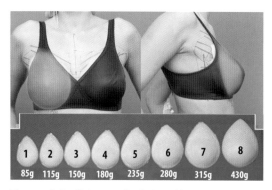
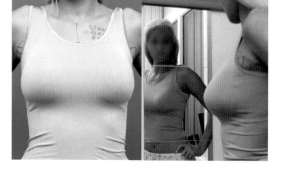

Figure 6.9 Outcome simulation with external sizers.

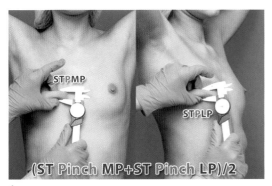

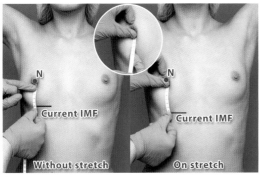

Figure 6.10 Evaluation of current soft tissue parenchyma. (A) Soft tissue pinch thickness medial and lateral pole (B) Current distance from nipple to IMF (under maximum stretch).

selection of an appropriate implant for an individual patient is based on the same staged process (Agarwal & Roy 2001). The first dimension to be selected is the base width of the implant. Once the desired breast width is selected, by shifting the breast medially and laterally, then the implant width is determined by subtracting the medial and lateral soft tissue thickness. For selecting the second dimension (height) we ask the patient, in front of the mirror, to simulate the desired appearance of the upper pole by pushing her breast up. The height of the implant is accordingly selected from three available height options.

The third dimension is the projection. Implant projection depends on current parenchyma projection, tissue elasticity, skin stretch and the desired cup increase (Figure 6.11). The most appropriate profile is then selected from available four implant projection options. Cohesive form stable implants are available in varying degrees of softness/firmness. It is important

to involve the patient in selecting an implant cohesivity that most appropriately simulates or complements her current breast consistency. In our proposed dimensional process of implant selection, each step is taken while asking for the patient's opinion. Every choice should be within acceptable aesthetic, individual anatomic and surgical limits. Desires, expectations and patient choices that are outside the limits of balanced device/tissue characteristics and will inevitably lead to an unstable and deteriorating result over time are dealt with by explaining the negative outcomes, complications and unpredictable long-term sequelae.

Following this concept of dimensional consultation helps create realistic patient expectations and makes the patient assume responsibility for her choices. Involving the patient in every step of the process increases patient satisfaction and decreases reoperation rate. The conversion rate from consultation to surgery using the 'biodimensional process' for patient evaluation and implant selection has increased from 25–80% in our series.

Pre-operative preparation

Once the appropriate implant has been selected, the surgical technique and operative planning became easier. The choice of incision site is more critical when using cohesive gel implants. The length of incision according the implant size and gel consistency must be longer and around 4.5–6 cm. A shorter incision in the fold or in patients with a small areola makes the introduction of the device into the pocket difficult, risking fracture of the cohesive gel causing a deformity in the device and in the breast.

While it is possible to introduce a form stable shaped implant through the axilla, it is more difficult. The vertical positioning of the implant and controlling the inframammary fold and upper pole are difficult and less accurate through this limited access route. It has been the senior author's experience, following 15 years of primarily using the transaxillary route, that the need for reoperations is prohibitively high when compared to the two other options. Our extensive experience shows that the inframammary incision is the best way to introduce form stable implants into breasts. A precise technical execution of a retromuscular, dual plane with internal soft tissue modifications (differential incision of the origin of the pectoralis major muscle at different heights according the breast type,

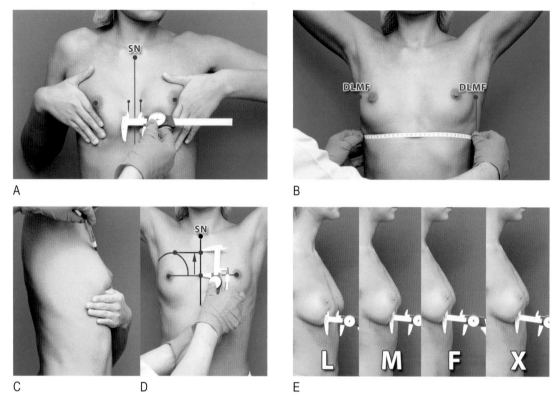

A

B

C   D

E

Figure 6.11   Patient dimensional evaluation of desired breast. (A) Desired intermammary distance (B) Desired lateral mammary fold (C,D) Desired upper pole position (appearance) (E) Desired projection increase.

anterior parenchymal release and fold control) requires an inframammary incision. Making an adequately long incision that is accurately placed in the new inframammary fold and stays there is important but easier said than done.

Too short an incision not only carries a risk of damaging the implant but also damages the skin edges and consequently increases the risk of local wound healing problems, infection and unattractive, hypertrophic, pigmented and visible scar. Good planning takes into account two important dimensional parameters: the vertical location of the implant's lower pole (vertical distance between the nipple to the new inframammary fold on the sternum mid line, generally half of the desired breast height), and the skin length from the nipple to the inframammary fold measured on the breast contour (under maximum stretch) (Figure 6.12). The calculation of this distance can be done using a more complex formula (Figure 6.13) or can be calculated in a simple way by adding 4 cm to the implant projection plus three-quarters of the current parenchyma thickness. It is at this distance from the nipple where the incision is made.

Skin length in cm from nipple to new IMF
   = implant projection + 4 cm

By defining the vertical and horizontal limits of the pocket, the implant rests in a stable, tailor made position, without internal deforming forces. Deciding on the site of cohesive implant placement is still unsettled and controversial (Figure 6.14). Traditionally, if soft tissue thickness in the upper pole is less than 3.5 cm, the implant is placed under the muscle. Others (Hammond 2008) feel that 2 cm and as little as 1 cm upper pole pinch enable a subglandular or subfascial placement. This may be possible due to the fine tapered design of the implant's edges as well as the reduced or minimal wrinkling on its surface.

Both authors of this chapter maintain that in order to achieve a long term stable result – that brings into the equation future quantitative and qualitative changes of soft tissues due to pregnancy, breast feeding,

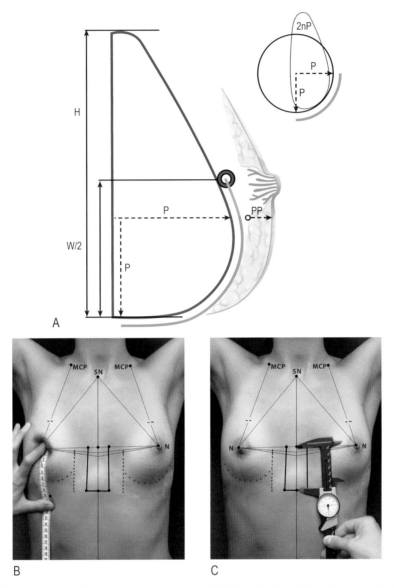

Figure 6.12 Pre-operative markings and pocket location. (A,B) New skin length from the nipple to the IMF (C) Implant lower pole position (vertical distance from the nipples line to the IMF on sternal medium line).

weight loss and aging – the implant should be placed under the muscle in a dual plane site in most breasts and patients (Tebbetts 2001).

Operative technique

Operative steps

A high cohesive gel implant, anatomically shaped and dimensionally selected needs a dimensionally accu-

rate planning and marking of the implant pocket placement and adequate skin envelope to cover tridimensional upper and lower pole without excessive stretching and expansion.

Generally, a good operative plan must provide:

- external markings.
- decision of implant location (submuscular or subglandular) considering the soft tissue thickness in the upper pole.

Semi-cohesive gel implants

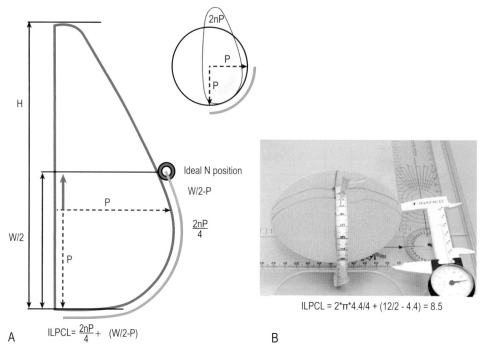

$$ILPCL = 2^*\pi^*4.4/4 + (12/2 - 4.4) = 8.5$$

A $\quad ILPCL = \dfrac{2nP}{4} + (W/2\text{-}P)$ $\qquad\qquad$ B

Figure 6.13 Geometrical formulas to accurately calculate (A) the ideal location of the nipple (at the level of half of the implant base width) and (B) implant lower pole contour length (ILPCL) (where P is implant projection, W is implant base width and H is implant base height).

- location of incision approach considering the best place to control the internal pocket dissection and adequate length to introduce the implants with minimal risk of implant deformation.

If selection of access incision is located in the IMF region (which is the preferred approach for the authors in 90% of the cases) the operative sequence is:

- incision of the skin, subcutaneous tissue and fascia superficialis at IMF, approximately 4.5–5.5 cm (according to implant size and gel consistency)
- subpectoral dissection of implant pocket with total release of infero-medial pectoralis major origin using mono RF dissection forceps as a unique instrument for cutting, releasing and prospective hemostasis of encountered structures (vessels, muscle fibers and muscle fascia)
- use of dual plane pocket dissection principles regarding the pectoralis major – glandular parenchyma interface in gradually higher position according to the breast type (dual plane type I, II, III)
- placement of selected implants in the subpectoral pocket starting with the implant introduction, placed

with the vertical dots perpendicularly on the vertical axis of the implant pockets. The final position of the implants, once placed in the pocket, must be close to the vertical location of the dots, with minimal further internal manipulation. With the implants in the pocket, the final adjustments regards pectoralis major release in the lateral or infero-medial parts to get the desired Intermammary cleavage, upper pole and lower pole shape and lateral protrusion.

- external reconstruction of the IMF with staged closure of the pocket and fixation of the IMF incision at the level of the desired, planned, implant lower pole.

The external markings and pocket dissection are aimed to provide a snug and fitted vertical and horizontal implant location as well as to enable a balanced redraping of the skin over the implant's lower and upper pole. An accurate pocket dissection reduces the risk of rotation and controls and determines the future breast shape. The breast parenchyma is modified to adapt over the implant and to keep the nipple and areola complex in a natural position at approximately half of the breast height, pointing slightly lateral and upward, in the mid axis of the breast.

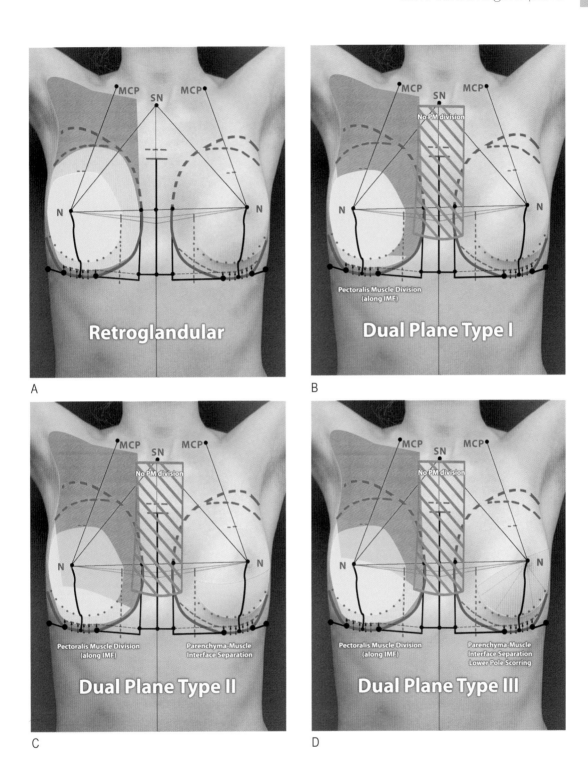

Figure 6.14 Pocket location in breast augmentation with stable shape/high cohesive gel implants (A) If soft tissue thickness upper pole is more than 0.5 cm, subglandular; (B–D) If soft tissue upper pole is less than 0.5 cm, dual plane technique.

Once the implant is introduced into the pocket under direct vision, the pocket is adjusted as necessary to have the implant in a smooth and optimal position without distortion and with a proper muscle tension. Suturing the inframammary fold with the anterior, the posterior lamella and the deep dermis to the thoracic fascia, fixes the fold, creates a stable pocket and keeps the incision hidden in the fold. A natural light ptotic appearance of the lower pole is thus obtained. The pocket dissection is done under direct vision using a head light and either a fine needle tip or a mono radio frequency breast forceps and 4.0 MHz dual Surgitron® (Ellman, Oceanside, NY) (Figure 6.15) The dry pocket facilitates recovery with less pain and reduces the risk of seroma and inflammation. Patients return to normal life within few days. Post-operatively, patients are instructed to refrain from massaging the breasts, restrain vigorous exercising for 3 months, gentle handling of the breasts during sexual activity and wearing a special bra for 1 month.

Pitfalls

Introduction of high cohesive gel, anatomical shaped implants with dimensional patient evaluation and implant selection represents a step forward in planning a proportional breast with long lasting result and minimal risk; however, the control of a lot of data became more difficult and the surgeon learning curve became more steep. Without a planning system which considers a patient dimensional evaluation with thorax/parenchyma/soft tissue limits, selection of the implants became an arbitrary process with non-predictable results and an adventurous surgical technique.

Dissection of the pocket must be done properly to adapt the implant as a hand in a surgeon's glove with controlled soft tissue–implant internal dynamic. In our experience with a large number of patients from the introduction of the new implant family and working with a lot of patient breasts we found some pitfalls which must be known in order to avoid the same mistakes.

- Selection of the implant in a dimensional system, larger than thorax frame (generally inside the limits of the two anterior axillary lines, right to left) creates the risk of inferolateral breast implant palpability and visibility.
- Using progressively larger projected high cohesive anatomical implants requires to know the appropriate skin length on the lower pole necessary to cover the new complex implant–parenchyma. In a large majority of small breasts this requires the modification of the IMF. Without an adequate and accurate reconstruction and fixation of the inframammary fold structures at the right vertical level of the implant creates large risks for implant malposition (Figure 6.16).
- The gel cohesivity (sometimes two gel cohesivities like Allergan 510 Dual Gel implants) creates problems when selection of the incision approaches and manipulation of the implant at the time of the introduction in the pocket. This is why, generally, the incision length must be larger than in classical low responsive gel implants and manipulation of the implant must be minimal with specific rules. Otherwise implant deformation can occur.
- Planning and dissection of the pocket implants must perfectly match the implant width, height and projection to reduce the risk of rotation (Figure 6.17). In case of lower height implants, the vertical extension of the pocket must be very precise otherwise the risk of rotation is larger in this particular implant shape.
- Any dimensional system for implant selection and surgical planning has limits and it is the surgeon's task to adapt intraoperatively the final adjustments to get the best results and to reduce unwanted outcomes.
- If parenchyma and skin–soft tissue can be dimensionally evaluated, the thorax asymmetry in the

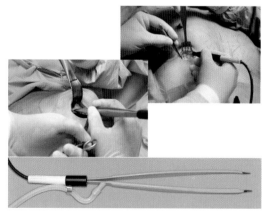

Figure 6.15   Pocket dissection with mono RF breast forceps and empire needle cut/coag (Ellman, Oceanside, NY).

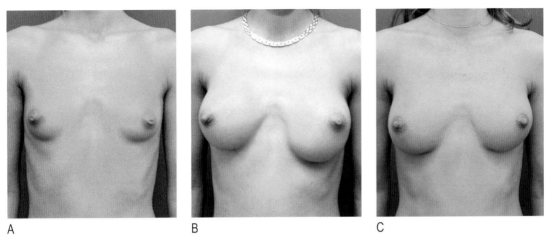

Figure 6.16   Pitfall: implant malposition in a 20-year-old woman. Implants: Allergan 410 Soft Touch™ MM245; dual plane type I; (A) before, (B) after 6 months (implant malposition in left breast); (C) After 1 year (solved).

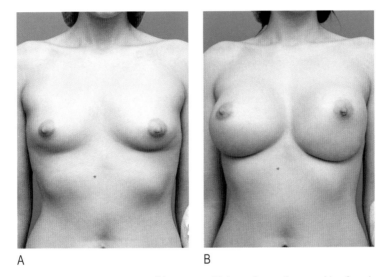

Figure 6.17   Pitfall: implant rotation. A 26-year-old woman with large thorax frame asking for a large implant base width and large thorax deformity in the area of the left breast's lower pole; Implants: Allergan 510 Dual Gel LX 475 dual plane type I; (A) before, (B) after 6 months.

future breast region is very difficult to evaluate before the surgery and the risk of asymmetry is definitely larger. In these cases the patient must be thoroughly educated about the limits and the possible postoperative asymmetries.

• If the anatomic high cohesive gel implants in a good surgeon's hands is able to provide good

results in large categories of breasts, in particular cases some pitfalls can create fear for the young starting surgeon in accepting these implants. Only a good evaluation of the patient before the surgery and an adequate custom implant selection and an adapted surgical plan can prevent many of these problems.

Semi-cohesive gel implants

Results

Case **1**

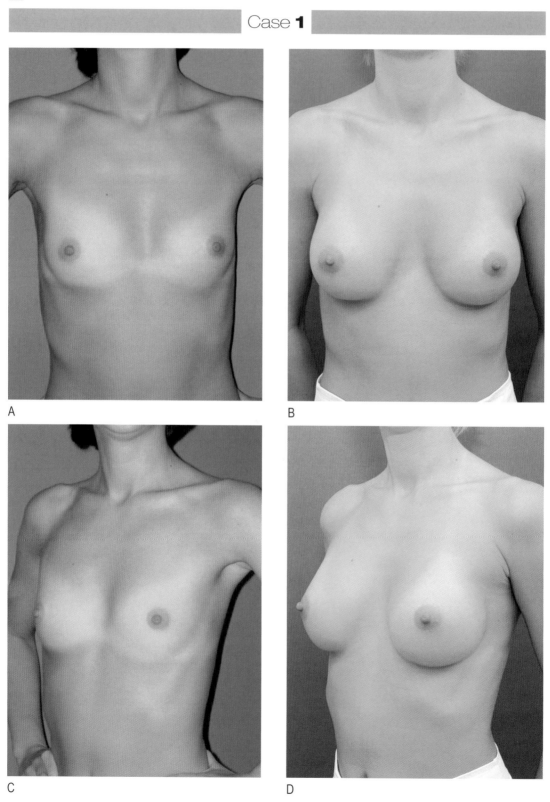

A

B

C

D

Figure 6.18 A 30-year-old woman. Implants: Allergan 410 Soft Touch™ MM 215 g in dual plane type I. (A,C) Before; (B,D) After 2 years.

Case **2**

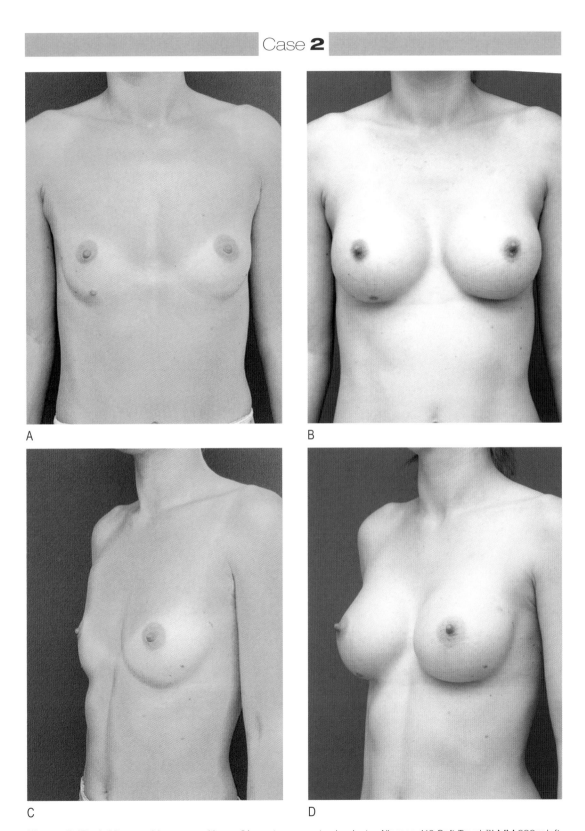

A

B

C

D

Figure 6.19 A 36-year-old woman with small breast asymmetry. Implants: Allergan 410 Soft Touch™ MM 220 g left breast and MMF 335 in right breast; dual plane type II. (A,C) Before. (B,D) After 1 year.

Case **3**

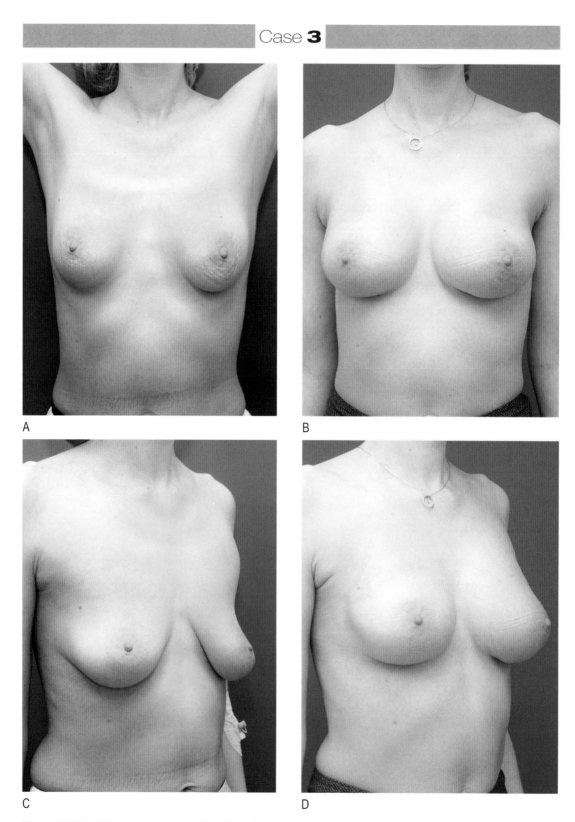

A

B

C

D

Figure 6.20 A 35-year-old woman with light ptotic breasts. Implants: Allergan 410 Soft Touch™ FM 310 g in dual plane type III. (A,C) Before, (B,D) After 6 months.

Case **4**

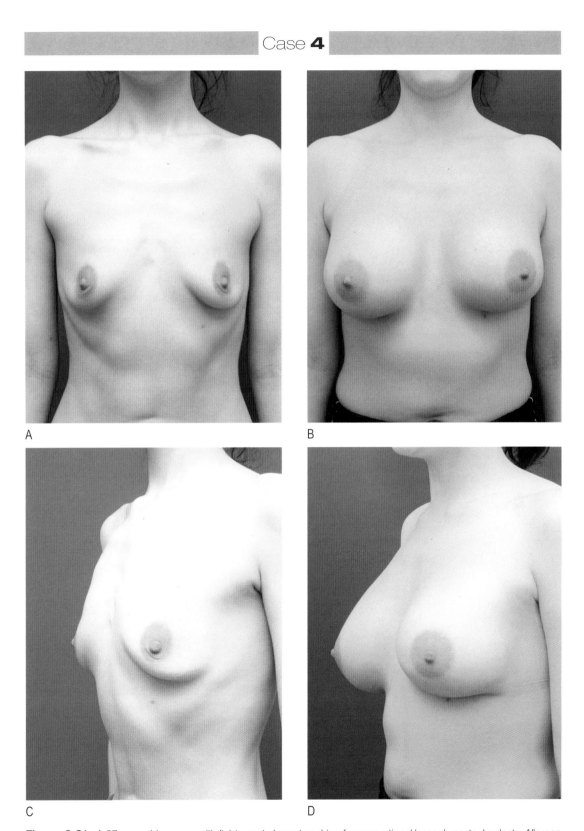

A

B

C

D

Figure 6.21 A 27-year-old woman with light empty breasts asking for proportional larger breasts. Implants: Allergan 410 Soft Touch™ FM 395 g in dual plane type III. (A,C) Before, (B,D) After 18 months.

Semi-cohesive gel implants

Case **5**

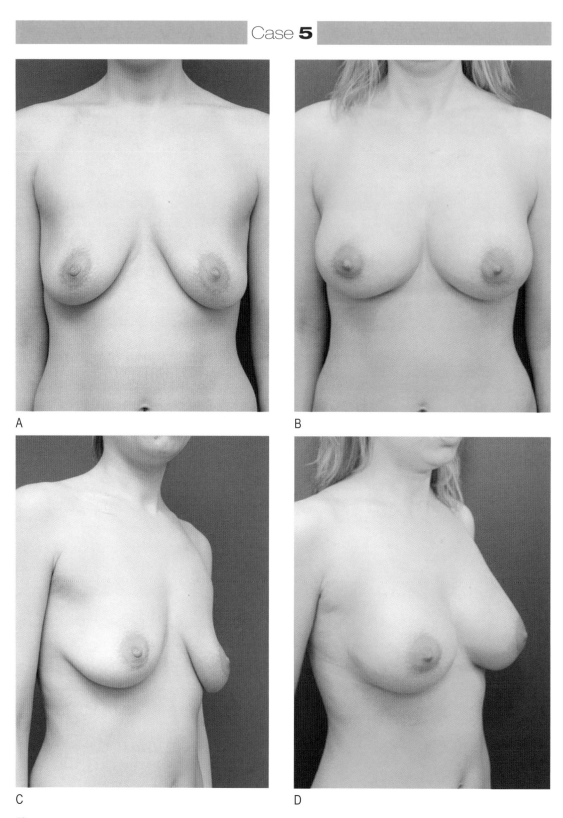

A

B

C

D

Figure 6.22 A 32-year-old woman with medium ptotic breasts asking for larger breasts with shape improvement without mastopexy. Implants: Allergan 510 Dual Gel MX 385 g in dual plane type III. (A,C) Before, (B,D) After 2 years.

Case 6

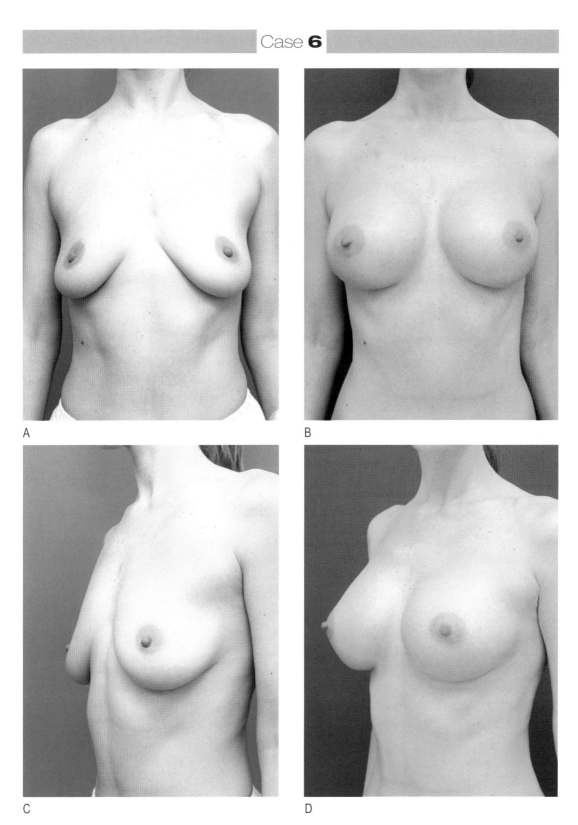

A

B

C

D

Figure 6.23 A 32-year-old woman with medium ptotic breasts asking for larger breasts with shape improvement without mastopexy. Implants: Allergan 510 Dual Gel MX 385 g in dual plane type III. (A,C) Before, (B,D) After 6 months.

Case **7**

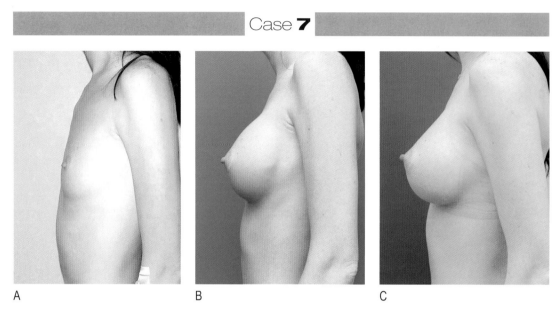

A   B   C

Figure 6.24 (A) Patient lateral view of breast before. (B) After 6 years with round, low responsive gel implant and (C) after implant exchange for a better shape and consistency (Allergan Matrix 510 Dual Gel).

Closure

The use of form stable, cohesive gel implants is more difficult, has a steep learning curve and requires a more involved process of patient education, information, consultation, physical examination and measurements and a more elaborate surgical technique. The final results however are more rewarding, the appearance is enhanced in a more natural and unoperated look, the results are more predictable and breast shape is stable over a longer period of time. The advent of the new era of breast enhancement using form stable implants and a dimensional selection process presents the modern breast surgeon with a challenge and an opportunity of creating better looking breasts in a more predictable way for a longer period than ever before.

Acknowledgments

The authors would like to thank Peter Damoc BME for the help he provided in the creation of the drawings, photos and photo post-processing.

Further reading

Agarwal RK, Roy D. Breast augmentation using McGhan's biodimensional silicone implants. Int J Cosmet Surg Aesth Dermatol 2001;3:211–214.

Bengtson BMD. Style 410 highly cohesive silicone breast implant core study results at 3 years Plast Reconst Surg. December Supplement 1, 2007.

Drever MJ. Cohesive gel implants for breast augmentation. Aesth Surg J 2003;23;405–409.

Friedman T, Davidovitch N, Scheflan M. Comparative double-blind clinical study on round versus shaped cohesive gel implants. Aesth Surg J 2006;26: 530–536.

Hamas RSM. The post-operative shape of round and teardrop saline-filled breast implants. Aesth Surg J 1999;19:369–374.

Hammond D. BodyLogic – new way of sizing, new tactical considerations in augmentation mammoplasty. Oral presentation SAM Congress, February 2008, Moscow.

Palidwar D. Allergan potential customer survey. Personal communication, Oct. 31, 2007.

Spear Sl, Mardini S. Alternative filler materials and new implant designs: what's available and what's on the horizon? Clin Plast Surg 2001;28:435–443.

Tebbetts JB. Dimensional augmentation mammaplasty, Using the biodimensional system. Santa Barbara, CA. McGhan Medical Corporation 1994:1–90.

Tebbetts JB. Dual plane breast augmentation: Optimizing implant-soft tissue relationships in a wide range of breast types. Plast Reconstr Surg 2001;107:1255.

Tebbetts JB. Breast implant selection based on patient tissue characteristics and dynamics. The TEPID approach. Plast Reconstr Surg 2002a;190:1396.

Tebbetts JB. An approach that integrates patient education and informed consent in breast augmentation. Plast Reconstr Surg 2002b;110;971.

Tebbetts JB. Achieving a zero percent reoperation rate at 3 years in a 50-consecutive-case augmentation mammaplasty premarket approval study. Plast Reconstr Surg 2006;118:1453.

Tebbetts JB, Adams WP Jr. Five critical decisions in breast augmentation using five measurements in 5 minutes: The high five decision support process. Plast Reconstr Surg 2005;116:2005–2016.

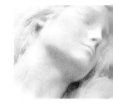

7

Subfascial transaxillary breast augmentation

Ruth M. Graf, André R.D. Tolazzi, Maria Cecília C. Ono

Key points

- The mainstay of transaxillary breast augmentation is the absence of a scar on the breast. It can be adequately performed using endoscopic instruments or even long lightened retractors.

- Subfascial breast augmentation offers some advantages over the submuscular placement, without the drawbacks of this approach.

- As pectoralis muscle fascia is a well-defined structure and very consistent in the upper thorax, it can be used to cover the implant and minimize visualization of its edges.

- Most lymphatic vessels in axilla can be preserved if some technical details of subcutaneous tunnel and pocket dissection were followed.

- Subfascial transaxillary breast augmentation has given a no-scar and natural look to the breast. It has also been a reasonable solution to the problem of acquiring adequate soft tissue coverage without distortion of the implant by the muscle contraction.

Breast augmentation has been a very common procedure in plastic surgery in the last few decades with multiple options for incision location, implant design and pocket plane. Implant position or pocket plane in breast augmentation has been the subject of some controversy because an implant can be positioned in a subglandular, retropectoral or subfascial plane (Graf et al 2000, 2008) (Figure 7.1). For an optimal result, the implant must have adequate soft tissue coverage, otherwise it can become palpable or visible. The position of an implant in a retroglandular space has significant disadvantages if the soft tissue coverage is insufficient.

In addition to implant palpability and visibility, incidences of fibrous capsular contracture, rippling and nipple sensation alteration and numbness are higher (Serra-Renom et al 2005). In order to get rid of the problems encountered with retroglandular placement, the utilization of the retropectoral space has become commonplace. The disadvantages of subpectoral placement include a more invasive procedure,

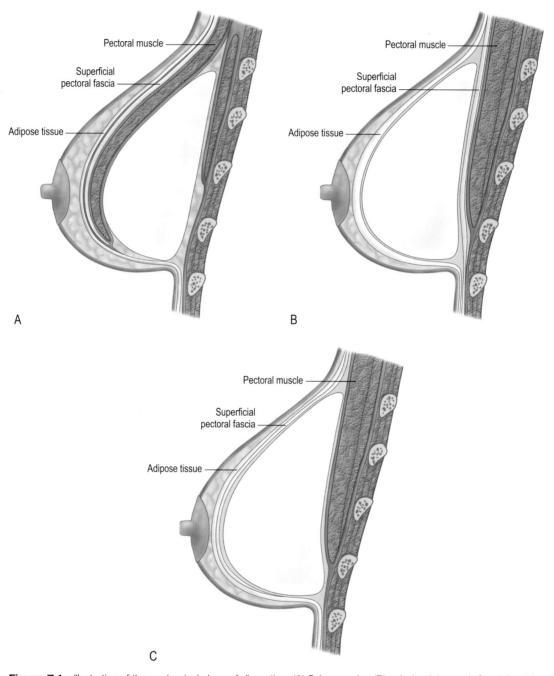

Figure 7.1 Illustration of the anatomical plane of dissection. (A) Submuscular; (B) subglandular; and (C) subfascial.

increased postoperative discomfort and visible flattening or distortion of the breast when the pectoral muscle is contracted (Serra-Renom et al, 2005). If the muscle is released inadequately medially the implant may ride too high or if the muscle is released excessively the implant may be displaced inferiorly and laterally.

A reasonable solution to the problem of acquiring adequate soft tissue coverage without distortion of the implant through muscle contracture has been the use of the subfascial plane (Graf et al 2000, 2008, Goes & Landecker 2003, Barbato et al 2004). As the pectoralis muscle fascia is a well-defined structure and very consistent in the upper thorax, it can be used to minimize the appearance of the edges of the implant on the skin, making them less noticeable. The integrity of the muscle is preserved and the implant is totally covered. The fascia supports the implant without requiring additional tissue to give a good aesthetic result. In the subfascial plane, there won't be any alteration to the breast shape or implant displacement caused by muscular contraction.

The pre-operative evaluation includes the analysis of breast tissue and thoracic shape, the elasticity of the breast, the presence of ptosis, and the distance between the nipple and the inframammary fold. Subfascial breast augmentation aims to offer a better and natural shape to the breast. There is an additional soft, but firm tissue between the implant and skin, which improves breast contour, especially in the upper pole, leading to a less noticeable implant edge.

Transaxillary breast augmentation presents many advantages over other techniques (Eiseman 1974). Its mainstay is the absence of a scar on the breast. The rationale for placing the implant submuscularly, and recently subfascially, is to reduce the incidence of capsular contraction in the late post-operative period and to avoid areolar sensation disturbances (Howard et al 1996). The use of endoscopic magnifying lenses and video amplifies the images and gives a better visualization of tissues and planes, allowing more precise dissection and hemostasis while using only a small axillary incision (Chachir et al 1994, Barnett 1990). This technique is not indicated for moderate and severe ptosis.

Breast endoscopic surgery has been used since 1987, for internal capsulotomy and to evaluate mammary implants (Beer & Kompatscher 1995, Dowden & Anain 1993, Höhler 1977). In 1993, Johnson and Christ (1993) first described the video endoscopic approach in transumbilical breast augmentation, and in the same year Laurence Ho published his experience with transaxillary endoscopic augmentation (Ho 1993). In 1994 Price reported endoscopic transaxillary subpectoral breast augmentation with good aesthetic results and no complications (Price et al 1994). He was followed by other authors (Papillon 1976, Regnault 1977, Tebbetts 1984, Biggs & Yarish 1990).

Anatomical considerations

The breast is essentially a skin appendage contained within layers of the superficial fascia. The superficial layer of this fascia is near the dermis and is not distinct from it. The deep layer of the superficial fascia is more

distinct and is identifiable on the deep surface of the breast when the breast is elevated in a subglandular augmentation mammaplasty. There is a loose areolar tissue between the deep layer of the superficial fascia and the fascia that covers the pectoralis major muscle (Würinger et al 1998) and continues to cover the adjacent rectus abdominis, serratus anterior and external oblique muscles (Figure 7.2).

This fascia has its origin on the clavicle and sternum, extending toward the lateral border of the muscle to form the axillary fascia. At the caudal border of the pectoralis muscle, the clavipectoral, pectoral, and serratus anterior fasciae become continuous and form suspensory ligaments that extend to the breast's inframammary fold (Hwang & Kim 2005). The deep fascia covering the lower aspect of the pectoralis major muscle is well defined, as is the fascia of the serratus anterior muscle. This deep fascia is continuous with the fascia of the external oblique and rectus abdominis muscles.

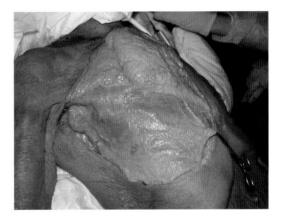

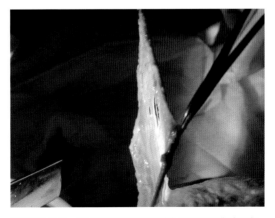

Figure 7.2 Anatomical study of the pectoralis fascia. Note that it continues with the serratus and rectus abdominalis fascia.

The upper portions of the external oblique and rectus abdominis muscles and their overlying fasciae are deep to the lower portion of the breast. The digitations (spreading) of origin of the external oblique muscle are associated with the lateral inferior fibers of the pectoralis major muscle and laterally with the serratus anterior muscular digitations (spreading). We have observed that the pectoralis major fascia tends to be thin and more fragile over the lower two-thirds of the muscle.

Operative approach

Operative steps:

- Skin markings with the patient in upright position.
- Important landmarks: inframammary fold (at least 5–7 cm below the areola); medial marking 1–2 cm from the mid sternum; anterior axillary line as the lateral limit.
- Subcutaneous infiltration (normal saline + epinephrine 1:300,000).
- Axillary incision in a natural fold, about 4 cm long, not extended beyond the lateral border of the major pectoralis muscle.
- Subcutaneous tunnel dissection should limit inferior-lateral undermining in order to preserve most of lymphatic vessels.
- Subfascial breast pocket is created by a blunt or electrocautery dissection.

Markings

Pre-operative marking is performed with the patient standing up. The design of the pocket for the implant is marked. The inframammary crease is marked, and if the distance between the areola and the inframammary fold is around 5–7 cm, the original inframammary crease is maintained. However, if this distance is shorter than 4 cm, a new inframammary crease is also marked 1 or 2 cm below the original one. The anterior axillary line is drawn on the lateral side. A line is drawn 1 or 2 cm from the mid-sternum line and extended cephalically to the level of the second intercostal space (Figure 7.3).

Technique

Epidural block associated with sedation is the preferred option for anesthesia, with the arms 90°

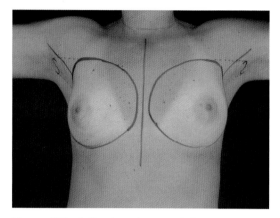

Figure 7.3 Axillary breast augmentation: preoperative markings. The pocket is undermined related to the landmarks.

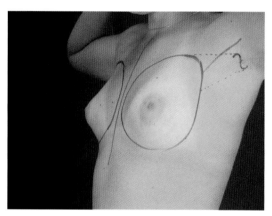

Figure 7.4 S-shape incision in the axilla 4 cm length and 1 cm behind the lateral border of the major pectoralis muscle.

abducted and the dorsum is slightly elevated. The axillary incisions are placed in a natural crease, in S shape, approximately 4 cm length, but never crossing beyond the lateral edge of the pectoralis muscle (Figures 7.4, 7.5). The incision lines are infiltrated with epinephrine, 1:300 000, using an average of 20 mL in each side (Figure 7.6). One stitch is done at the anterior incision to avoid disruption of the incision during the surgery (Figure 7.7). Careful subcutaneous dissection (Figure 7.8) exposes the lateral border of the pectoralis muscle where the fascia is incised. Subcutaneous tunnel dissection should limit inferior-lateral undermining in order to preserve most of the lymphatic vessels (Figure 7.5).

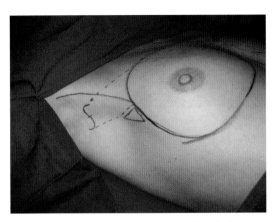

Figure 7.5 Close of the S shaped incision in the axilla, the lateral border of the major pectoralis muscle and the triangle inferior-lateral to the muscle border.

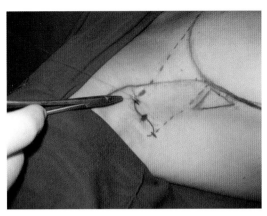

Figure 7.7 One stitch is done anterior to the incision to avoid disruption of the incision during the surgery.

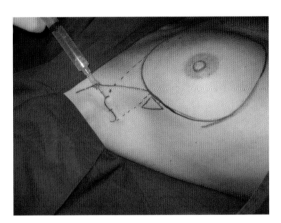

Figure 7.6 The incision line and the tunnel are infiltrated with saline solution and epinephrine, 1:150000.

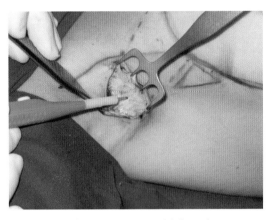

Figure 7.8 Subcutaneous careful dissection.

The subfascial breast pocket is created by blunt or electrocautery dissection, using endoscopic or long lightened retractors (Figures 7.9, 7.10). The thickness of the fascia increases from approximately 0.1 mm in the inferior part to approximately 0.5 mm in the upper third of the pectoralis muscle, with good coverage of the implant. In the cephalic portion, the fascia is more defined and resistant. Its inferior portion is thinner and more friable. This undermining should be done very carefully to avoid fascia injury and if there is doubt about the plane, some muscle fibers may be lifted with the fascia. The limits for blunt dissection are the third intercostal space superiorly, 1.5 cm from the midline medially, 7 cm below the areola to the

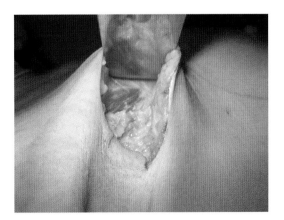

Figure 7.9 The lateral border of the pectoralis muscle is exposed where the fascia is incised.

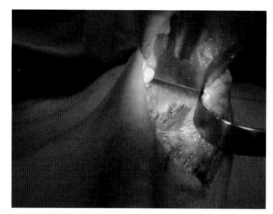

Figure 7.10 The plane between the pectoralis muscle and its fascia is undermined by direct vision and the subfascial pocket is created, by endoscopy retractor or direct view. The fascial septa can be observed from the fascia to the muscle.

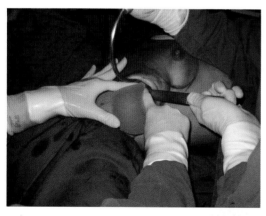

Figure 7.11 The implant is inserted into the pocket.

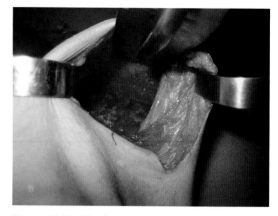

Figure 7.12 The implant at the subfascial plane.

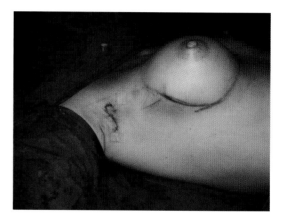

Figure 7.13 The incision is closed with a running suture.

Post-operative care

It is recommended to use a bra and an elastic band on the upper pole of the breast for 1 or 2 weeks to help maintain the implant in the correct position. Regular movements of the arms are allowed after that. To avoid hypertrophic scars silicone sheets can be used. Walking is allowed in the first post-operative day and physical activities can be started after 1 week.

Complications

Malposition of the implant is one of the complications of breast augmentation. Low displacement of the implant can be encountered in the postoperative period in patients with skin laxity prior to the surgery. Other complications have been modest, as capsular contracture, hematoma, brachial hypoesthesia, breast

original inframammary fold and the anterior axillary line laterally. The distance between the implants should be approximately 2–3 cm and the distance between the areola's medial border and the midsternal line should be about 9–10 cm (Figure 7.3). Once dissection is completed, a meticulous evaluation for bleeding is carried out, and the implant is inserted into the pocket (Figures 7.11, 7.12). Breast sizers may be used. The incision is closed with a running suture (Figure 7.13).

asymmetry, seroma, axillary fibrous banding and infection. As described by Stoff-Khalili and colleagues (Stoff-Khalili et al 2004) comparing the results of the subglandular, subpectoral and the subfascial augmentation, the total rate of complications diminished significantly in the last group.

Some complications can be avoided with some technical maneuvers including careful hemostasis. Using gauze in the pocket is not advised because of the possibility of a foreign body (gauze tread) might cause reaction. If needed, suction may be used. Using a no touch technique for handling the implant will also minimize contamination. In addition, the patient is advised to minimize arm mobilization for a week. We found no increase rate in capsular contracture with

the subfascial technique relative to the submuscular technique. No patient submitted to subfascial breast augmentation developed implant distortion due to pectoralis muscle movement. The implant edges were not noticeable, even in the large size implants.

Results

Utilizing the subfascial technique results in a more natural look of the breasts with good soft tissue coverage to the implants and no possibility of implant distortion during pectoralis major muscle contraction. It also showed a similar complication rate compared with other techniques.

Case 1

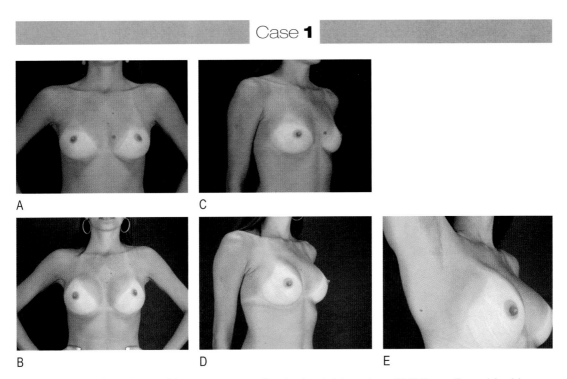

A

C

B

D

E

Figure 7.14 (A,C) A 22-year-old woman pre-operative, front and oblique views. (B,D) Transaxillary subfascial technique, 3 years post-operatively. (E) Close-up view of the S-shaped axillary scar 3 years post-operatively.

Case **2**

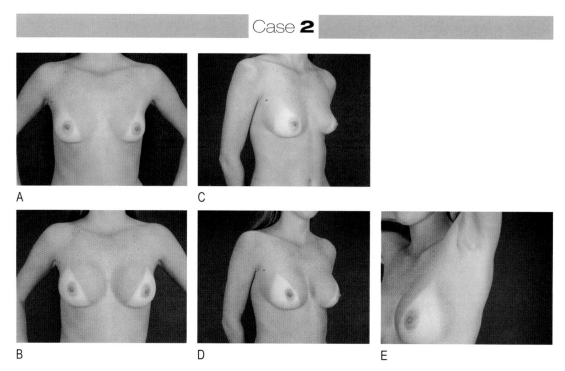

A   C

B   D   E

Figure 7.15   (A,C) A 19-year-old woman pre-operative, front and oblique views of a hypoplasic breast. (B,D)
Subfascial transaxillary breast augmentation, 4 years post-operatively. (E) Close-up view of the S-
shaped axillary scar with good quality, 4 years post-operative.

Conclusion

The subfascial placement has become the preferred
technique for breast implants in our practice. Because
the pectoralis muscle fascia is a well-defined structure

and very consistent in the upper thorax, it can be used
to minimize the visualization of the implant edges,
making them less noticeable. Compared with the
subpectoral insertion, the subfascial implant gives the
breast a better and more natural contour. Long-term
complication rates have been decreased.

Further reading

Barbato C, Pena M, Triana C, Zambrano MA. Augmentation
mammoplasty using the retrofascia approach. Aesth.
Plast. Surg 2004;28:148–152.

Barnett A. Transaxillary subpectoral augmentation in the
ptotic breast: Augmentation by disruption of the
extended pectoral fascia and parenchymal sweep. Plast.
Reconstr. Surg 1990;86:76.

Beer GM, Kompatscher P. Endoscopic plastic surgery: The
endoscopic evaluation of implants after breast
augmentation. Aesth. Plast. Surg 1995;79:353.

Biggs TM, Yarish RS. Augmentation mammaplasty: A
comparative analysis. Plast. Reconstr. Surg 1990;85:368.

Chachir A, Benzaquen I, Spagnolo N, Lusicic N.
Endoscopic augmentation mastoplasty. Aesth. Plast. Surg
1994;18:377.

Dowden RV, Anain S. Endoscopic implant evaluation and
capsulotomy. Plast. Reconstr. Surg 1993;91:283.

Eiseman G. Augmentation mammaplasty by the
transaxillary approach. Plast. Reconstr. Surg 1974;
54:229.

Goes JCS, Landecker A. Optimizing outcomes in
breast augmentation: seven years of experience with
the subfascial plane. Aesth. Plast. Surg 2003;27:
178–184.

Graf RM, Bernardes A, Auersvald A, Damasio RCC. Subfascial endoscopic transaxillary augmentation mammaplasty. Aesth. Plast. Surg 2000;24:216–220.

Graf RM, Canan LW Jr, Romano GG et al. Re: implications of transaxillary breast augmentation: lifetime probability for the development of breast cancer and sentinel node mapping interference. Aesthetic. Plast. Surg 2007;31:322–324.

Graf R, Pace DT, Damasio RC et al. Subfascial breast augmentation. In: Innovations in Plastic and Aesthetic Surgery. Chapter 50: 406–413, Springer, New York, 2008.

Ho LCY. Endoscopic assisted transaxillary augmentation mammaplasty. Br J Plast Surg 1993;46:332.

Höhler H. Further progress in the axillary approach in augmentation mammaplasty: Prevention of incapsulation. Aesth. Plast. Surg 1977;1:107.

Howard PS, Oslin BD, Moore JR. Endoscopic transaxillary submuscular augmentation mammaplasty with textured saline breast implants. Ann. Plast. Surg 1996;37:12.

Hwang K, Kim DJ. Anatomy of pectoral fascia in relation to subfascial mammary augmentation. Annals of Plastic Surgery 2005;55:576–579.

Johnson GW, Christ JE. The endoscopic breast augmentation: The transumbilical insertion of saline-filled breast implants. Plast. Reconstr. Surg 1993;92:801.

Papillon J. Pros and cons of subpectoral implantation. Clin. Plast. Surg 1976;3:321.

Price CI, Eaves FF 3rd, Nahai F et al. Endoscopic transaxillary subpectoral breast augmentation. Plast. Reconstr. Surg 1994;94:612.

Regnault P. Partially submuscular breast augmentation. Plast. Reconstr. Surg 1977;59:72.

Serra-Renom J, Garrido MF, Yoon T. Augmentation mammaplasty with anatomic soft, cohesive silicone implant using the transaxillary approach at a subfascial level with endoscopic assistance. Plast. Reconstr. Surg 2005;116:640–645.

Stoff-Khalili MA, Scholze R, Morgan WR, Metcalf JD. Subfascial periareolar augmentation mammaplasty. Plastic and Reconstr. Surg 2004;114:1280–1288.

Tebbetts JB. Transaxillary subpectoral augmentation mammaplasty: Long-term follow-up and refinements. Plast. Reconstr. Surg 1984;74:636.

Würinger E, Mader N, Posch E, Holle J. Nerve and vessel supplying ligamentous suspension of the mammary gland. Plast. Reconstr. Surg 1998;101:1486–1492.

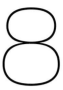
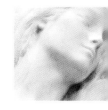

8

Secondary augmentation

Steven Teitelbaum

Key points

- Over time, more revisions of breast augmentations will ultimately be done than primary augmentations.
- All problems should be evaluated for the contribution of: (1) parenchyma/tissue coverage; (2) skin envelope; (3) capsule; (4) pocket position; and (5) the device.

- Optimizing soft tissue coverage is the first priority in all primary and revisionary breast augmentation surgery.
- Informing a patient that another operation is not indicated and refusing to operate when there is little likelihood for substantial improvement is an option that must not be forgotten.

Introduction

A requirement of the product labeling on all breast implants is to inform potential patients that a breast implant is not a lifelong device and will inevitably need replacement. This means that each of the nearly 500,000 women a year undergoing breast augmentation in the United States is destined for a revision. In the meantime, the millions of women who have undergone an augmentation since the inception of the modern operation in the 1960s have already or will require a revision in the future. Many women will live long enough to need or want more than one routine revision; others will need more than one operation to correct a complex problem; while others will have revisions in pursuit of a physical perfection unattain-

able for their underlying anatomy. It is therefore a fact that more secondary breast augmentation procedures will be done than primary procedures.

We must be as diligent in our understanding of secondary augmentation as primary augmentation. In fact, the frustration and dissatisfaction that some revision patients experience casts a pall over our entire specialty, reducing demand not just for primary augmentation, but for other aesthetic surgical procedures as well. As a specialty, it is incumbent upon us to do our utmost to satisfy, to the greatest extent possible, the dissatisfaction of previous augmentation patients. Furthermore, experience with secondary augmentation improves our results with primary augmentation. Every secondary augmentation patient has their own story, and each patient encounter is an opportunity to learn more about what might have been done differently in that patient's past to have either reduced the extent of their dissatisfaction, physical deformity, or merely to have increased the time interval between operations.

Every patient considering secondary breast augmentation surgery has some complex interrelated issue between her tissue, the device, and her expectations. Each of these parameters needs to be considered for every patient complaint. While the situation can be simple in the case of a patient with a saline deflation who otherwise was perfectly pleased with all aspects of her surgery, the process can be extremely complex in the case of a patient with multiple past surgeries, thin tissue coverage, stretched skin, asymmetry, contracture, palpable implant edges, and high expectations for her outcome.

Each of these categories: tissues, device, and expectations, have within themselves a vast number of potential problems and complaints, creating literally hundreds of permutations that drive patient consultation for secondary breast augmentation surgery. Therefore, it is implausible for a single chapter or even an entire book to detail management for the myriad of possible presenting scenarios. Fortunately, there is a way to organize a secondary patient's presenting complaints in a way so that they can be methodically organized, allowing the surgeon to create a thorough and thoughtful management plan. A sound philosophical approach rather than a series of algorithms or recipes will provide for the optimal management of our future secondary augmentation patients.

This chapter will focus on long-term problems following breast augmentation, rather than managing short-term issues such as infections and hematomas as these really fall under the purview of management of complications from the primary surgery. As we will see, most long-term adverse outcomes of breast augmentation result either from suboptimal surgical planning decisions, imperfect execution of the initial operation, or failure to set appropriate patient expectations prior to the initial surgery, therefore allowing the uninformed patient to continuously pursue a series of reoperations in pursuit of the unwise or anatomically impossible outcome.

So too is a detailed treatment of each of the surgical procedures and sequences commonly used to treat secondary augmentation deformities beyond the scope of the chapter. The reader instead will learn to analyze the complex variations of implant problems in order to provide the patient with thoughtful and definitive management.

Scope of the problem

More concerning than the general notion that an augmentation does not last a lifetime, is that more than one in five women undergoing a breast augmentation undergoes a second breast surgery within 3 years. That number is unacceptable for a purely elective, cosmetic operation. Worse yet, is that some of these women enter a cycle of revision procedures, in which they endure the expense, risk, and anguish of repeated surgeries in an effort to fix their problems. And some of these problems can never be remedied. There are many women even in their late 20s several years following their augmentation who feel more self-conscious about the appearance of their breasts than they did prior to their initial augmentation.

Most surgeons do not believe that the 3-year reoperation rate is as high as it is, but it has been repeatedly validated by multiple PMA trials by different manufacturers, different implants, and different surgeons. Unless a surgeon had their personal data CRO reviewed in a PMA study, then it would be hubris to suspect their rate to be any lower. There is another hidden lesson that is proved by the similarity in reoperation rates seen in studies of different implants: that the predominant cause for reoperation is not the device, but it is how we educate patients, make surgical choices, and conduct the surgery. This fact is further validated by data from a single surgeon isolated from the remainder of surgeons in the same PMA study, in which that one surgeon had lower reoperation rates than the pooled average of the other doctors in the study. This striking disparity in outcomes with the same device again proves that results are less related to the device than to other factors. As a competitive breast implant manufacturing industry touts the relative advantages of their devices, an unintended consequence is that patients and surgeons alike have come to believe that the device is an important determinant of the result. However, the totality of data suggests that this is false; the largest documented improvements in patient outcomes have come from improved processes rather than any implant.

Surgeons may doubt the extent of this problem due to a natural tendency to remember our happy patients. Moreover, many of our dissatisfied patients have lost confidence in us and have gone elsewhere if they needed a revision. Sometimes, problems are not visible for years after the first surgery, and the patient has moved, the doctor has retired, or the patient has even forgotten the original surgeon's name. At best, we are only aware of our known personal revision rate, but it is the patient's revision rate that matters.

How long do implants last?

This is frequently asked by potential breast implant patients but is a very different question from 'When will I likely need another breast implant surgery?' Understanding the difference between these two similar but rhetorically different questions offers important insights into the issue of secondary breast augmentation. From a purely statistical point of view, this issue can be rephrased in the following way: 'If devices fail at a rate of about 1% per year, why is the 3 year reoperation rate nearly seven times that?'

The presumption in asking how long implants last is that device failure will be the likely causative reason for their secondary breast surgery, but in fact it is not likely to be. Most revisions are the result of issues with patient tissue or patient expectations. Weight gain and loss, pregnancy, lactation, gravity, hormonal fluctuations, sun damage and time itself will inevitably make even the non-augmented breast change with time, and with the added weight and pressure of an implant, these senescent changes of the breast can be more rapid and more pronounced. Ptosis, soft tissue atrophy, implant visibility and palpability, skin stretch and capsular contracture are all issues of the patient's own tissues and not actually of the device. Of course, some devices may be less likely to cause contracture or to be visible with a given degree of tissue thickness, but the role of the device in these issues is almost always less contributory than the patient's tissues and biology.

Just as the primary augmentation patient presenting today may have sought consultation a year earlier or a year later than they did, so too is there no absolute time frame at which a patient seeks consultation for a secondary surgery. The same problem that would lead one woman to seek an immediate revision may not bother another woman at all or she may not want to undergo surgery. More difficult to define is to understand disparities that occur between the potential offered by a patient's tissue and the cosmetic goal that she pursues. This process was often set into motion at the time of the first surgery, in which a thorough or honest assessment of her tissue and the limitations it posed may not have been realized or discussed. For instance, patients with such thin tissue that their ribs are visible should not present for secondary surgery wondering why their implants are visible.

A lack of thorough pre-operative assessment and setting of appropriate expectations can lead multiparous women and weight loss patients to not understand why their implants do not stay high and round. Women with subtle forms of pectus carinatum do not understand why they do not have more cleavage. Patients with subtle volume, ptosis, or IMF (inframammary fold) asymmetries may seek revision for issues that are within normal limits. These issues can bring women in for revision surgery before really necessary. Recognizing the limitations of patient's tissues and informing the patient is an important role for the physician seeing the secondary augmentation patient. These sorts of issues become central in the evaluation of a secondary augmentation patient. The surgeon must assess the interplay of patient tissue and biology with device, surgical technique, and patient expectation.

Know the normal ideal augmented breast

Gillies's first principle of plastic surgery, 'know the normal', is as important with secondary breast augmentation surgery as with any other reconstructive procedure. And the differences between the unoperated ideal normal and the augmented ideal normal should also be understood. Many plastic surgeons fashion themselves as 'artists', opposing efforts to characterize surgical aesthetics by any canons of beauty. These concepts never deterred artists such as Da Vinci. And without documenting measurements, we cannot learn from ourselves or from one another. There are only three critical parameters that define the ideal augmented breast: (1) base width and its relationship to N:IMF; (2) amount and distribution of fill within; and (3) implant-soft tissue relationships, including palpability of the implant.

Base width and nipple: inframammary fold distance

There are many different breast measurements that have been described, but none is as powerful as simply looking at the ratio of the base width to the nipple to inframammary fold distance. If these ratios are not optimal, there will be a deformity. Ideally, this relationship should be 11 cm : 7 cm; 12 cm : 8 cm; 13 cm : 9 cm. This holds true in a wide variety of breast types, whether augmented or not. Determining the root cause of variances from these ratios in the secondary patient can be challenging, as it requires defining differences between inframammary fold height on the chest wall, implant height and nipple height. In nearly all cases of a suboptimal appearing breast, there will either be asymmetries in these measurements between the breasts, or an inappropriate relationship relative to the dictates of these canons.

Amount and distribution of breast fill

In the AP view of the ideal non-augmented breast, there is a clear line of demarcation between the breast and the surrounding tissues only from about 4 o'clock to 10 o'clock, when looking at the right breast; the remainder of the breast tapers off gradually without a visible step-off, blending into the surrounding tissues. At the lower portion of the breast, this is what we call the inframammary fold. The only exception to this in the non-operated breast is in the rapidly growing adolescent breast in which the skin has not yet stretched to accommodate the increasing volume, the engorged lactating breast, and in the constricted lower pole breast, which for the same reason, forces the envelope of the upper breast to excessively fill, creating a marked step-off between the implant and the surrounding tissues. In the lateral view, the same breast would be relatively straight or empty in the upper pole, depending upon how full that patient's breast skin envelope is. It is never convex in the non-augmented breast.

In the augmented breast with ideal implant volume, one that fills the breast but does not stretch the breast, these relationships are still largely preserved. A progressively larger implant will create a more visible delineation of the perimeter of the breast than a non-augmented breast. This may or may not be desirable to a particular patient, but all patients should understand than an implant that creates increasing degrees of this appearance is objectively not natural, and also risks pressure atrophy of the breast parenchyma and progressive stretch of the overlying skin.

Similarly, the ideal upper pole in an augmented breast should also be straight. An upper pole convexity is indicative of over-fill; a concave upper pole indicative of under-fill. Some patients desire that upper 'bulge' or 'shelf', With nulliparous, young, and tight lower pole skin, there may be situations in which upper convexity is maintained, but with time lower pole skin (unless there is a contracture or mild degrees of inferior pocket closure), will give way to the weight and pressure of the implant, allowing this early upper bulge (whether desired or not) to dissipate as the implant filler redistributes itself towards the bottom of the shell. True 'drop' of an implant, as defined by the implant shifting caudally on the chest wall and coming to rest in an inferiorly displaced position, is uncommon and considered a deformity. There are many patients with small and tight breasts who want to achieve a large size and cannot understand why this is unattainable without the upper bulge, and they need to be educated. Similarly, patients with lax envelopes who want only a small increase in volume often do not understand why they still have upper pole convexity, and they similarly need to be educated. Thus the amount of distribution of fill within the breast envelope, consisting of both implant and native tissue, is of paramount importance in determining breast aesthetics.

Implant–soft tissue relationships

Obviously, the non-augmented breast has no implant visibility or palpability, and in the augmented breast, the goal is to make the implant as indetectable as possible. Any woman receiving a breast implant should expect that her implant will in some way and in some positions be detectable. The extent of this is dependent somewhat on the type of the implant, but, moreover, is a function of tissue coverage relative to the size of the implant. A small bag of pebbles would be relatively undetectable if used to augment a 'small D' to a 'mid D', but no implant on the market today can augment a very small breast to a very large breast and not be obvious. Capsular contracture and implant overfill/underfill all contribute to excessive implant perceptibility. No patient or surgeon should ever expect to eradicate this. The goal is to make this as subtle as possible, and the indication for surgery to correct this is not that the implant is detectable, but whether it is likely to make the implant less detectable in the long run. Nearly as important as the thickness of tissue coverage and the thickness of the capsule, but harder to define, is the dynamic relationship between the implant with the capsule, and the capsule with the overlying tissue. Any study that will enable better prediction of these phenomenon will profoundly help in the avoidance and correction of dissatisfaction following breast augmentation.

Consultation with the secondary augmentation patient

Whether or not you were the original operating surgeon, you must assess the state of the patient's condition, the limitations posed by their biology or tissue, and the likelihood for improvement. I have seen a tendency for surgeons to be more circumspect about reoperating on their own patients than they would be about operating on a new secondary patient entering their practice. In fact, however, the indications for surgery should be the same. Why would there be this difference? Other than medico-legal issues, clearly there is a tendency when it is your own dissatisfied primary augmentation patient to be more suspicious of changing patient expectations than a shortcoming in the surgical plan or execution. When the patient comes from another surgeon, one can be too quick to be sympathetic to the patient's requests and to blame the previous surgeon's poor planning or technique.

Every effort must be made to secure all previous operative records. Incisions, pocket locations, implant type and fills, use of drains, recovery, changes in cup size, lactation and weight loss history, and satisfaction/dissatisfaction with each procedure should be documented. Patients should be asked to give a complete laundry list of complaints or wishes for the revision surgery. One by one, the surgeon must assess the validity of their complaint about each issue, seek the cause or source for the problem, and determine whether or not, and to what extent, each problem might be fixed. It is important to recognize not just requests that are unfulfillable, but also those that are contradictory. For instance, a patient may at the same time ask to be larger, yet have edges that are less visible. A patient may ask to be smaller, yet want to have greater upper fill and not want a mastopexy. Examples of this are numerous, and it is important to consider trade-offs inherent in fixing a particular problem.

The surgeon must always be detailed and conscientious in assessing a patient's tissues and the limitations they impose on a result, and never is this truer than in the secondary patient. Many of these patients are seeking secondary operations because their expectations were not properly set in the beginning or procedures were done in an effort to attain an unattainable result. With the passage of time and damage to their tissues, they may even be farther from the possibility of achieving their goal than before their first procedure. It is critically important to assess their tissues and their goals, and reconcile the two. This can be a disappointing conversation for many patients, but the sooner they learn the limitations of their tissue, the less suffering they will ultimately endure. In fact, most patients actually appreciate the candor of a physician willing to engage in an honest and direct discussion, even if the content is ultimately disappointing to them.

And for purely selfish reasons, it would behoove the surgeon to discuss limitations of outcome posed by the patient's own tissues. The dissatisfied secondary augmentation patient is certainly a litigation risk. But short of that, the more realistic the expectations the surgeon sets with the patient, the more likely it will be that the surgeon fulfills the expectation they have given that patient. A common situation with both primary and secondary breast surgery is that there can be a disparity between what the patient wants or is willing to do as opposed to what the surgeon thinks is best. Certainly, the surgeon must never do something they think is inappropriate. But the reality is that sometimes patients just will not do what the surgeon thinks is best. In these situations, it is very important that the patient be informed of the specific trade-offs inherent in their decision, and they must physically sign off on their acceptance of them. Not only does this medico-legally help in transferring responsibility to the patient, the boldness of such a document further encourages patients to accept what their surgeon is encouraging them to do.

While patients in these complex situations may often not select the therapeutic course that their surgeon recommends most highly, a surgeon should never proceed with any course that they feel is not in the patient's best interest. In fact, to justify doing so by arguing that 'this is what she wanted' may be indefensible in court. Plastic surgeons are sometimes pulled in two directions: the demands of the patient and the requirements of her tissues. No other surgical specialty is expected to pay heed to patient requests to the same extent. Ultimately, however, patient demand should not be permitted to press a surgeon toward proceeding with anything they think is inappropriate.

Secondary augmentation

Declining to operate on a patient eager to schedule is a key option that the busy reoperative breast surgeon will need to resort to on a frequent basis. It is probably true that the patient will go elsewhere and find a surgeon to meet their request, but that does not make it right.

Secondary breast augmentation surgery runs a spectrum from fairly straightforward surgery to situations that are not only complex, but also even unsolvable. In order to create a treatment plan and to predict the likelihood of improvement, the surgeon must begin by organizing and categorizing each patient's problems. Only after assessing all of the contributing factors to the deformity can solutions be found.

Not fixing a problem or removing without replacement

No discussion of secondary augmentation is complete without making a serious note of the possibility of suggesting that a patient either accept a problem as it is or undergo removal without replacement. This is far easier said than done, as patients typically have set in their minds a particular appearance they hope to achieve with another revision, or they have enjoyed their augmentation so much that they are loathe to be explanted. Many of the worst problems I have seen have been as a result of a single surgeon repeatedly trying to make things a little better for the patient, only instead to have the patient develop ever-worsening tissue problems. It is nearly impossible to tell our own dissatisfied primary augmentation patients that their situation is not likely to be improved, and that all their money, discomfort, time, and expectations were for naught, and that they should either just accept the current situation or actually pay yet again, but this time to have their implants permanently removed.

It is easier, but also very difficult, to say the same thing to a patient whose previous operations were done elsewhere. A combination of hope that we may help them and wanting to avoid disappointing them has led many a surgeon to offer an operation to a patient whose situation is unlikely to be substantially improved. Unfortunately, if we are to make any serious gains in reducing reoperations, we need to be stricter in defining the circumstances in which we will operate, and the situations in which removing without replacement best serves the interests of the patient.

The only way to achieve success in this regard is if these criteria are discussed and understood by the patient prior to their first surgery. It is nearly impossible to make these issues understood and accepted after the patient has paid for and completed their first surgery with certain expectations in their mind. The situation will not be substantially improved until plastic surgeons as a group all educate their patients. Tebbetts introduced the concept of defining specific 'out point' criteria prior to the first operation. His patients must sign off understanding that their surgeon will not perform elective size change unless medical indications or surgeon agreed aesthetic compromises are present, nipple asymmetries <1.5 cm, IMF asymmetries <1.5 cm, and contractures less than a Grade III. The additional benefit of defining these and having the patient sign off on them preoperatively is that it defines a margin of imprecision that the surgeon and patient consider tolerable. Finally, understanding these issues before the first operation further incentivizes surgeons and patients to perform the operation and make the decisions and choices that are most likely to yield an excellent long term result. Similarly, no revision other than explantation without replacement is offered to patients with recurrent capsule contracture after one revision in which all measures were followed that could prevent a recurrence of the contracture, and patients with implant visibility and palpability with tissue pinch <5 mm at the thinnest area.

Causes for reoperation

In PMA studies for both Mentor and Allergan, operation on capsular contracture remains the most common reason for secondary surgery, followed by patient request for size change, scarring, implant malposition, asymmetry, ptosis, and suspected implant rupture. It is interesting to note that actual implant rupture was not listed amongst the top ten reasons for revision of a breast augmentation. It behooves the surgeon to recognize that this list reiterates the importance of patient tissues, surgeon and patient decision making, and surgical technique as a cause of the second operation as opposed to the device itself.

The most complex situation can always be broken down into five causes, each of which has a discrete set of potential solutions: in priority they are parenchyma/tissue coverage, skin envelope, capsule, pocket position, and the device. As the surgeon assesses each patient, they should carefully consider each of the five key components that may contribute to the problem, even if the complaint does not at first specifically seem to require consideration. Sometimes there is a problem that the patient had not noticed that the surgeon might overlook, only to be noticed after the revision. Most importantly, none of these can be considered in isolation, as issues in each of these categories can cross over and affect the others, and the correction of one problem may reveal an otherwise masked problem in another category or exacerbate what had only been a mild problem in yet another category.

Manufacturers, patients, and even surgeons have excessively focused on the device as a cause of and solution for problems in breast augmentation patients. While there are undeniably substantial benefits in using various implants in specific situations, by and large the causes and solutions of problems are predominantly related to the patient and surgeon decision making, which is often flawed due to inadequate education of the patient at the time of the initial operation. There is obviously interplay between all of these – and that makes the situation more difficult.

Breast augmentation for surgeons and patients initiative (BASPI)

In 2004, a group of plastic surgeons gathered to consider solutions to concerns that were voiced by the FDA during the 2003 panel hearings. There was concern over reoperation rates, amongst others. This group put together algorithms to establish best practice approaches to several clinical situations that are relevant to secondary augmentation. These flow charts did not define a standard of practice, but rather presented a range of options that are available and need to be considered. They demonstrate how a reasoned approach that considers all options, benefits and tradeoffs, one in which the patient participates, can succeed in reducing the cycle of reoperations that some patients experience.

Specifically, there were algorithms for management of concerns of shell disruption or a leaking silicone gel implant, management of stretch deformities and implant malposition, management of size exchange,

and management of capsular contracture. Each of the possible alternatives at each point of the decision making process were posed, and the patient had to initial each point in the decision making tree.

Classification of secondary augmentation problems

The following Teitelbaum classification of breast augmentation problems (Table 8.1) not only inventories all of the problems, but it suggests solutions, and the likelihood for improvement. It reminds the surgeon of all possible causes and solutions.

They are listed in their order of priority:

- Parenchyma/tissue coverage
- Skin envelope
- Capsule
- Pocket position
- Device.

A patient is given two scores: one for their appearance at the time of consultation, and another for the patient's expected result following surgery. Like the Glasgow coma scale, the lowest score indicates the greatest deformity and the highest score indicates the ideal normal. The highest score of 15 would come from the maximum score of 3 for each of the 5 categories. The lowest score of 5 would come from a score of 1 for each of the categories. Each of the five categories is given a score between 1 and 3 according to the following scale:

1. Significant deformity
2. Minor deformity
3. No deformity.

A patient is first scored according to the appearance at the time of presentation. All of the information derived from the history and physical examination are culled and analyzed within the structure of these 5 categories, in order to give a preoperative score. After scoring each of these five categories in the patient's current condition, a second scoring is predicted for the various surgical plans being considered. This helps patients to select which option best meets their needs, and even whether the costs and risks of surgery are enough to justify surgery. This system forces surgeons to look at each of the relevant categories of the surgery and make an assessment of the likelihood of improvement for each. Without such systematic thinking, it is all too easy to inadvertently neglect a pertinent issue or trade-off.

This system also helps to reconcile trade-offs and secondary deformities, e.g. the submuscular patient with adequate soft tissue coverage who elects to go submammary who preoperatively has a '3' for the soft tissue score, may go down to a '2' for that in an effort to raise a '2' for minor ptosis to a '3'. The complexity of these situations requires an organized and coherent approach with which to attempt to quantify the advantages and disadvantages of the various options.

Parenchyma/soft tissue coverage

Assuring optimal soft tissue coverage for a patient's lifetime is the highest priority in secondary breast augmentation, just as it is in primary breast augmentation, and the lack of it is the most prognostic sign of

Table 8.1 Teitelbaum classification scheme of breast augmentation problems

Minimum score: 5	
Maximum score: 15	
Parenchyma/tissue coverage	
Significant deformity and/or lack of tissue coverage (pinch <1cm)	1
Moderate deformity and/or lack of tissue coverage (pinch <2 cm)	2
No deformity from lack of tissue coverage	3
Skin envelope	
Significant ptosis; N:IMF>11 or APSS>4 (with implants in place)	1
Moderate Ptosis, N:IMF>9.5 or APSS>3	2
No disorder of skin envelope	3
Capsule	
Severely distorting or painful contracture	1
Moderately distorting contracture	2
No clinically significant contracture	3
Pocket Position	
Significant deformity from implant malposition	1
Moderate deformity from implant malposition	2
No deformity from implant malposition	3
Device	
Significant device-related deformity	1
Moderate device-related deformity	2
No device-related deformity	3
TOTAL SCORE	15

an unsatisfactory outcome. If there is enough tissue coverage, subtle implant malposition can go unnoticed, severe implant folding can be undetectable, stretched and thin skin can still be kept full, and even capsular contraction can be hard to feel. We can change implants; we can move implants; we can reduce skin with mastopexies; we are often successful at treating capsular contracture. But unless the implant is submammary and we can switch to submuscular or dual plane, we do not yet have a way to consistently and significantly augment the soft tissue of the breast. So if a patient has a problem related to very thin tissue coverage, no implant or perfectly executed surgery can fix all of the patient's problems.

If a patient has abundant soft tissue, there rarely is a problem that cannot be substantially improved. On the contrary, there is a rarely a patient with very thin and inadequate tissue for whom a perfect result can be achieved. This truth can be extremely difficult for patients to accept – particularly in a culture in which excessive thinness is so celebrated – and actually can be difficult for surgeons themselves to recognize and accept as well. Obviously, many augmentation patients initially presented because of having small breasts with thin parenchyma. Large implants can further put pressure on the parenchyma, causing increasing soft tissue thinning from pressure atrophy. Tissue can further atrophy following lactation subsequent to the original augmentation. Some patients have had parenchyma removed along with capsular tissue when undergoing previous capsulectomies. In the era of mass silicone fear in the 1990s, many other women unfortunately underwent significant resection of otherwise normal parenchyma and even muscle.

In fact, some secondary breast augmentation patients have soft tissue that is so thin that they are best thought of as if they were subcutaneous mastectomy patients. Some of these patients still bring in photos from the Internet of women with substantial parenchyma thickness as examples of how they want to look. It is very difficult, but important to inform them that their expectations should be based more on the appearance of a subcutaneous mastectomy reconstructive patient than the elective cosmetic patients whose appearance they wish to emulate. There is a paucity of photographs of thin-tissued secondary augmentation patients available, so it should come as little surprise that few if any of these patients are at all aware of how difficult a situation they are in. In fact, subcutaneous mastectomy patients can even be in a better situation than some secondary augmentation patients, as repeated augmentation surgeries and pocket changes can result in a pectoralis that has been partially resected, avulsed off of the sternum, or in some other way allowed to window shade so far cephalad such that it is no longer can cover the implant as well as an undamaged pectoralis can cover the implant in a subcutaneous mastectomy situation.

Patients and surgeons must be reminded that breast implants are at their best when they serve as a platform for the existing breast tissue, projecting it forward, thereby allowing the existing parenchyma to be seen and felt. But when coverage is thin and the implant is large, the implant is not augmenting the existing breast so much as it becomes the breast. To date, there is no device that can mimic the natural soft tissue of the breast. An implant should be viewed not as a soft tissue replacement. Tissue coverage and implant size go hand in hand: coverage inadequate for a large implant may be adequate for a smaller implant. But for this section, we will consider the thickness of the coverage; finding an implant of the appropriate size will be addressed in the device section.

Assessing tissue coverage and the parenchyma

Tissue coverage should be assessed in all breast augmentation patients, both in primaries and secondaries, even if the patient's complaint at that moment does not specifically relate to coverage issues. Tissue coverage always becomes the most important issue affecting the appearance and long term result in a breast augmentation, and it should be assessed before planning any surgery. Caliper pinch thickness at the superior, inferior, medial, and lateral poles should be documented, as well as the visibility of the implant edge. The position of the implant relative to the muscle must be assessed. The patient should contract her pectoralis by pushing her hands together in front of her chest while the surgeon observes the motion of the chest and palpates the attachment of the pectoralis to both the sternum and the ribs along the medial inframammary fold. Usually, one can determine whether the implant is in front of or behind the pectoralis muscle.

In some situations in which the implant is purportedly retromuscular, this exam can reveal that there is actually little or no coverage. This can be seen in cases of severe ptosis, in which case the implant sits so far caudally, that even its superior border sits beneath the

inferior border of the pectoralis. It is also seen when the pectoralis was dissected off of the sternum, allowing it to window shade superiorly, slipping over and above the implant. This is possible with every incision, but it is most commonly observed with the periareolar incision, often in cases of very small areolas. This may be due to poor visualization, or a loss of landmarks in which the surgeon, while dividing pectoralis muscle origins along the medial inframammary fold, continues up too far along the sternum until level with the point of access at the areola, exacerbated by the destruction of fibrous attachments between the superficial surface of the pectoralis and the deep surface of the gland, some extent of which is nearly unavoidable with the peri-areolar approach. Interestingly, this is the opposite of the pattern typically seen with a blunt transaxillary approach, in which the muscle is frequently not adequately taken down along the IMF, leaving an implant positioned too high.

While coverage is the main consideration with parenchyma, other significant issues exist. Some patients with lower pole constriction may have a deformity from inadequate release and may still require release. This can be seen in the tuberous or constricted breast. Conversion of a subpectoral to a dual plane type II release can allow access to the deep surface of the gland for scoring to allow expansion. Animation deformities can exist with dual plane, total retromuscular, or partial retropectoral coverage. Total muscular coverage is virtually impossible without wide exposure and lifting the serratus off of the chest wall, which can be bloody, painful, and prolong recovery. Animation deformities decrease significantly with dual plane compared to traditional partial retropectoral pockets.

Management of coverage/parenchyma issues

The only reliable method of increasing soft tissue coverage is to convert from a retromammary to a retromuscular pocket. If the implant is already truly retromuscular, there is often little to do to add substantial tissue coverage.

When retromammary

One must recognize that there may be difficulties and trade-offs when converting to a retromuscular position. If there is lower pole stretch, the new implant may still sit so low that little if any of it will end up behind the muscle. If N:IMF is greater than ideal for the given implant size (7 for 200, 8 for 300, and 9 for 400), the surgeon must be circumspect about how much of the implant will gain coverage. If there is coexisting ptosis, then the surgeon should consider whether conversion to a partial retropectoral or dual plane pocket risks exacerbating the ptosis. Conversion to a dual plane pocket by dividing pectoralis origins along the medial inframammary fold can help obviate the problem of exacerbating ptosis, but if the envelope was very thin or stretched, it will not look as full as when submammary.

Furthermore, if tissue pinch along the IMF is <5 cm and maximal coverage is necessary inferiorly, one may have to consider whether the benefits of a dual plane pocket outweigh the sacrifice in tissue coverage from division of the pectoralis origins along the inframammary fold. And when the muscle is taken down along the fold following a previous submammary augmentation, it often will window shade up higher than it would in a primary augmentation. That is because in a well-executed dual plane pocket created in a primary augmentation, the attachments of the pectoralis to the overlying gland help hold the muscle down to cover the inferior pole of the breasts. With these attachments completely eliminated by a subglandular pocket, there is nothing to hold the muscle down after division of the pectoralis inferiorly.

In fact, even without an inferior release, the caudal edge of the pectoralis can pull up superiorly in some cases. It can even create a band of tension over the implant, compressing the implant superomedially where there is coverage, with the implant then bulging out inferolaterally where there is no muscle. These problems can sometimes be controlled by suturing the muscle up to the overlying gland. However, attempts at pulling the muscle down and holding it far inferiorly by tacking it to the overlying gland often result in significant deformity. An alternative therefore is to use marionette sutures as described by Spear. Finally, another option may be to use dermal grafts, such as AlloDerm® or Strattice™. Attached to the caudal edge of the pectoralis, these dermal substitutes are being used as an interposition between the muscle and the inframammary fold, not only increasing coverage through its own thickness, but moreover drawing the muscle down to maximize muscle coverage.

One must also consider the potential for animation deformities when converting to a retromuscular pocket. It is difficult to assess, but it is my impression that these problems are more noticeable in the secondary patient switched from submammary to dual plane than in the primary dual plane patient. While one must consider a change to submammary pockets in any patient with significant deformity, one must reassess the litany of advantages of muscular coverage for that particular patient before embarking on a pocket switch, being certain that the advantages outweigh the disadvantages for that patient. In particular, it appears that the patients who most notice animation deformities, in particular deformities of dimpling and retraction of the skin, frequently have tissue pinch <2 cm, so the decision to change the pocket must be made judiciously. Patients frequently complain about inferolateral implant palpability and rippling, particularly when leaning forward or bending over. While conversion to a retromuscular pocket may be indicated for other reasons, the patient should be reminded that there is no pectoralis muscle in this area, and that this zone would not be expected to improve following a switch to a retropectoral pocket.

Particularly when coverage is very thin, and in all cases, for that matter, one must consider whether the implant size is appropriate for the patient's available soft tissue. There are times in which the coverage may be inadequate for the current implant size, but would be adequate for an implant of a smaller size. Unfortunately this is not always easy to determine. In the ideal situation, the primary surgeon documented the critical measurements to determine implant size pre-operatively (STPTUP, STPTIMF, APSS, PCSEF). These measurements can then be used to evaluate whether the patient's current implant size is appropriate for her tissues. It is uncommon to find even such basic information in previous records. The importance of these objective measurements in revision surgery is so great that it behooves all surgeons to document them before a primary patient's first operation. One can assess whether the base width of the augmented breast is being defined by the base width of the implant, or whether the natural base width is wider than the implant. If it is the former case, then visible edges or a lack of adequate coverage may be improved by selecting an implant that fits within the footprint of the breast.

When retromuscular

A great many patients with severe soft tissue inadequacy are already 'behind the muscle'. How can that be? Pectoralis coverage is dependent upon three things: its origins along the sternum, from the ribs along the IMF, and from its overlying attachments to the gland. When the origins along the IMF are divided, the attachments to the overlying gland hold the pectoralis down, allowing it to pull upwards only a centimeter or so from the IMF. However, if those attachments between pectoralis and the overlying gland are released excessively, the muscle will window shade superiorly, substantially sacrificing coverage. This can intentionally be done in a precise and selective manner so that the muscle can rise to the lower border of the areola in a Dual Plane Type II, or to the upper border of the areola in a Dual Plane Type III, in response to specific clinical situations, such as glandular ptosis or a constricted lower pole.

It occurs quite frequently, however, in an unintentional manner during routine breast augmentation from one of two maneuvers. With the periareolar approach, there is disruption of these attachments as a result of the dissection path that may be taken from the areola to the IMF. Even with the best of intentions, even careful PA techniques can result in excessive vertical elevation of the pectoralis, thereby sacrificing coverage. It can also happen with the inframammary incision, if excessive dissection is done on top of the pectoralis before finding a way under it. Disruption of what seems like just a centimeter or two can result in massive window shading of the muscle after the origins along the IMF are released and the muscle is put under stretch by an implant underneath. This sort of problem is usually non-existent with the transaxillary approach; while frequently one finds incomplete division of the pectoralis origins along the IMF with the TA approach, it would take tedious, intentional, and difficult retrograde dissection from the axilla to disrupt the connections between the pectoralis muscle and the overlying gland. It is therefore unlikely to ever see significant loss of muscle coverage following a previous transaxillary augmentation.

The submuscular patient with significant implant visibility problems represents the most difficult problem to correct in all of secondary breast surgery. If the pectoralis muscle is known to be fully intact, then there might not be anything to do. Perhaps in the future, tissue augmentation with fat or other injectables may be de rigueur, but at this point they are still being explored. If the pectoralis can be felt to have window-shaded superiorly so that the patient does not

have adequate muscle coverage, the goal must be to pull the muscle back down over the implant. In some cases this may be exacerbated by the implant sitting low, and a procedure to either raise the pocket itself or a mastopexy may necessary in those situations.

The pectoralis muscle may often be thin and not a stout structure with which to place sutures. But every effort must be made to move it inferiorly to add coverage. The dermal substitutes Alloderm® and Strattice™ are also described for this purpose. By sewing them along the caudal edge of the pectoralis muscle, they can then be sewn down to the inframammary fold. The point is not so much to gain coverage from the material as to pull the muscle down as far as it will go, thereby increasing the surface area of the implant covered by the patient's own muscle.

Other parenchymal issues

In addition to lack of coverage, parenchymal maldistribution can create deformities. The ones most notable are the so-called double-bubble and constriction of the lower pole.

Double-bubble   The double-bubble occurs when the implant sits below the old inframammary fold. The presence of parenchyma above this line and the absence of parenchyma below it gives the step-off characteristic of the double bubble. This problem is more pronounced with pre-existing 'tight' inframammary folds, as such folds denote a sudden demarcation between the thick breast and much thinner upper abdominal tissue. What is double is the perception of the breast mounds: there is a mound from the device, and the original breast mound is perched on top of it, shifted superiorly to some degree.

The first issue is to assess whether the implant is of the right size for the breast. The larger the implant, the more the fold has to be lowered. If the implant is too large, switching to a smaller implant will allow the IMF to be raised, reducing exposure to the lower mound. Even a small raise of the IMF can dramatically reduce the perception of this deformity. If the implant must be lower than the original IMF, it is released with as many vertical scores on the deep surface of the parenchyma as necessary. One can feel when the release is enough, but sometimes this requires going all the way through to the dermis. It is easy to 'buttonhole' through the skin with this maneuver, so one must be very careful. But even with a maximal release, if the difference in thickness between the subcutaneous tissues immediately above and below the fold are great, and the transition sudden, there will likely always remain some visibility of the old inframammary fold.

If the implant is the correct size, one should check to be sure that the N:IMF distance is appropriate for that implant. Sometimes, one needs just to raise the IMF (see section on pockets). But if the implant still needs to be lower than the old IMF, extensive scoring of the parenchyma to allow its redistribution may be necessary.

Lower pole constriction   Developmental constriction of the lower pole is quite common. Sometimes there is a true tuberous breast, but more commonly there may be horizontal tightness of the lower pole or maldistribution of the parenchyma centered just deep to the areola, resulting in an excessively projecting breast. Unless the implant was dual-plane or submammary and the parenchyma was scored, these problems often persist after the first augmentation. Such patients need to be converted to a dual plane from a partial retropectoral or total submuscular pocket, and extensive scoring of the lower pole of the gland needs to be undertaken.

Scoring:
1. Significant deformity and/or lack of tissue coverage (pinch < 1 cm)
2. Moderate deformity and/or lack of tissue coverage (pinch < 2 cm)
3. No deformity of tissue coverage.

Skin envelope

The problem

Many patient complaints and needs for secondary surgery relate to the state of the skin envelope. While there are some cases of skin deficiency related to constricted breast deformities or excessive prior mastopexy, the most common skin issues in the secondary breast augmentation patient are stretch deformities with skin excess and/or ptosis. These include generalized laxity of skin with no ptosis (essentially an underfilled envelope), increased nipple to inframammary fold length with appropriate positioning of the nipple areola complex on the breast mound (bottoming out),

and true ptosis (nipple–areola complex positioned low on the breast mound).

Small breasts age better than large breasts whether they are natural or augmented. The small A cup breast will frequently be as pert on a 70-year-old as it was when she was 20, albeit small. But almost every naturally D cup woman develops some ptosis by her late 20s, and the situation is frequently similar in the augmented breast. Whether breasts were initially sized by volume or dimension, each implant has a weight to it, and that weight exerts an effect on the breast skin that is often unpredictable. Though it would be impossible to ever expect to demonstrate this statistically, it is clear to every surgeon experienced with secondary augmentation that increased breast implant size is associated with greater stretch of the skin envelope. This is due to both the increased pressure of the projection of the implant and stretch on the lower pole of the breast due to the weight of the implant.

Women whose first operation was done following involution and/or glandular ptosis post partum or following weight loss are frequently found in this group. With skin stretched or thinned before their first operation, they frequently requested to be full again. Oftentimes their skin was not just stretched from lactation, but it developed striae and thinning, and lost some elasticity. The weight of the implant against their thinned skin can result in accelerated stretch. Many of these patients report that in hindsight their original surgeon initially suggested a mastopexy, but that they didn't want the scars. Instead, in order to fill their envelope, they may have received a larger implant than they wished, and in any case, any additional weight further stretched their skin.

The secondary mastopexy augmentation patient is a category of secondary augmentation patients that deserves its own chapter. This subgroup of augmentation patients has a higher reoperation rate than primary augmentation patients alone, and the reason is obvious. Though it is done frequently, and is done for appropriate indications, it nonetheless is an operation that at its core is inherently illogical. By definition, the mastopexy-augmentation candidate has skin that failed to hold the pre-existing weight of the breasts. Even if due to a relatively short term event like nursing, permanent changes frequently occur to the skin. Skin is removed with a mastopexy, but the skin that remains is the same skin that gave out once, and under the influence of greater weight, it can be expected to stretch again.

Assessment of the skin envelope

In the primary augmentation patient, measurement of skin stretch by pulling forward on the medial border of the areola to see the maximum amount the skin can be distracted has been described and is de rigueur for many surgeons. This can also be done in an identical manner on the augmented patient and documented. Absent quantified, documentable numbers, information cannot be recorded for the benefit of the patient, and surgeons cannot discuss amongst themselves in order to further medical knowledge.

It is important to assess the quality of the skin and its potential to stretch. It is unfortunate that we do not yet have an accurate way to either quantify or predict that potential. But even rough assessments are important. For instance, it is important to point out striae and obviously thin tissues to patients, so that they specifically understand that these are issues inherent to their tissue that the surgeon cannot improve. One of the most important parameters to be measured and documented is nipple to inframammary fold distance. The rule of 7 cm, 8 cm, and 9 cm has been published and is a reliable indicator of the ideal distance for implants of 200, 300, and 400 mL respectively. A special note must be made about patient request for upper pole fullness. A common request of the secondary augmentation patient is to have more upper pole fullness. Unless the patient's lack of upper pole fullness is due to placement of an implant that is small relative to the patient's breast tissue – which is uncommon – the problem is likely due to a stretched lower pole.

The breast fills from the bottom up, just like a bucket being filled with water. The greater the lower pole laxity, the greater the volume it will take to fill the upper breast. But the surgeon should rarely expect to gain long lasting upper pole fill by filling the lax breast with an ever-larger implant. This poor decision is frequently made. While this can gain short-term improvement in upper pole fill, if the lower pole is stretched, it frequently restretches even worse than it was before, resulting in a one-step forward and two-step backward situation.

Sternal notch to nipple is also a helpful measure of asymmetries, but is not an absolute indication of whether a nipple needs to be moved superiorly. In the augmentation patient, the issue is the position of the nipple–areola complex relative to the breast mound and its axis relative to the horizon. If a nipple–areola complex is low on the breast mound or pointing down, one must determine first whether the breast mound is in the right place, or if the mound is high. A high riding implant can simulate ptosis; similarly an implant that is positioned too low can give the nipple–areola the appearance of being too high. Capsular contracture can also pull an implant superiorly, giving the illusion of a low nipple–areola complex, and treating the contracture at times can create a proper relationship of the nipple to the breast mound. A partial retropectoral pocket that holds an implant too superiorly can similarly make the nipple look low on the mound, as can too large an implant for the N:IMF distance. One must be alert to all of these possibilities when assessing the skin envelope of an augmented breast.

Solution

Patients rarely like the solution for skin envelope problems, which is typically some sort of mastopexy. Many pursued augmentation for cosmetic reasons, and accepting significant scars on the breast are anathema to them. If they are necessary in the surgeon's judgment, the surgeon must document this advice clearly, and explain to the patient the ramifications of forgoing the mastopexy. Legal documentation aside, it would behoove the surgeon to either not operate on someone unwilling to undergo the proper procedure, or at least be certain that the patient really understands the limitations of not undergoing the entire procedure as the surgeon sees fit, as the disappointed secondary augmentation patient can become quite a significant emotional liability. But there are many patients who prefer to have 'somewhat droopy' breasts to having perkier but scarred breasts. It seems that many patients who need a mastopexy frequently fail to see what their breasts will look like without a mastopexy. It is important to make it clear to them that they will have larger breasts that hang lower on the torso. The importance of discussing these issues with patients cannot be stressed enough.

It is often very difficult to assess the extent and pattern of skin redundancy when there are implants in place. There may be asymmetry, and it is often unclear whether this predated the surgery or is a result of it. Oftentimes, patients with stretch deformities are post-partum, and their baby may have favored nursing on one side and this contributed to the asymmetry. Coexisting capsular contracture can make

Secondary augmentation

assessment of the skin envelope difficult, as contracture can draw the implant up, itself causing a difference in SNN and N:IMF measurements. Asymmetry in contracture can create an apparent asymmetry in nipple height. One should embark on correcting both of these in one stage only if you are extremely experienced and confident that you can deliver a result that will meet that patient's expectation. There are some patients who are tolerant of some asymmetry in N:IMF distance, nipple height, or upper fullness. Others will only be happy if it is perfect. One should always at least consider first correcting the contracture, and then allowing skin to settle and redrape before assessing for and planning mastopexy. This is particularly true if there is a volume disparity or a disparity in the extent of contracture, which can make planning a precise mastopexy very difficult. It is true that patients can be sat up on the operating table for marking, but in my opinion, these markings are sometimes not as precise as if they were made with a patient standing preoperatively, with the surgeon able to stand back and assess, mark, and remark as necessary. If nothing else, this also provides a greater margin of safety for the blood supply to the nipple–areola complex.

A very useful technique for assessing ptosis in saline patients is to do a preoperative deflation. Used when one knows that there is ptosis, but is unable to assess its extent, it is simple to use an angiocath to drain both implants. The underlying asymmetry of both volume and of the skin envelope can then be revealed. Without the pressure of the implant, the skin will rebound to a varying degree. Though most patients want to be deflated as close to the time of surgery as possible, the rare patient who is willing to go deflated for several weeks or more often sees a greater degree of rebound contraction of the skin, allowing for a more precise preoperative planning of the mastopexy, or in some circumstances reveal that a mastopexy is not even necessary. It is certainly acceptable to not deflate these patients and do the surgery all in one stage. But by informing the patient that a staged approach can be safer and more accurate, the surgeon has legitimately transferred responsibility for a less than perfect result to the patient. Given the difficulty in creating a perfect result in these patients, this is a very important thing to do.

Treatment options

The first priority is to define whether or not the breast mound is in the proper position. Deciding whether the implant needs to be moved up or down must be considered before one considers tightening the envelope or raising the nipple–areola complex. When determining the appropriate type of mastopexy, one must be specific about the area of excess of the skin envelope and resect accordingly. There is no mastopexy that is ideal in all situations. Start by defining what needs to be changed, and that will guide you to selecting the proper mastopexy.

If the N:IMF is long relative to the breast width, then a horizontal scar will likely be necessary to adequately shorten it. Periareolar and vertical mastopexies have only a limited ability to shorten the N:IMF distance. By definition, any patient that has implants and needs a mastopexy has skin that is compromised. Though the mastopexy removes skin, that which remains is the same skin that stretched the first time. I have seen many mastopexy augmentations with the periareolar or vertical scars, and though there are situations in which these may be satisfactory choices, they do appear to stretch vertically more with time in these circumstances than does the inverted T pattern mastopexy.

If the breast is wide or needs projection, it will need a vertical scar. A periareolar scar reduces projection; in fact, that it why it is so useful in a tuberous breast. But when applied to the typical atrophic and ptotic augmented breast, it overly flattens the already flat breast, reducing often-needed projection. Sometimes the nipple position is adequate for the mound, and so no circumareolar incision is necessary. In rare cases, it is possible to just do an elliptical incision along the inframammary fold to shorten the N:IMF distance, though this typically cannot shorten it more than several centimeters without creating an excessively long inframammary scar, as well as reducing breast projection. If there is horizontal laxity or if more projection is needed, then a vertical scar will be necessary. Though this is typically done together with a circumareolar incision, it is possible to make the vertical limbs converge at 6 o'clock on the areola, eliminating the periareolar incision.

In the augmented breast, one would be wise to restrict the use of the donut mastopexy to cases in which the areola just needs to be reduced, there is a minor amount of generalized skin envelope laxity without ptosis, or for correcting ptosis in small, light breasts, with small implants. This incision is not adequate for significant excisions or raising of the nipple–areola complex in most situations. The most important aspect of this discussion is to recognize the risks involved in doing a mastopexy on the augmented breast. Even a submuscular implant reduces blood supply to the nipple–areola complex, and a submammary implant probably reduces it even more so. Always assess the thickness of the skin envelope. Augmentation patients who need mastopexy frequently have extremely thin tissue, and one must be exceedingly cautious in preserving the blood supply. While it is tempting to undermine freely in order to maximise tissue draping, undermining should be kept to as little as necessary to pull the skin together.

If a capsulectomy is being done at the same time, one must be exceedingly cautious in performing a mastopexy. While there are times in which this must be done, the surgeon must be aware that each procedure can damage the blood flow to the nipple–areola complex from both the superficial and deep surface. Handel's landmark paper on this subject is a must read for any surgeon performing this surgery. Markings should also be made much more conservatively than they would doing a mastopexy in a similar sized breast that is not augmented, as the tissue over the implant does not mobilize and slide to the same extent as it does in the non-augmented breast. Occasionally patients with contracted implants but who do not want a capsulectomy request a mastopexy. This can be an extremely challenging situation, as the overlying tissue is often very restricted in its movement, and mobilizing enough laxity to allow closure of even a conservative mastopexy excision can be problematic.

Scoring:
1. Significant ptosis, N:IMF > 11 or APSS > 4 (with implant in place)
2. Ptosis, N:IMF > 9.5 or APSS > 3
3. No disorder of skin envelope.

Capsular contracture

While capsular contracture remains the most common reason for revision surgery in published data, the use of antibiotic irrigation solution and relatively bloodless surgical technique have made this an increasingly uncommon phenomenon. Patients and surgeons must understand that Grade II 'contractures' are non-pathologic, and do not require revision. Only III or IV contractures that are distorted or painful require or warrant surgery. There should be no expectation that a II can ever be converted to a I over the long term,

and patients without distortion or pain should not have surgery only for reasons of the capsule.

Assessment

In an era in which many American patients had augmentation with saline implants, which were commonly overfilled, one should be cautioned to be mindful of implants appearing distorted and feeling contracted which in fact are merely over-inflated saline implants. In particular, over-filled high profile saline implants can quickly adopt a very spherical shape and feel quite firm, which can be indistinguishable from a Grade III contracture on physical examination. The McGhan Style 468 implant was designed with published fill volumes that were themselves adequate, and so the implant was not intended to be overfilled. If overfilled, this implant also became particularly hard, mimicking a contracture. One may not be able to discern this until the capsule is exposed at surgery, and though the surgeon may still choose to do a capsulectomy, in fact any improvement in shape or feel may be due less to the removal of the capsule than converting to an implant that is itself less spherical and less firm.

One must also be aware that a capsular contracture can act somewhat like an internal bra, pulling the breast tissue up and in, concealing a true state of ptosis. Many a dissatisfied high, hard, and round contracted patient has been converted to a much more dissatisfied low, soft, droopy and even rippled patient after satisfactory correction of the contracture, but with reveal of the previously occult ptosis. It is impossible to describe exactly the patient in whom this is a risk, but it is most commonly noticed in patients in their 50s or older who have lactated, lost weight, and have sun damage or striae on their breast skin. Whether or not this is the case, and the extent to which a patient might droop after the capsulectomy is too unpredictable for one to choose to do a mastopexy at the time of capsulectomy, as well as the fact that it may be hazardous to the blood supply of the breast.

In assessing the patient for improvement in capsular contracture, one must look to see what can be done differently than the last operation that led to a capsular contracture; if plan A failed, make sure that plan B is different than plan A. In order to improve capsular contracture, each of the following must be considered: bloodlessness and overall skill set of initial surgeon; use of antibiotic irrigation; textured vs smooth implants; premuscular vs retromuscular; periareolar vs

IM or TA incisions; history of infection in the breast; whether previous implants are or are not either saline or low-bleed silicone implants with a barrier shell; if it is a tertiary, whether previous capsule was given a complete capsulectomy and drained. If every one of these things was executed in the previous surgery, and the surgeon has nothing different to offer, the patient should be advised that they should either live with the implant as it is, or to be explanted without reimplantation. Patients and surgeons should be loathe to embark on a revision for capsular contracture if there is no room to do something different than has been done before.

Treatment

The workhorse treatment for capsular contracture is the complete capsulectomy. Since a substantial body of evidence suggests an infectious etiology to contracture, a capsulotomy, which leaves capsule behind, should not be viewed as a definitive treatment for capsular contracture. Capsulotomy should not be viewed as a definitive treatment for capsular contracture; it is best reserved for opening up areas of either closed off or underdissected pocket that are preventing an implant from occupying its intended position.

Capsulectomy for capsular contracture should be done as bloodlessly as possible, and the new implant should not be placed until fastidious electrocautery hemostasis and antibiotic irrigation has been completed. The superolateral portion of the capsulectomy almost always tends to be the most difficult to dissect with excellent hemostasis, owing probably to a combination of reduced visibility in that area and an abundance of muscle perforators. One must avoid the temptation to use excessive distracting forces on the capsule at this point which can result in tearing of blood vessels which stain tissues with blood, leading to a difficulty in visualizing the vessels, as well as increased post-operative pain and potentially inflammation that can lead to a recurrence of the capsular contracture.

The pocket should be thoroughly washed of all debris with antibiotic solution, and the antibiotic solution should be allowed to sit within the breast in an attempt to sterilize it. If there is any fluid observed around the implant, it should be sent for culture for aerobes, anaerobes, acid fast and fungi, with instructions to hold the culture for at least 3 weeks and con-

sider plating on enriched media if there are PMNs on the Gram stain or the surgeon has a suspicion that there may have been a contamination, perhaps owing to a slightly inflamed capsule, or the quantity or color of fluid. If cloudy fluid is found, the surgeon should consider not placing any implant. All implants carry labeling that restricts them to single-use. An implant that develops a capsular contracture should therefore not be reused, even in the same patient. Furthermore, since bacterial contamination is a possible etiology, it would be illogical to use the same prosthesis again. And the shell may have been weakened from the contracture or trauma at the time of the initial surgery, and it makes sense to use the opportunity of having a patient asleep with the capsule opened to start afresh with a new device. This has always sounded inherently logical to me, but I continue to see patients who had their implants removed and the same ones replaced in the setting of capsular contracture.

Retropectoral capsulectomy

If the previous implant was already retromuscular, one must be very cautious dissecting the posterior wall of the capsule. The posterolateral wall usually can be dissected easily, owing to the pectoralis minor and serratus muscles, which are deep to it. This creates an easy plane of dissection in which there is not a lot of adherence, as well as being a layer of protection over the rib cage. The inferomedial portion is usually the most adherent to the chest wall, unless the capsule itself is extremely thick or calcified. While a pneumothorax is a risk even with the most carefully executed capsulectomy, the surgeon should remind him or herself that no additional removal of capsule warrants increasing the risk of pneumothorax. In the case that safety requires a subtotal capsulectomy, then the remaining capsule should be desiccated with a cautery in an effort to maximally sterilize it. When dissecting over the anterior wall of the capsule, one usually finds that the dissection becomes more difficult when one dissects deep to the muscle, as often the capsule seems to thin or becomes more adherent to the muscle than it had been to the parenchyma inferior to the caudal free edge of the muscle. That muscle coverage may be very important to that patient, so one must use great caution in preserving all the muscle fibers possible, taking pride in submitting a specimen to the pathologist as free from muscle as possible.

Neoretropectoral pocket

Another option to consider with submuscular capsules is to do a neoretropectoral pocket dissection. By dissecting behind the muscle and in front of the anterior wall of the pocket capsule, the implant does not come into contact with the interior of the old capsule, and has fresh tissue around it. I have done this when the capsule is restrictive enough that I want to create a new space, but where the dissection of the posterior wall off of the chest would not be technically feasible without entailing risk of damage to intercostal muscles, or when the capsule is too intimately associated with the ribs to actually be removed from them. This has also proved valuable in the uncommon but hardly rare situation of a capsular contracture in a medially, laterally, or inferiorly malpositioned implant. If a complete capsulectomy is done in such patients, there is often little tissue left behind of sufficient durability to hold capsulorrhaphy sutures. But the neoretropectoral pocket allows for both the creation of a new space for the implant that is perhaps less contaminated with bacteria than the old pocket, as well as closing off the previous malpositioned space.

Submammary capsulectomy

Subglandular capsulectomies tend to be much easier, perhaps because these capsules often seem thicker, but more importantly because their anterior wall does not need to be freed from adherence to the deep surface of the pectoralis and the posterior wall is protected from the intercostal musles by the pectoralis, allowing an easier and safer plane of dissection; the posterior wall of a subglandular capsule is rarely as adherent to the superficial surface of the pectoralis as is the anterior wall of a submuscular capsule to the deep surface of the pectoralis. Again, one must avoid resecting muscle fibers along with the posterior wall, and surgeons should pride themselves on avoiding as much muscle as possible with the specimen.

If the contractures occurred with subglandular pockets, the patient should be urged to consider retromuscular pockets. One must be aware when converting from subglandular to submuscular pockets, there is no overlying parenchyma attached to the muscle that can hold the caudal edge of the muscle inferiorly. Particularly if the pectoralis is released along the inframammary fold, which often is necessary, the pectoralis can window-shade high superiorly, often reducing the

extent of muscle coverage to a small superomedial area. If the lower pole of the breast is stretched, one can do all of this and find the patient with the muscle completely above the implant. Since the attachments along the inferomedial fold are critical to holding the muscle down, one must be more judicious about dividing them than in a primary augmentation, discussing with the patient possible implications for a high-riding implant or greater animation deformity. In particular, there must be no separation of any pectoralis fibers off of the sternum in this situation. Even the smallest division of pectoralis off of the sternum can permit excessive cranial malposition of the caudal border of the pectoralis. One must also consider marionette sutures to hold down the muscle as described by Spear, tacking the muscle up to the overlying parenchyma to maintain coverage, or using Alloderm®, Strattice™, or another tissue matrix, as an extension of the caudal edge of the muscle to be sewn along the inframammary fold, thereby preventing excessive window shading of the muscle and maintenance of optimal muscle coverage of the lower pole of the breast.

The role of devices

New devices may themselves offer some improvement in reduction of capsular contracture. Saline and low-bleed silicone with barrier shell technology seem to have roughly similar contracture rates, below those of earlier-generation silicone gel technology. The lowest rates have been shown with the highly cohesive form stable implants, but no direct comparison in similar groups has been done between them and responsive silicone. Surface texturing may offer some advantage over smooth-surfaced implants, perhaps most significantly if the implant is placed in the submammary position. So long as the issue of texturing remains unresolved, the option of placing a textured implant should probably be at least discussed with any patient having an operation for capsular contracture.

Pharmacologic agents

Much has been made of montelukast and zafirlukast, but as of this date, there is not enough conclusive data to suggest what would be an off-label use of these agents for this use, particularly in light of significant risks associated with them. However, for the properly informed and consented patient who wishes to try everything without surgery, these may still be reasonable management options. While the risks are uncommon, they are very severe. Even their advocates suggest their use in early capsules only; the treatment for an established capsule is surgery.

Incision choice

Periareolar incisions usually require transecting the breast parenchyma, which contains the same bacteria that have been implicated in capsular contracture. Many patients with previous PA incisions refuse IM incisions, and the possible trade-off in avoiding bacterial contamination should be discussed with them. The evidence is not compelling enough at this point to make PA incision at all unacceptable, but theoretical considerations are sufficient for patients to be suggested to consider the IM incision, particularly if they have been plagued with severe or recurring capsular contractures.

Antibiotic solution

I use Adams formula whenever performing breast augmentation (50 mL povidone iodine, 1 g cefazolin, 80 mg gentamicin in 500 mL physiologic saline). FDA product labeling restricts povidone iodine contact with implants, so patients sign an off-label consent. The data clearly shows this solution to be extremely powerful in reducing capsular contracture. For the surgeon who does not want to use povidone iodine, 50,000 units of bacitracin can be used as a substitute. Either solution should be used liberally for irrigation throughout the operation.

Drains

Most surgeons suggest draining even the driest capsulectomy, as a significant amount of serous fluid can accumulate in these cases. If nothing else, removal of this fluid makes patients comfortable by limiting the swelling they have, but it stands to reason that removal of blood and debris around the implant may help in reducing contracture in patients who are likely to ooze following a capsulectomy.

Sterility

Capsular contracture is the end result of inflammation. There are many causes of inflammation, but there are several we can reduce. Probably the most potent source is low-grade bacterial contamination. Blood, debris, and unnecessarily traumatic technique all contribute to inflammation. All implant surgery must be done with this in focus in the surgeon's mind.

Scoring
1. Severely distorting or painful contracture.
2. Moderately distorting contracture.
3. No clinically significant contracture.

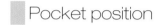

Pocket position

It is of course impossible to know exactly the position of a pocket by observing a patient externally. This division puts into one category all causes of implant malposition. Since an implant sits wherever the pocket is, implant malpositions can best be thought of as pocket malpositions. Implants can be malpositioned inferiorly, superiorly, medially, or laterally.

Medial malposition

A mild medial malposition can be seen as one implant sitting closer to the midline than the other. In the most severe case, the implant can cross the midline and the presternal skin can be lifted off of the sternum, creating symmastia or the so-called 'uniboob' deformity. This is often associated with an inferior malposition. Medial malpositions almost never occur passively; they usually are the result of excessive medial dissection, with the notable exception of patients with pectus excavatum, the angle of whose chest wall allows gravity when the patient is supine to cause excessive medial migration of the implant.

Inferior malposition

Inferior malpositions are frequently referred to as 'bottoming out,' though for clarity I prefer to use the term 'bottoming out' to describe lower pole stretch deformities as characterized by an increased N:IMF distance with appropriate fold position. This can coexist with inferior implant malposition or can exist alone. However, many surgeons use 'bottoming out' to describe inferior malposition, and there is no standardized nomenclature with which to set the record straight. It may be the result of improper determination of the inframammary fold, or of the implant lowering beneath the intended fold. No matter the terminology used by the surgeons, the approach to treatment and expectations for correction are different between N:IMF stretch problems and an inferiorly displaced IMF.

Superior malposition

Superior malpositions are of several types. Capsular contracture itself frequently causes the contracted implant to displace superiorly, resulting in an inadequate fill of the lower pole of the breast and a prominent upper bulge. Failure to adequately dissect the lower pocket can also result in a superior malposition. One of the frequent causes of this is failure to accurately take down the pectoralis along the inframammary fold. Though this can happen with any incision, it seems to happen frequently with the transaxillary incision, particularly if it is done blunt and blind. The triad of upper bulge, animation deformity, and high inframammary fold is almost pathognomonic for a transaxillary augmentation with imprecise release of the inframammary fold.

Another cause of superior malposition is failure to lower the inframammary fold appropriately for the size of the implant that was placed. But it is possible for even the most perfectly dissected pocket to fill with fluid in the early post operative stage and close itself off. There is a dead space at the bottom of every pocket, and it can close off, causing a 1-1.5 cm superior displacement of the implant. A tight or misplaced bra may contribute to this problem. Constricted lower poles that were not properly expanded at the first operation by dual or subglandular plane positioning with parenchymal scoring can result in inadequate lower pole expansion and fill, resulting in what appears to be a high-riding implant. Finally, one must remember that a breast fills from the bottom up. Any device that is too large for the breast envelope or is too large relative to the N:IMF, will appear high riding for that breast. Whenever assessing a breast bulge for its cause, whether intraoperatively or in the examination room, always look for underdissection at the area of the bulge or at 180 degrees from the bulge. Finally, while excessive medial, lateral, and inferior pocket malpositions are treated by closing the pocket in that dimension, true superior malpositions do not require closure of any excess superior dissection. So long as the N:IMF distance is long enough for the chosen implant, the device will fall inferiorly to lay in its proper position.

Lateral malposition

Lateral malpositions can be the result of dissecting an excessively wide pocket, but it can happen passively over time due to the shape of the chest wall. For this reason, lateral dissection in primary augmentation should never proceed lateral to the lateral border of the pectoralis minor. Far too often, surgeons dissect to the lateral border of the breast. Dissecting to the lateral border of a 14-15 cm wide breast makes an excessive lateral pocket almost every time. Other than a symmastia patient, no patient ever complains of too much cleavage, and even small incremental increases in lateral dissection at the primary augmentation can result in significant lateralization with time. For this reason, patients will frequently describe this problem as increasing over time. It is often associated with somewhat of a barrel- or pectus-carinatum-like shape to the chest, in which the sternum is far anterior to the anterior axillary line, creating a steep slope along which the implant falls laterally when the patient is supine, stretching the lateral tissues and even gradually enlarging the pocket laterally. Patients must be reminded that their implants do not sit on a flat surface; in fact, for all patients, but to varying extents, when they lie on their back. The two sides of their chest are like the roof of a house. The natural tendency is for the implants to fall to the sides when they are supine, and even to some extent when they are upright.

Some patients with implants complain that when they lie supine, their implants do not fall laterally in the same way as do natural breasts. Yet, other patients with implants that do fall laterally complain that their breasts do not maintain anterior projection when they are supine. Much of this is due to the shape of their chest, and patients in both camps need to be counseled as to the reality of their situation.

Treatment

Start by marking where the pocket should be. I usually start by determining the ideal N:IMF distance for that breast width, and then draw over the breast were I want the borders of the implant pocket to be. There may be zones where the new pocket extends beyond the existing pocket, and there may be areas in which the existing pocket extends beyond where the new pocket should be. So there will be areas where you will want to close off the pocket, and perhaps others where you will want to open the pocket. Opening the pocket is the easiest, as it usually only requires a capsulotomy. Closing off an area of undesired pocket is more difficult, and this requires either a capsulorraphya site change, or creation of a neosubpectoral pocket. Releasing the capsule often in and of itself often allows more pocket to open up than one might anticipate. After the capsule is incised, try placing a sizer before dissecting, as there is frequently enough stretch for the pocket to open adequately without significant dissection.

Capsulorraphy

The capsulorraphy is the gold standard for reduction of one or more dimensions of the pocket. External markings of the desired extent of the pockets are transposed to the anterior wall of the capsule by using angiocatheters along the proposed borders of the pocket. A cautery device is used to mark each of the sites of the angiocatheter and then to connect them into a smooth curve. This line is then transposed onto the chest wall. Depending upon the quality of the tissues and the amount of space to be eliminated, the area to be obliterated can be sewn to itself or a capsulectomy of the proposed area of the pocket to be closed off can be resected, with a running permanent suture placed along the entirety of the new pocket. A capsulorraphy can provide excellent results, but so too can it be tedious, requiring the suturing of thin tissues, particularly inferiomedially along the chest wall. Sutures often need to be placed, removed, and repositioned. One must be careful when transposing the marks on the inside of the anterior wall of the capsule to the chest wall, as there is a tendency to transpose these marks superiorly, resulting in superior implant displacement. There can be early irregularities and over correction following a capsulorraphy.

Neoretropectoral pocket

The neoretroepectoral pocket was original described by Heden as a means to reduce the dimensions of a submuscular pocket to fit an anatomically shaped implant in order to reducet he likelihood of rotation in a secondary augmentation. Spear and Maxwell have popularized the use of this procedure for reduction of enlarged pockets in difficult secondary augmentation situations.

This procedure works when the implant is already subpectoral, the space is over-dissected in one or more dimensions, and the surgeon wishes to remain in the subpectoral position.

The operation starts with marking of the proposed new borders of the pocket. Dissection starts along the anterior surface of the implant, much the same as one might begin a capsulectomy. However, in this case, dissection stops when the surgeon reaches the preoperative markings. The pocket is therefore only as large as the surgeon wishes it to be, and the limits of it are limited by the dense fusion between the capsule and overlying breast. The implant is removed, the anterior wall is tacked to the posterior wall and everal small capsulotomies are made in the now collapsed anterior wall to prevent accumulation of fluid in the old pocket.

This powerful tool works wonders for medial, inferior, and lateral implant malposition. The advantage over capsulorraphy is the speed and ease of dissection, the avoidance of the need to place multiple sutures into areas of often weakened tissues, and what appears to be a smoother and more accurate pocket border. Perhaps because of the absence of multiple sutures, these patients also seem to have less pain than capsulorraphy patients. It deserves emphasis that most patients with inferior, medial, or lateral malpositions have a thin and non-restrictive capsule. It is often difficult to perform a capsulectomy on such thin capsules, and such capsules, particularly posteriorly, are often too thin to provide the surgeon confidence that their capsulorraphy sutures will hold. In contrast, with the neosubpectoral pocket, it is the "lamination" of the capsule to the breast that determines the limits of the pocket.

Neosubglandular pocket

If there is an enlarged pocket in the subglandular position, the surgeon would typically make a submuscular pocket. But if there is some reason that it is elected not to do this, then a neosubglandular pocket can be made.

This follows the same principles as the neosubpectoral pocket, except that in this case the new pocket is between breast and anterior wall of capsule, rather than between muscle and anterior wall of capsule.

Site change

The easiest way to deal with a pocket malposition is to create a new space, e.g. converting from submamary to dual plane or dual plane to submammary. But oftentimes there was good reason to have initially made a submuscular pocket, and if the surgeon wishes to preserve that pocket location, then a capsulorraphy or neosubpectoral pocket must be done. More frequently, there is less reason to maintain a submammary pocket, and conversion to a dual plane pocket can help correct pocket malpositions. One should be reminded, however, that there is no muscle at the lateral border, so conversion of submammary to submuscular, or submusuclar to submammary, will not in and of itself correct lateral pocket malposition. In the case of inferior malposition, one must be careful when converting from submammary to submuscular what is done with the origins of the pectoralis along the inframammary fold. These precious fibers are what will hold up the implant, and they typically should not be divided in this situation.

Scoring

1   Significant deformity from implant malposition.
2   Moderate deformity from implant malposition.
3   No deformity from implant malposition.

 Device

This is listed as the final cause of revisions as PMA studies consistently demonstrate similar rates of revision surgery across various implant types. If clinical trials of quite different devices yield similar revision rates, then the causes of the revisions have more to do with surgeons' processes and patient's expectations than it does with the devices themselves. Just by the statistics, soft tissue coverage, skin stretch, implant malposition, and capsular contracture are far more common causes of secondary breast surgery, and addressing them at the time of revision surgery is far more important than device changes. It is important for surgeons, patients, and manufacturers to distinguish problems that are caused and solved by the device as opposed to other factors.

But since we are talking about revision of breast implant surgery, there is understandably significant focus on the breast implant itself. While frequently there are issues related to the breast implant, and sometimes the breast implant itself can be the driving force for the operation, the surgeon should think about optimizing all of the other factors in every revision

case. No device change should ever be relied upon to fix an unsolved problem in any of these other arenas.

Scope of device-related issues

Size

Revision for size is the most frequent device related issue reported in clinical trials. Fortunately, this is a problem that is easily solved, if, at the time of the first operation, patients are made to understand that the goal of the operation is to fill their breast envelope rather than to achieve an arbitrary size determined by their whims, then operation for size exchange will always be inherently illogical.

If sizing at the time of the original surgery was based upon subjective criteria only, e.g. 'how big do you want to be?' then that patient has been set-up to reconsider her size repeatedly in the future. When a prospective primary augmentation patient is taught to ask for and expect whatever size she wants, then she thinks that size selection is arbitrary, and that all sizes are possible. If dissatisfied with her size later, she can always blame herself or her surgeon for her size, and reconsideration of her size choice is a matter that is always on the table for her.

Any sizing method that requires a patient to make a choice based upon her wishes rather than her tissues requires her to second guess her later choice. Any sizing method that relies upon the surgeon's intraoperative impression of what most fulfills his or her understanding of the patient's wishes rather than her tissues, further extends the concept that sizing is subjective, which opens the door for future reconsideration of the initial size choice. Parenthetically, intraoperative sizing risks putting responsibility for the implant size on the shoulders of the surgeon, risking that the patient blames the surgeon for her final size.

If a patient is taught that there is an ideal implant size for each breast, and if she selects that size, then theoretically reoperation for size exchange should never happen. Prospective patients do understand the concept that there is a limited range of volume that can be accommodated in their breasts, and that a smaller volume results in an empty upper pole, and that a larger volume results in a bulging upper pole, an unnatural look, and more parenchymal atrophy and skin stretch with time. When patients understand and sign off on this at the time of the primary operation, they rarely will request either a downsize or an upsize at a later time. In reality, however, few patients are taught this or understand this at the time of the first operation, so the surgeon performing secondary augmentation will frequently see patients requesting size changes who did not understand these issues prior to the first surgery. It is the secondary surgeon's role to educate them about these issues.

Unfortunately, there is a pervasive myth that patients always wish that they were larger, and as a result, they are told to request an even larger size than they desired at the first operation. Nothing can be further from the truth. There are many patients distressed that their implants look larger and more fake than they had originally wanted. In fact, feeling self-conscious about size and feeling leered at by others is much more emotionally disconcerting than being happy with enlarged breasts, but merely wishing that they had been enlarged even more.

And the women who wish that they were larger have not suffered any permanent damage to their tissue. But women who were made larger than ideal for their tissues frequently have parenchymal atrophy, skin thinning, concavities in their rib cage, and skin stretch that may not be at all correctable, may require several surgeries, or may require significant mastopexy scars to correct.

Assessing the potential for size change

One of the difficulties is that breast measurements from the time of the first operation rarely can be found; and at times, even records of the implant size are difficult to find. While there are methods to accurately determine ideal implant size at the time of the first operation, there are no such methods described for assessing the appropriateness of size of an implant for a breast that has no preoperative measurements. This is critically important. The secondary operating surgeon must take into consideration the patient's request to be either larger or smaller, and assess the breast for the appropriateness of current fill, and the possible response of the breast to a greater or lesser amount of fill.

The first priority in this matter is tissue coverage. If visually the implant borders are already visible through the skin, then coverage with the current volume is already inadequate; such a patient should be considering a decrease in size, if any change is being considered. If coverage anywhere over the upper pole of the implant is <2 cm and anywhere along the medial border or IMF is <1 cm, the patient should be informed that their tissue coverage is already thin, and that a further increase of implant size would thin this coverage even more.

Next, the degree of fill of the existing breast envelope should be assessed. A concave upper pole would suggest the potential for adding more volume, and a convex upper pole would suggest that the breast envelope is already over-filled. Skin stretch can be measured and documented exactly as in the primary breast augmentation patient. Stretch <1 demonstrates that there is no additional capacity for volume, but stretch >2 does not necessarily mean that there is usable capacity; it might indicate that the skin is damaged and already excessively stretched and without good elasticity. In fact, many breasts with implants already >500 have >2 cm of stretch due to underlying damage to their skin either from pregnancy or weight loss, or from the device itself.

One of the most critical measurements is N:IMF. A frequent complaint of patients asking to go bigger is not size per se, but wanting to achieve more upper pole fill. A larger implant is rarely the proper means for creating more upper fill. The breast fills from the bottom up, so even a slightly increased N:IMF distance creates a volume capacity in the lower breast which can steal volume that otherwise would have filled the upper breast. Using the ratios already mentioned (7,8,9 : 200,300,400), if a long N:IMF is encountered, the solution should be shortening it rather than increasing volume. In some cases this may be due to an inferiorly malpositioned IMF necessitating superior pocket repositioning, or it may be stretch of lower pole skin, which requires a mastopexy. Though the theoretically correct fix for such a problem, the skin of a patient that has once stretched enough to require a mastopexy is at significant risk for restretching following the procedure. The extent to which the skin will restretch is difficult to predict, but the patient considering mastopexy in this situation must be told that upper pole fill cannot be guaranteed as the skin may stretch again to an unpredictable extent.

Patient wishing to go larger

If we have the records and realize that the patient was properly sized, then the patient requesting to go larger should be counseled about the effects such a choice might have on her tissue. Sometimes, however, a patient chose to go smaller than was calculated as ideal for her tissue for fear of being too large; this is the one situation in which going larger is indeed appropriate. Unfortunately, the most frequent request for going larger seems to be from patients who have already gone too large for their tissues, and their goal is often not just size per se, but filling up their ever-increasingly stretched skin envelope. Such patients are on a slippery slope, not unlike the pattern we have all experienced when we pushed a sweater up our forearm and the elastic of the wrist gave out; we push it progressively higher and it stays tight for a short time, but ultimately we keep pushing it up higher and higher, until it is above our elbows and unwearable.

Some surgeons argue that they will only do a size exchange if it is for a change of more than a certain amount of volume, arguing that a small change isn't worth the surgical risk. Others argue that it is more logical to make the least change possible to an implant that is already appropriately sized. While it may not seem worth the risk and expense to add 30 or 50 mL to a breast, that may actually be more logical than adding 100 mL or more to an already full breast, increasing all the tissue trade-offs already discussed. In either case, this relatively simple decision can be one of the most difficult ones in all of secondary breast augmentation surgery. A large number of these patients seem unhappy following revision surgery to increase their implant size: if they do not see a big change, many patients are happy. If they do see a big change, with time tissue consequences increase. Careful documentation of all discussions and decisions must be made, and the surgeon should only proceed after being convinced that the patient understands the consequences of the untended plan.

Patient wishing to go smaller

Years after their augmentation, there are many patients who wish to go smaller. Some say that they were always larger than they wanted to be; others say that while the size was appropriate for them at a younger age, at this point it seems too large. Unlike size exchange to go larger, this carries with it no specific new adverse soft tissue consequences, other than perhaps revealing stretch deformities that were masked by the fill of the larger implant. It is difficult to predict who will and will not need a lift following exchange with a smaller implant, but it is a subject that should be discussed. The only drawback is less upper pole fill and a greater degree of emptiness. Patients often ask whether they will droop, and once again the N:IMF distance is the

most accurate predictor of this phenomenon. If the N:IMF is longer than ideal for the new implant size, the surgeon should consider whether it is due to an inferiorly displaced inframammary fold, or if it is due to a stretched lower pole, and deal with those issues accordingly. Sometimes a patient requests to go smaller not so much because of volume per se, but because of the breast having too much upper bulging. In such a situation, evaluation of the N:IMF should be evaluated to see if it is short, and the origins of the pectoralis along the medial inframammary fold should be evaluated to see if they are intact. If the N:IMF is proportional for the current implant, and the patient is going smaller, one should consider raising the IMF to suit the smaller implant in order to create a proportional breast. For instance, the BW 11 breast that was overaugmented to 400 mL and is now being properly sized down to a volume of 250 mL may need the N:IMF reduced to 7.5 cm, from what might be as much as 9 cm. Failure to do so will result in excessive lower pole fill and perhaps an upturned nipple–areola complex.

There are many patients in this category who are good candidates for implant removal without replacement. Sometimes a patient had a proportionally sized implant and has gained weight over time Sometimes tissue pinch of >5 cm is easily palpable around the entire periphery of the implant, and such a patient may want to be substantially smaller. Frequently, in order to make the patient's breasts the size they want, the device size becomes so small that it makes sense just to be explanted. If an implant is very small relative to the overall size of the breast, then it will do little to augment it. What's more, the dimensions of such an implant would render it to sit down in the lower pole of the breast, contributing to a perception of ptosis and adding nothing to upper pole fill.

Severe rippling

If a hypothetical patient had adequate soft tissue coverage over a small bag of pebbles, the 'implant' would still be non-visible and non-palpable. Put in more common terms, a large implant with thin coverage will frequently yield problems of some sort, while a small implant with substantial coverage will almost always be relatively undetectable. While the device gets blamed for rippling problems, the problem is far more often an inadequacy of soft tissue coverage. Patients and surgeons alike believe that a device will solve these problems. While it is true that some devices have this tendency less than others, no device can solve the problem of inadequate soft tissue coverage, and it is important that the surgeon sets this expectation with the patient.

The first priority in the patient with rippling is to assess the thickness of the parenchyma as described in the first section. Only after every effort to improve coverage has been made, and a plan to maximize tissue coverage has been discussed, should the patient and surgeon look to the implant as the possible solution to the problem. When saline implants (except the McGhan Style 468) were filled to manufacturer's recommended fill-volumes, they were invariably underfilled and rippled. Overfilling beyond that risked voiding warranties and made implants increasingly firm in feel and round in appearance. If filled further still, they developed stippling or scalloping around their periphery. While the minimal added thickness of the textured shell should theoretically not contribute significantly to rippling, in clinical experience the presence of texturing seems to make rippling more pronounced. This was rarely seen with the McGhan Style 468, probably because this implant was properly filled (though it is consequentially firmer than the typically underfilled round saline implant, whether smooth or textured). Perhaps the texturing makes the shell a bit less pliable, making the fold a little stiffer with less of a tendency to dissipate with gentle pressure. Even silicone implants can ripple, as almost all silicone implants that have been made are still underfilled relative to mandrel volume. Like saline implants, this phenomenon seems more notable with textured implants.

The profile of a round implant may also make a device more or less prone to rippling. Many feel that higher profile implants tend to ripple less, but this has never been demonstrated. But it is logical that since a higher profile implant has less shell surface area relative to volume, it would have less of a tendency to collapse and therefore fold. Or the phenomenon may be related to the fact that lower profile implants are often selected that are wider than the pocket will be, mandating that the wider implant fold on itself in order to fit within the pocket. It should also be pointed out that some degree of folding can always be expected on gentle palpation along the inframammary fold, particularly when tissue pinch is <1 cm. Inferolateral rippling palpable when the patient bends over should even be considered a normal phenomenon, as there is

no pectoralis with which to cover the implant in this area and the tissue tends to stretch and thin in this area with time.

Solution

The solution for implant folding is first to optimize the soft tissue coverage. Second, the envelope needs to be considered, as an implant unconfined by a loose envelope will tend to fold on itself more than it would with the same degree of coverage in a tighter envelope. In such a situation, mastopexy should be considered. Finally, consideration should be made of the implant that will best be suited for the situation. In order, the implant that has the greatest tendency to fold to the least tendency to fold would be textured saline (other than 468), smooth saline, textured gel, smooth gel, and finally highly cohesive form stable gel would be the least likely to fold. Many patients and surgeons believe that the cohesive implant is the quick fix for these situations, and it is not. The shaped form stable devices are at particular risk for rotation in a revision. These risks can be reduced if a new pocket is made that will be tight around the implant, but this often cannot be achieved. And round form stable devices will indeed look quite round. This may be an acceptable trade-off in these situations, but this needs to be understood ahead of time.

Rupture

We tell all patients that no device is a lifetime device, presupposing that all are destined to ultimately fail. In fact, we do not know whether this is true, as changes to the soft tissues or patient desire for replacement with a new implant prior to actual failure of the previous implant makes truly long term studies impossible to ever complete. With saline implants, the rupture is usually obvious, with one breast decreasing in size in a matter of days or weeks. With silicone implants, rupture can be diagnosed because the patient develops swelling, distortion, or newly developing capsular contracture (though there are other causes of this). Or rupture can be presumptively diagnosed by radiological imaging studies.

Scoring
1 Significant device-related deformity.
2 Moderate device-related deformity.
3 No device-related deformity.

Results

Case 1

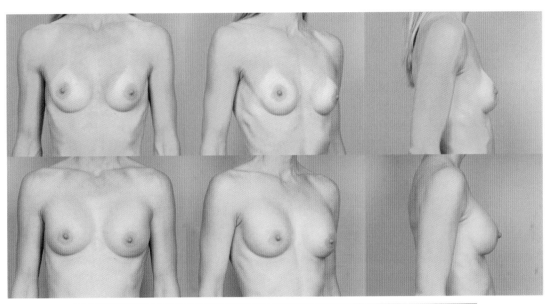

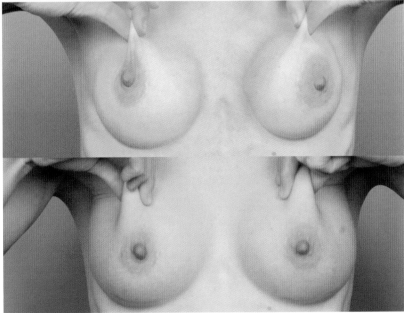

Figure 8.1   A patient demonstrates skin pinch of upper pole of breast to determine the soft tissue coverage. This patient demonstrates the inadequacy of her submammary coverage. This woman is shown four years after a subglandular augmentation with a high profile implant. While at first she appears to have a capsular contracture, she actually just has very thin tissue. Her preoperative score was 12, with 1 for parenchyma/tissue coverage, 3 for skin envelope, 3 for capsule, 3 for pocket position, and 2 for device. Following change to dual plane to offer more coverage and to a wider and taller full height anatomic form stable implant, her score increased to a 14, with 1 point still lost for tissue coverage.

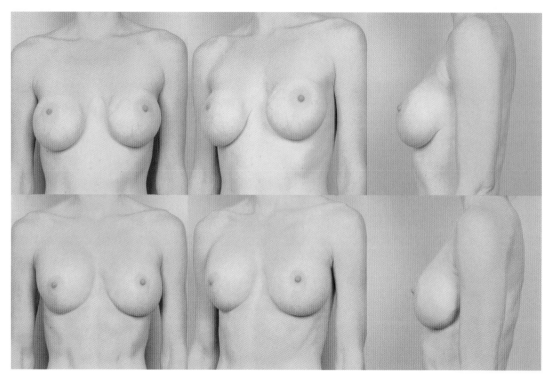

Figure 8.2 This multiparous woman is seen 2 years after an augmentation. She complained of her implants being too large, visible, fake, and droopy. She was advised to get a mastopexy at the time of her first procedure, but she did not want the scars. Her pre-operative score was 9, with 1 for parenchyma/tissue coverage, 1 for envelope, 3 for capsule, 2 for pocket position, and 2 for device. After conversion to dual plane, a mastopexy, and switching from saline to silicone, her score became 13 , with 2 for parenchyma/ tissue coverage, 2 for envelope, 3 for capsule, 3 for pocket position, and 3 for device. While her tissue coverage is better dual plane and the envelope is better after skin reduction, neither can become a 3.

Case **3**

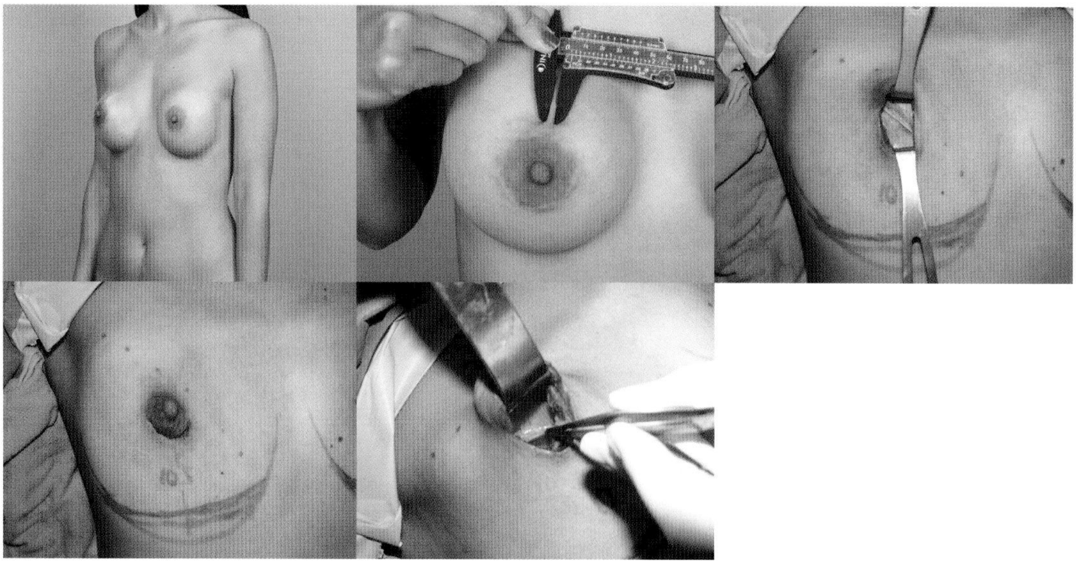

Figure 8.3 This patient said that her high profile saline implants are behind the muscle. If so, why is so much rippling visible in (A)? Why is so little coverage in (B)? Examine the caudal edge of the muscle in (C): it is retracted beyond the upper border of the areola, more than a Dual Plane Type III as shown by the dotted lines in (D) marking the course of the muscle. And given her long N:IMF distance, little if any of the implant was behind the muscle. In fact, one can see in (E) that there is capsule both in front and behind the cephalad migrated edge of muscle, such that this patient never benefited from true muscle coverage.

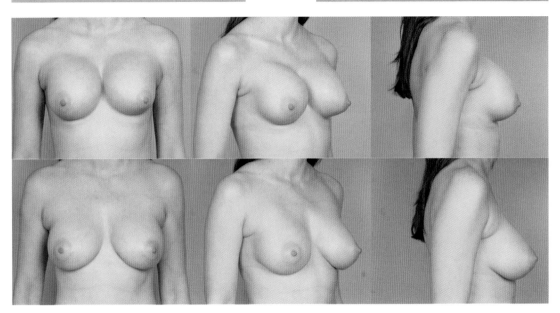

Figure 8.4 This patient felt too big, hard, fake, and uneven. Her implants were too large, and her pockets were medially malpositioned and the right was inferiorly malpositioned. Her pre-operative score was 12 with 3 for parenchyma/tissue coverage, 3 for skin envelope, 3 for capsule, 1 for pocket position, and 2 for device (because of size.) A neosubpectoral pocket succeeded in placing the implants in proper position, raising and lateralizing each pocket such that her score went to 3 for pocket position. Placing in a smaller implant raised her device score to a 3. Through all examples in this chapter, note that so long as there is good parenchyma and skin envelope scores, the result is usually beautiful. Nothing within control of today's surgeon can obviate significant deficiencies in parenchyma/tissue coverage and skin envelope.

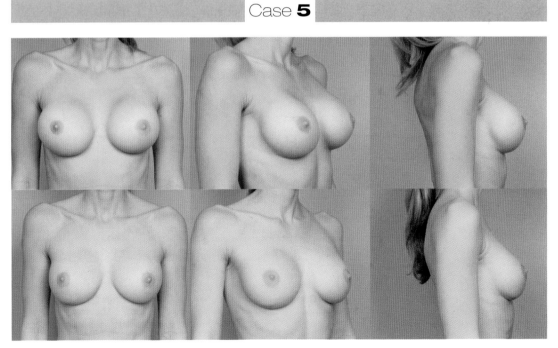

Figure 8.5 This woman complained of being too fake, too large, and not having a pretty shape after placement of subglandular saline implants. Her preoperative score was 12, with 2 for parenchyma/tissue coverage, 3 for skin envelope, 3 for capsule, 2 for pocket position, and 2 for device. After conversion to dual plane and a smaller silicone implant, her score went to a 15, with 3s for all categories.

Case **6**

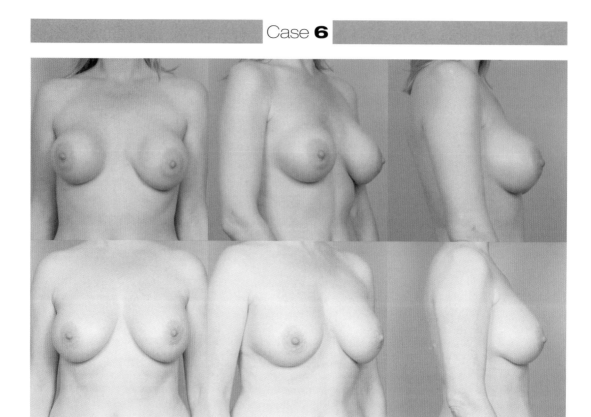

Figure 8.6 Classical appearance of a subglandular capsular contracture: round, firm, and visible implant edges. Her preoperative score was 13, losing 2 points for the capsule. Postoperatively, her score raised to 15 following complete capsulectomy and conversion to dual plaine full height anatomic form st5able implants.

Case **7**

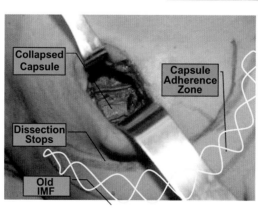

Figure 8.7 This patient had an inferiorly malpositioned infrmammary fold and was corrected with a neosubpectoral pocket. The most caudal blue line is her preoperative inframmary fold; the red line shows where the new inframammary fold was meant to be. Dissection was carried down to the capsule, and a space was developed superficial to the anterior capsule wall, stopping at the new inframmary fold height. The yellow indicates how much higher the new IMF is. Instead of being limited by a capsulorrapy, the dense adherence between the capsule and the overlying parenchyma prevents the implant from falling caudally.

Case **8**

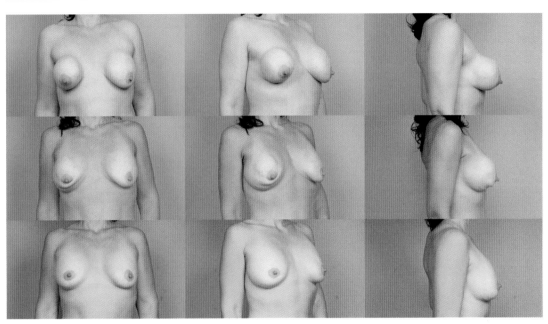

Figure 8.8 This patient had capsular contractures of prepectoral high profile saline implants, along with skin excess, nipple asymmetry, and parenchymal atrophy. She was given a preoperative score of 8, with 1 for parenchyma/tissue coverage, 1 for skin envelope, 1 for capsule, 3 for pocket position, and 2 for device. Her tissue was very thin, so it was felt a single stage mastopexy/capsulectomy would be risky. (All readers are advised to study the landmark paper of Handel listed in the references for a prescient discussion of these issues.) Also, given the asymmetry of her implant sizes, nipple positions, and contractures, it was felt that a two stage procedure would allow for greater accuracy. The top line shows her pre-operatively; the middle line shows her after a premuscular capsulectomy and placement of dual plane silicone implants. Her score rose by 1 for parenchyma/tissue, 2 for capsule, and 1 for device to a score of 11. While the plan was to do a Wise pattern mastopexy, she had sufficient rebound tightening of her skin over the 3 month waiting period for the mastopexy, such that she underwent a periareolar mastopexy. Her skin envelope score raised by 1 to give her a total score of 12; had she undergone a complete mastopexy, she would have had more projection (albeit with more scar), giving her perhaps a higher score for skin envelope. But thin parenchyma precluded her from having a higher score and better result.

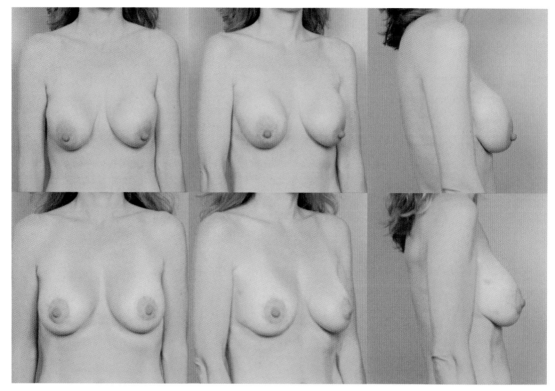

Figure 8.9 This patient has capsular contractures in the subglandular position along with an underlying skin stretch deformity. Her pre-operative score was 9 , with 1 for parenchyma/tissue coverage, 1 for skin envelope, 1 for capsule, 3 for pocket position, and 3 for device. Switching to Dual Plane raised the coverage to just a 2 (her tissue is too thin to qualify for a 3.) The circumareolar lift increased her skin envelope to a 2; a Wise pattern mastopexy may have increased it to a 3, but she preferred the more limited scar, even at the expense of less of a correction of the skin envelope, and the capsule remained soft raising her capsule score to a 3. Her post-operative score was therefore a 13.

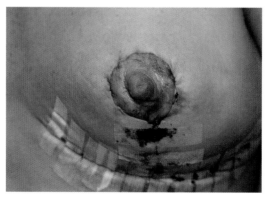

Figure 8.10 The viability of this nipple-areola complex appears threatened in this patient who had a simultaneous capsulectomy and mastopexy. While this can be safely performed in certain circumstances, one should remember that in such patients, the previous implant/capsulectomy has disrupted the blood supply to and from the nipple areola complex beneath the areola, and the skin pattern and undermining further disrupts the remaining blood supply. One must consider the thickness of the parenchyma, the amount of intended undermining, the extent to which the nipple areola complex will be transposed, etc., before deciding whether to attempt this in a single stage.

Case **11**

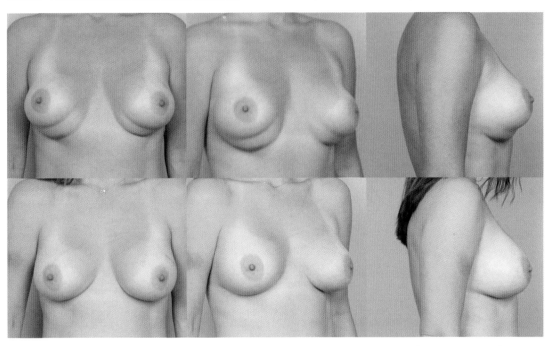

Figure 8.11 The inframammary folds in this patient have been caudally displaced far inferior to her natural inframammary folds. Her pre-operative score was 13, losing 2 points for pocket position. With capsulorraphy to close off the lower portion of the inferiorly malpositioned pocket, her post-operative score rose to 15. This deformity is inferior malposition of the implant; bottoming out is a stretch deformity of the lower pole envelope, increasing N:IMF length with a properly positioned inframammary fold.

Case **12**

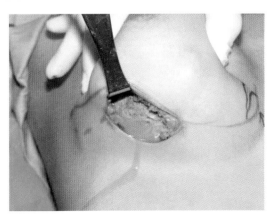

Figure 8.12 While undergoing a capsulectomy, this patient was found to cloudy fluid around her implant. Gram stain revealed multiple PMNs, and a decision was made not to replace an implant. In hindsight, on physical exam preoperatively, her capsule was quite adherent to the surrounding tissue and there was a feeling of bogginess, suggestive of an active, inflammatory process.

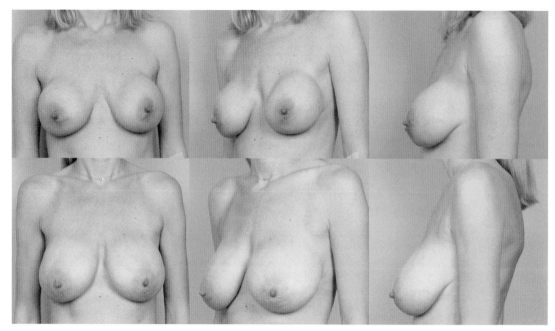

Figure 8.13 This patient had subglandular capsular contractures. But she also had significant skin stretch, though the capsular contractures made it less apparent. Her preoperative score was 10, with a 1 for parenchyma/tissue coverage, a 2 for skin envelope, a 1 for capsule, a 3 for pocket position, and a 3 for device. If she were converted to Dual plane, she would have raised her parenchyma/tissue coverage score, but we were concerned that it would exacerbate her skin envelope laxity. We thus just did a capsulectomy with replacement in the subglandular space. Her score increased by 2 for correction of the capsular contracture, but it dropped 1 point for the rippling and 1 point because the removal of the capsule revealed the extent of the true, underlying skin envelope laxity, which was hidden by the capsule pulling on the breast envelope from the inside. So her pre- and post-operative scores were each a 10. Many unhappy hard and smooth contracted patients have been converted to very unhappy soft and rippled patients. Technically speaking, the problem was capsular contracture, and the operation done this way would have to be deemed a success, with the shortcomings due to the inadequacy of the patient's tissues. Still, anticipating this ahead of time and discussing it with the patient is important.

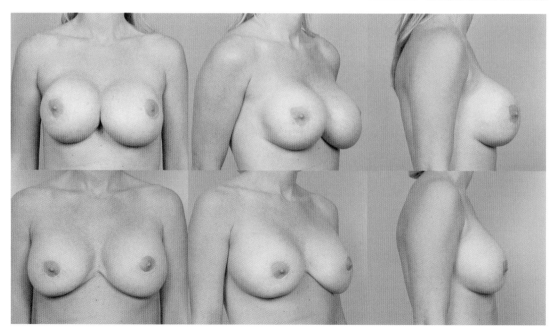

Figure 8.14 This multiparous woman has severe longstanding synmastia with 600 mL partial retropectoral implants. Her preoperative score was 9 with 1 for parenchyma/tissue coverage, 1 for skin envelope, 3 for capsule, 1 for pocket position, and 3 for device. After capsulorraphy and placement of a smaller implant, her score rose just by 2 in the pocket position category, increasing her score to 11. But because her thin tissue coverage was unchanged and she did not want a mastopexy to reduce her skin envelope, her score was not higher than an 11.

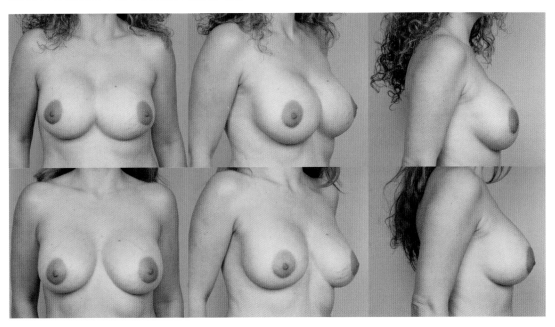

Figure 8.15 This woman also had severe symmastia with a pre-operative score of 12 with 3 for parenchyma/tissue coverage, 3 for skin envelope, 3 for capsule, 1 for pocket position, and 2 for device. After creation of a neosubpectoral pocket and placement of a smaller silicone implant, her score rose to 15. Why does she look so much better than Case 8? Because she has so much more parenchyma and less stretched of a skin envelope. Parenchymal atrophy and skin damage may sometimes be improvable, but they cannot corrected in a fundamental manner.

Case **16**

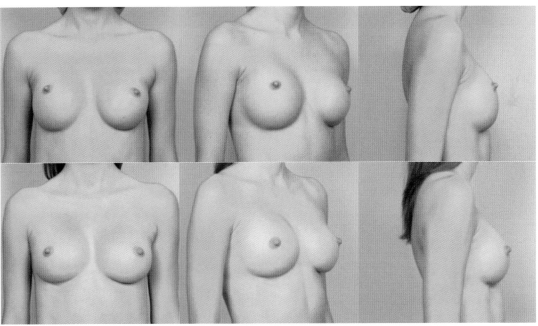

Figure 8.16 This patient had inferiorly displaced inframammary folds, with a N:IMF distance of 13. Her old scar is visible all the way down at 13 cm below the IMF, meaning that if the IMF is placed where it needs to be, her scar would be visible in her upper abdomen. Her preoperative score was 13, losing 2 points for pocket malposition. After correction with a neosubpectoral pocket, her score raised to 15. Note in particular how her low implant made her nipples appear high. But once the implant height was corrected, the nipple position was seen to be correct. A high implant can make nipples look low, and a low implant can make nipples seem high; make sure the implant position is correct before proceeding with a nipple repositioning procedure. In the intraoperative photo, notethe extent of depression of her chest wall from a large, high profile implant. This should serve as a reminder that breast size cannot be increased with impunity; just like Chinese used footbinding to mold bones, so too can excessively sized implants mold the ribcage, creating permanent and uncorrectable deformities. Whenever a surgeon sees a problem such as this, they should consider taking intra-operative photographs to show the patient post-operatively the prevailing circumstances that limited their ability to give a perfect result.

Secondary augmentation

Further reading

Adams Jr WP. The process of breast augmentation: four sequential steps for optimizing outcomes for patients. Plast Reconstr Surg 2008;122:1892–1900.

Adams WP, Bengston, BP, Glicksman CA et al. Decision and management algorithms to address patient and Food and Drug Administration concerns regarding breast augmentation and implants. Plast Reconstr Surg 2004;114:1252–1257.

Adams Jr WP, Rios JL, Smith SJ. Enhancing patient outcomes in aesthetic and reconstructive breast surgery using triple antibiotic breast irrigation: six-year prospective clinical study. Plast Reconstr Surg 2006;118(Suppl 7):46S–52S.

Adams Jr WP, Teitlebaum S, Bengson BP et al. Breast augmentation roundtable. Plast Reconstr Surg 2006;118(Suppl 7):175S–187S.

Handel N. Secondary mastopexy in the augmented patient: a recipe for disaster. Plast Reconstr Surg 2006;118(Suppl 7):152S–163S.

Handel N, Jensen JA. Capsular contracture: results of 3002 patients with aesthetic breast augmentation: Reply. Plast Reconstr Surg 2006;118:1500–1502.

Handel N, Hayden BB, Jervis WH, Maxwell PG. Revisions in breast augmentation. Aesth Surg J 2000;20:141–148.

Maxwell GP, Gabriel A. The neopectoral pocket in revisionary breast surgery. Aesth Surg J 2008;28:463–467.

Spear SL. Reoperations or revisions. Plast Reconstr Surg 2007;119:1943–1944.

Spear SL, Bogue DP, Thomassen JM. synmastia after breast augmentation. Plast Reconstr Surg 2006;118(Suppl 7):168S–171S.

Spear SL, Carter ME, Ganz JC. The correction of capsular contracture by conversion to "dual-plane" positioning: technique and outcomes. Plast Reconstr Surg 2006;118(Suppl 7):103S–113S.

Tebbetts JB. Discussion: breast capsulorrhaphy revisited: a simple technique for complex problems. Plast Reconstr Surg 2005;115:302–303.

Tebbetts JB. Wishes and tissues: a concern about dimensional planning systems that lack volume restrictions and do not prioritize long-term soft-tissue coverage. Plast Reconstr Surg 2006;117:318–320.

Tebbetts JB. Achieving a zero percent reoperation rate at 3 years in a 50-consecutive-case augmentation mammaplasty premarket approval study. Plast Reconstr Surg 2006;118:1453–1457.

Tebbetts JB, Adams WP. Five critical decisions in breast augmentation using five measurements in 5 Minutes: The high five decision support process. Plast Reconstr Surg 2006;118(Suppl 7):35S–45S.

Teitelbaum S. The inframammary approach to breast augmentation. Clin Plast Surg 2009;36:33–43.

Wiener TC. The role of betadine irrigation in breast augmentation. Plast Reconstr Surg 2007;119:12–15.

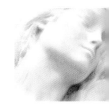

Breast reconstruction and augmentation using pre-expansion and autologous fat transplantation

Roger K. Khouri, Daniel A. Del Vecchio

Key points

- Fat grafting to the breast can be used for aesthetic and reconstructive applications with reliable long-term results.

- Harvest of the fat should be performed in a manner that maximizes survival of the fat grafts in order to reduce the amount of resorption or fat necrosis.

- The recipient site requites preparation and use of the BRAVA should be considered.

- Careful pre-operative and post-operative screening for early detection of breast cancer should be performed and the risk of calcifications caused by fat transfer should be discussed.

- Multicenter prospective trials should be performed in order to document the safety and efficacy of fat transfer to the breast given the baseline risk of breast cancer.

Introduction

This chapter aims to define the current concepts, techniques, outcomes and controversies that surround autologous fat grafting to the breast. Although this is an area of great interest, it must be stressed that we are only beginning to unravel its full potential and limitations. The reader is advised to use the information herein in this spirit.

History of fat grafting to the breast

In 1895 Czerny first described transplanting a lipoma to reconstruct a breast defect (Czerny 1895). In the early part of the 20th century, Lexer openly used resected fat to treat bilateral breast defects (Hinderer & Del Rio 1992). Because of limited success and the significant donor site defect of en bloc fat harvesting, these techniques were not adopted. In 1983, Illouz published his large experience with liposuction confirming our ability to remove fat cells from small port incisions using a cannula connected to vacuum (Illouz 1983). This offered surgeons a new ability to address body contour. The ease of fat removal by liposuction also created an opportunity for its use as an autologous filler. However, because many of the variables important to fat grafting were not well understood, early results were disappointing. At the same time, the silicone breast implant was experiencing rapid growth over its prototype saline counterpart. The popularity of silicone further weakened interest in fat grafting for breast augmentation.

In 1988, Bircoll published his experience with the autologous grafting of liposuctioned fat for breast augmentation (Bircoll 1988). At the same time a series of opinion letters to the editor culminated in the American Society of Plastic Surgeons issuing a position statement questioning the safety of fat grafting to the breast (ASPRS 1987). The statement suggested that fat grafting would compromise breast cancer detection and should be prohibited. Because of this unprecedented strong ban and because early results were neither impressive nor reproducible, the technique was largely abandoned for more than 20 years.

The controversy of silicone breast implants in the United States in the 1990s and the subsequent moratorium on silicone breast implants until 2007 stimulated the potential for autologous tissue as a means of breast augmentation and reconstruction, and certainly this has been an undercurrent supporting the advance of this technique. Recently, there has been a resurgence of interest in fat grafting to the breast. In 2006, at the Annual Meeting of the American Society for Aesthetic Plastic Surgery, Thomas Baker presented a series of 20 patients augmented with liposuctioned fat with 90% graft survival and 180 mL growth documented by serial MRI and 3D volumetric analysis.

None of the women had difficult-to-interpret findings on mammogram (Baker 2006). At the latest update of this series, with over 40 women followed up for at least 6 months and for an average of 30 months, there were still no issues with breast imaging and difficult to interpret masses. The average breast volume augmentation increased to 200 mL, while the percentage survival deceased to 80% (Baker 2008).

In 2007, Coleman published his review of 17 patients who were grafted using autologous fat and were followed up with serial photography (Coleman & Saboeiro 2007). The results were overall successful with maintenance of volume over 7–12 years of follow-up. This publication helped stimulate renewed interest in this technique. Coleman generally used serial grafting sessions instead of injecting larger volumes in a single session in a pre-expanded recipient breast like Baker et al. Following this renewed enthusiasm for the technique and with the realization that the radiographic arguments behind the ASPS-imposed ban may no longer be valid, many surgeons across the world have started publishing their own experiences with fat grafting to the breast (Delay 2006).

General concepts and advances in fat grafting to the breast

There are multiple variables involved in fat grafting, but conceptually, fat grafting is comparable to sowing seeds in a field. To yield a good crop we need: (a) good seeds; (b) a large recipient field with good soil; (c) skilled planting techniques; and (d) optimal post-grafting nurturing of the planted seeds. The significance of these factors becomes even more critical when dealing with mega-volume grafting.

Donor graft ('the seeds')

The quality of the donor fat graft seems to depend upon donor age, donor site, harvesting technique & processing techniques.

Donor age (and therefore recipient age)

Age is thought to be a factor in the success of fat grafting. Animal studies in nude mice suggest this to be the case (Bucky 2002). Human donor fat over a range of ages was injected subcutaneously into nude immuno-compromised mice. The data suggested higher volume retention in the recipient with fat from younger donors. In practice, autologous fat grafting does not afford us the opportunity to control for this variable and this may only serve as a pre-operative prognosticator.

Donor site

There have been anecdotal reports that fat harvested from some areas in the body survives better than fat from others. This may be an effect related to the size of adipocytes in various locations of the body. For example, fat harvested from the neck during a facelift may contain smaller adipocytes than larger fat cells harvested from the anterior abdomen. Smaller fat lobules have a better surface contact to volume ratio and therefore a higher likelihood of revascularizing. There also may be less trauma and cell damage when smaller fat cells are harvested. However, in practical terms, especially for large volume grafting, there is no demonstrable evidence that fat harvested from any area is better than another.

Harvesting techniques: the role of vacuum

Pressures utilized vary greatly in liposuction and certainly impact cell survival and graft take. Several studies have demonstrated that for optimal adipocyte viability, vacuum pressures should remain below one half atmosphere (<15 inches mercury, while regular liposuction is >30 inches of mercury) and that the lower the suction pressures, the more viable the adipocytes. Liposuction aspirator machines dialed down to very low pressures may be used to aspirate the fat. This technique, however, has many limitations as it requires: i) a rigid collection containers (lest they collapse under vacuum); ii) a stable stand away from the surgical field to keep the container upright (lest the aspirate continues straight into the suction machine); iii) long sterile tubing resulting in significant dead space loss. Another drawback of using liposuction aspirators is the sudden high airflow gushing through the tubing whenever a side hole of the liposuction cannula loses the vacuum. This causes sudden violent splashing of fat into the collection containers and desiccation of the graft through the long tubing.

Generally, hand-held, smaller size (<10 mL) syringe methods are thought to generate lower vacuum and be less traumatic and are therefore recommended to harvest fat. They have the inconvenience of being much more time, resource, and personnel demanding. A more recent advance is the constant pressure syringe that maintains a constant 280–300 mmHg (11–12 inches of mercury, about one-third atmospheric) vacuum throughout the excursion of the plunger.

The role of the liposuction cannula

When Illouz described liposuction and in the early days of fat grafting, the most commonly used cannulae were 10 mm in diameter. These large bore cannulae harvested large tissue chunks. Because of the resultant low surface to volume ratio when grafting these larger grafts, there is significantly less revascularization potential. The preference now is to harvest with cannulae less than 3 mm in diameter with side holes less than 1 × 2 mm in size. The smaller fat graft droplets thus harvested have much better chance of surviving. We also showed that harvesting efficiency per 10 liposuction strokes increased as we increased the number of side holes, and that increasing the number of openings up to 12 holes allowed us to efficiently harvest fat at pressures well below the ones described in the literature (Figure 9.1). In addition, the lipo-aspirate obtained by these smaller gauge cannulae with smaller aspiration holes has a much lower tendency to clump and clog and is easier to re-inject.

Ostensibly, one might think that fat surgically resected en bloc, which is then diced with minimal trauma, would maintain cellular integrity better than suctioned fat by any method, and might result in better graft take (Kononas et al 1993). Ongoing studies are being performed in this area to better understand the role of minimizing graft trauma (Guyuron & Majzoub 2007) and there is an opportunity to validate this question and to potentially improve instrumentation in this area.

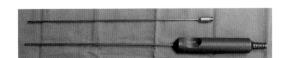

Figure 9.1 A 12 gauge multiple small hole cannula used in fat harvesting for grafting.

Processing techniques

There have been multiple reports of 'percent graft take' by volume (Billings & May 1989). Because of lack of standardization in grafting technique, we must consider re-thinking the results of many of these studies. For example, 60 mL of aspirated fat using the tumescent technique will decant to a variable aliquot of fat and serum, including blood and crystalloid. 60 mL of aspirate may decant to 30–40 mL of fat. When this fat is then centrifuged or rolled on a Telfa pad, two techniques used to further concentrate fat, the resultant fat may reduce to 20 mL by volume. It is, therefore not surprising that when fat is grafted, even if all the fat survives, if one does not effectively process the fat and remove crystalloid effectively, one has already committed to at best a 30–40% volume take, because that is the actual amount of fat that has been inserted by volume.

The controversy of centrifugation vs decantation

Separation by decanting (Figure 9.2) involves simple gravity to separate higher density blood and crystalloid from adipocytes. A high speed centrifuge uses much higher gravitational forces (3–5 g) and separates fat from crystalloid extremely well. These centrifuges also require transfer of fat into multiple individual 5 mL or 10 mL syringes. However, it has been demonstrated that subjecting adipocytes to 3–5 g of centrifugation results in a higher degree of cell death (Kurita et al 2008). Therefore, a compromise between these two techniques, used by several practitioners (Betti 2008) is manual centrifugation. Prototype devices, similar to the geared concept used in salad spinners, can subject larger volumes of adipocytes to 1.5 g forces to better separate out unwanted crystalloid, without subjecting the fat to excessive (3–5 g forces) trauma or excessive syringe manipulation (Figure 9.3).

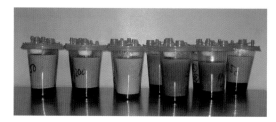

Figure 9.2 Simple decanting of fat from crystalloid.

Straining and filtration

Some separation methods advocate filtration of the lipo-aspirate. With this method, smaller fat droplets, pre-adipocytes, and other precious tissue such as platelets pass through the filter and are lost while the larger less useful clumps remain. Straining, as a method of preparation has the same drawbacks as filtration with the added disadvantage of decreasing adipocyte survival by exposing them to air. Air exposure, extensive manipulation and transfer from syringe to syringe increases the chance of contamination and the duration of hypoxia and has a potentially further deleterious effect on adipocyte survival.

In addition to potential cellular damage, centrifuged, strained or filtered lipo-aspirate delivers grafts in coalesced concentrated clumps with less chance to revascularize by interfacing the recipient bed than the loosely dispersed decanted fat. This is important for the large volume grafts required for the breast and is less of an issue in the well vascularized face where the smaller volumes usually grafted still have enough recipient contact and where more accurate control of the contour correction is mandatory.

Concentration of 'stem cells'

Recently, there has been a great deal of excitement and many claims made over the role of stem cells or the 'pre-adipocyte' present in high concentration in the lipo-aspirate. In order to separate out pre-adipocytes, several well-known processes exist. Crucial steps in separation techniques utilize enzymatic digestion of

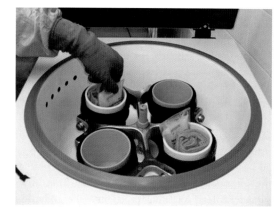

Figure 9.3 Manual centrifugation in closed IV collection bag system.

the lipo-aspirate tissue and centrifugation. In the current clinical trial protocols, stem cells isolated from half the lipo-aspirate are mixed with the remaining unprocessed raw aspirate and re-injected as a stem cell enriched lipo-graft. At the time of this writing, it is still unknown whether this practice represents a significant contribution from stem cells versus adult adipocytes alone. This is an exciting area of potential research both in the physiology of the stem cell and in its ability to be separated from viable adipocytes, and hopefully this will be delineated over the next decade.

Such concerns support the argument that fat grafting in large volumes (unlike those performed for lip or nasolabial folds) might best be accomplished with a team approach. Ostensibly, it is recommended that an assistant or several assistants process fat simultaneously while surgical liposuction harvest is performed. On the other hand, a standardized, simple and efficient, closed system for non-traumatic low pressure aspiration, processing of the aspirated material, and easy re-injection of the preserved active slurry with minimal dependence on assistants has the highest potential for use in this type of surgery.

Recipient site: 'preparing the field'

Recipient site management has only recently been suggested as an important variable in fat grafting that could be potentially manipulated and improved. The size, quality and pressure compliance of the recipient site are the most prominent components.

Recipient site size

In the familiar two-dimensional skin grafting of wounds, the surface of the wound determines the maximal limit of skin graft that survives, and over grafting does not help. Similarly, in three-dimensional grafting, the volume of the recipient bed sets the maximal limit to the volume of graft that can survive, and over grafting will lead to necrosis and oil cysts. Geometrical models of optimal dispersion of the individual fat droplets in the three-dimensional recipient matrix dictates that to preserve the three-dimensional vascular stromal interconnections of the matrix, anything more than a two-thirds ratio of donor volume

to recipient volume filling (assuming recipient stromal cell islands are approximately same size as the fat droplets) will lead to overcrowding and by worsening the graft-to-recipient contact drastically increase the amount of necrosis.

Using the 'seeds in a field' analogy, and with everything else optimized, the size of the field sets the upper limit of the crop size. Overfilling the recipient space with more grafts will lead to crowding, will reduce graft to recipient interface and will result in massive necrosis. This opens up an opportunity for positive intervention. For mega-volume grafting in a tight space, temporarily expansion of the recipient loosens the extracellular matrix and creates many more interstices where many more individual fat droplets can optimize their graft to recipient interface and survive (Figure 9.4).

Recipient site quality

It is well established that muscle tissue with its high capillary density is an excellent graft recipient and that the more vascular the recipient, the better the graft survival. Furthermore, a number of cytokines and growth factors can accelerate the process of graft neo-angiogenesis and improve survival. Thus attempts at priming the recipient site by increasing its vascularity and stimulate angiogenic cytokine production should improve engraftment. Tissue expansion is well known to be angiogenic and to stimulate the production of the potent angiogenic cytokine VEGF.

Recipient site filling pressure

From the general surgery trauma literature and from hand and upper extremity trauma, the importance of compartment pressure and the grave consequences of high interstitial pressure are well understood. If it were possible to pre-stretch the recipient space prior to fat grafting, it would make it more compliant and allow the injection of larger volumes of graft into the recipient site before reaching prohibitively high interstitial pressures.

Advances to improve the recipient site

The Brava® bra was initially developed in the 1990s as an external soft tissue Ilizarov expander to enlarge the breast. The device consists of a pair of semi-rigid domes with silicone gel rim cushion that interface

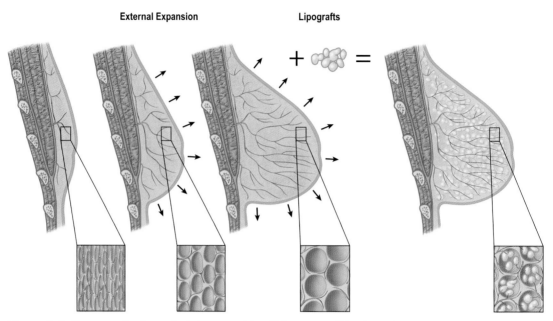

Figure 9.4 Pre-expansion theoretically increases interstitial space and blood supply.

with the skin and that are worn around the breasts like a bra. A small pump maintains inside the domes a low negative pressure that does not interrupt capillary flow and that imparts on the breast surface a constant gentle isotropic distraction force. Studies have shown that when the device is worn in an uninterrupted fashion for 10–12 hours per day, true and long lasting breast augmentation ensues over a period of weeks to months (Khouri et al 2000). Forty thousand women have used Brava over the past 7 years, but compliance with the cumbersome treatment and the slow pace of real tissue growth has limited its popularity. However, within a few weeks of use, substantial temporary swelling of the breast develops. This was found to be an ideal way to prepare the breast for large volumes of fat grafts. The three to four fold increase in volume that can be attained over 4 weeks of wear allows a proportionate increase in fat graft amount without crowding. The expansion effect is also angiogenic as has been documented by MRI.

Experience with the VAC as a means of wound management has proven that microangiogenesis is a direct result of negative mechanical pressure (Morykwas et al 1997). The extensive VAC data on vascular in-growth and improvement in skin graft take coupled with the MRI findings from Brava expanded breasts

support the authors' thesis that increased microcirculation, combined with the larger interstitial space created by the expansion may both contribute to the potential for increased graft volumes and increased diffusion gradients. This is substantiated by Baker et al, who reported 80–90% long-term survival of grafts with volumes in excess of 250 mL.

Grafting technique

Injection technique also varies and plays a major role in fat grafting survival. Cellular transplantation by injection, be it transplanted pancreatic islet cells or transplanted fat cells, requires cells to survive by diffusion in the initial 3–5 days till neoangiogenesis restores blood supply. In this early phase of graft survival called 'plasmatic imbibition'; the better the diffusion gradient, the higher the potential for the transplanted cells to survive. Thus, only the smallest graft droplets with larger surface to volume ratio and with best graft to recipient interface will survive to engraft. The central zone of localized deposits larger than 2–3 mm in diameter will undergo necrosis prior to being revascularized. Injections into a cavity or a lake and bolus injections are to be condemned as they usually result in fat liquefaction, necrosis and oil cysts.

The mapping technique

Donor cells have the highest chance of survival with the technique that best ensures an even, three-dimensional dispersion of the fat as tiny droplets in as many small interstices as possible while avoiding any localized deposit or lake formation. The 'mapping' technique involves the use of small (3 mL) syringes handheld and connected directly to a 14 gauge blunt cannula. Markings are made in the recipient areas (Figure 9.5) to aid in a systematic, diffuse and even injection of the entire recipient. An exact amount of fat (1–2 mL) is then injected slowly upon withdrawal of the 15–20 cm long cannula. The cannula is then inserted into another adjacent tunnel and the process is repeated in a fanning 3D weave to evenly crisscross cover the recipient space. This technique is deliberate and exact but does take time. In addition, it requires the operator to deploy the plunger and withdraw the needle at the same time.

Fallacy of the overcorrection technique

Because many reports suggest at best 30% fat take, one controversy in fat grafting has been whether to overcorrect or not (Kaufman et al 2007). Overcorrection seemed alluring as one might reach a desired endpoint knowing a significant amount of adipocytes would not survive. However, the increased crowding and interstitial pressure result in lack of diffusion to most of the grafted tissue and potentially to necrosis of all the graft. It is only reasonable to match the amount of graft to the volume of the recipient space. With the maximal graft to recipient ratio of 2:3 described above, a typical mastectomy defect or an A cup breast with a recipient volume less than 100 mL will at best, and with the most even graft dispersion, successfully engraft around 70 mL. Therefore, in ideal conditions, 70 mL is the largest amount of fat that can survive in a mastectomy defect or an A cup breast. With everything optimized, 70 mL of well dispersed fat might result in 100% survival. Overcorrecting to double that graft volume will decrease the graft survival by more than half and lead to much less than 50% graft take.

Indeed, some of the best clinical results in fat grafting have been demonstrated by those who promote small serial volume sessions of fat grafting (Delay 2006, Coleman & Saboeiro 2007). It is possible that this approach is successful because it respects the graft to recipient size ratio and the interstitial pressure limitations of the recipient site and in doing so, promotes diffusion during the initial critical days post grafting.

Post-graft care

Post-operatively, skin grafts are immobilized to promote secure apposition of the donor cells to the recipient wound bed. This promotes an adequate diffusion gradient and greater likelihood that angiogenesis will occur. Searing of the graft or movement of any type in this initial 3–5 days can prove fatal for a skin graft and similarly for a fat graft. It is felt that immobilization of the transplanted adipocyte can best be accomplished with mild external negative pressure. Not only does the mild negative pressure serve to immobilize the fat in its interstitial space, it may also help with angiogenesis as has been demonstrated with the VAC. The domes of the external expander Brava unit help protect the newly grafted tissue from external movement and trauma. Lastly, sustained Brava expansion effect post grafting might provide further growth by stimulating stem cells, which are well known to respond to mechanical stimulation.

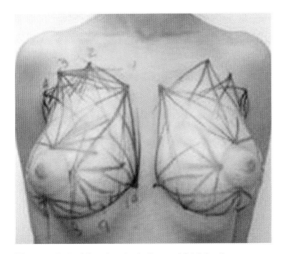

Figure 9.5 Mapping technique of fat injection.

Breast reconstruction and augmentation with fat grafts and external expansion

Mastectomy surgery in the United States

Annually in the USA, there are currently approximately 182 000 newly diagnosed cases of breast cancer that require some type of surgical procedure (YME 2008). These are generally some form of mastectomy or lumpectomy. On the other hand, there are approximately 57 000 breast reconstructions performed a year in the USA (ASPS 2008). If we assume that all these reconstructions are performed for immediate (or in the same year as the mastectomy) reconstruction, at best only 31% of patients are receiving some form of breast reconstruction. This number is probably lower as many of the reconstructions are performed on cases diagnosed and surgically treated in prior years. This also means that every decade, approximately 1.2 million women are electing to do nothing about their post-surgical breast deformity. Why do such a high percentage of breast cancer surgery patients elect to do nothing following lumpectomy or mastectomy? One postulate is that the degree of morbidity of the reconstruction outweighs the perceived aesthetic improvement over the existing deformity. These already disfigured women are reluctant to undergo more surgery and incur more scars, even if it is to restore their feminine figure. In this orphaned population, a low-morbidity procedure to reconstruct breast defects that results in significant aesthetic improvement to the breast, but also provides a 'bonus' liposuction represents a large opportunity.

Breast augmentation surgery in the United States

An adequate discussion of augmentation with breast implants is beyond the context of this communication. However, it is interesting to consider the risk-reward analysis similar to that outlined in the patient after breast cancer surgery. Reviewing available statistics there were approximately 348 500 cosmetic breast augmentations performed in the United States in 2007 (ASPS 2008). In addition, retail data suggests that at least 34% of women in the United States own padded bras. Based on standard assumptions about the US population and the percent of women of adult age, for every women who undergoes a cosmetic breast enhancement, there are over 100 women who, for whatever reason, would like their breasts to appear larger in some way. The same rational for non-surgery (padded bras) may also exist as it does for breast reconstruction. Besides financial issues, concerns over artificial implants, and other personal concerns, a remaining variable is that that the degree of morbidity of the augmentation does not outweigh the aesthetic improvement over the existing aesthetic concern. As in the case of reconstruction, a low-morbidity procedure to augment breasts that results in significant improvement represents a large number of potential patients, much larger than the reconstruction population. As an indication of its appeal, lipo-augmentation of the breast would be combining together the number one and two most commonly performed aesthetic surgical procedures.

Patient evaluation: medical

The patient presenting for breast reconstruction/augmentation with autologous fat grafting should be evaluated for associated medical conditions that might otherwise exclude them from safely undergoing a liposuction procedure. Acutely, the liposuction aspect of the intervention is probably higher in morbidity than that of the breast fat grafting. Smokers with their impaired microcirculation are not candidates for breast reconstruction with pre-expansion and fat grafting. Potential fat donor sites fat are evaluated for their likely availability. Irradiated patients have been treated using Brava® pre-expansion, and there is evidence that negative pressure and fat grafting improves the cyclical process of post irradiation fibrosis and chronic ischemia (Rigotti et al 2007). In irradiated reconstructions, the skin envelope expands more slowly and serial expansion/injection sessions are required. It is generally advised to begin breast reconstruction in non-irradiated mastectomy patients and first becoming familiar with these techniques before embarking on treating irradiated defects. The assessment of the opposite breast is addressed with the same principles as for any breast reconstruction.

Patient evaluation: the role of compliance

There are two compliances; the patient and her tissues. Breast pre-stretched by pregnancy or weight loss are more compliant breast than younger nulliparous breasts, especially if the latter are also constricted or tuberous. The post mastectomy, densely scarred and irradiated chest is also less compliant than softer, loose and non-irradiated defects. Compliance of the breasts determines their response to external expansion. As far as the patient's compliance goes, there is no substitute for sustained moderate to high negative pressure pre-expansion to maximize pre-fat grafting volume of the recipient site. Indeed, the earliest versions of the negative pressure pumps were low voltage battery operated devices that exerted a low negative pressure. These patients exhibited less dramatic pre-grafting expansion when compared to more powerful pumps currently used. These pumps are similar in negative pressure and in terms of size, portability as the VAC pump, and have demonstrated a 'dose response curve' with regards to both pre-expansion volume, and to overall fat volume results post grafting.

Based on the experience with the dose response data, the authors believe there is no substitute for adequate pre-expansion. The degree and extent of pre-grafting expansion is directly proportional to the amount of grafting possible to maintain a physiologic interstitial pressure. Last minute cramming on part of the patient has been experienced and does not result in successful preparation. It is ultimately the responsibility of the surgeon to adequately select, educate, coach and troubleshoot their patients to ensure adequate and optimal pre-expansion.

In conventional tissue expansion and flap reconstruction, the more expanded the tissue, the better the advancement and the better the resultant reconstruction. And in instances where expansion is not tolerated or possible, serial excision with multiple flap advancement procedures can achieve the same result after over a longer period of time and a few more procedures. The same concepts apply to external expansion and fat grafting. Adequate (>3 times volume increase,) external expansion will allow the grafting

and survival of the large fat volumes required for augmentation and reconstruction, while lesser expansion will only allow lesser volumes and no expansion at all, much less. Delay has shown that is possible to achieve primary breast reconstruction with fat grafting alone (Delay 2006). However, the procedure is only satisfactory for the smaller, non-ptotic breasts and it requires multiple repeat operations over a prolonged period of time.

Patient evaluation: baseline volume considerations

The more breast/subcutaneous tissue there is to begin with, the easier it will be to volume expand with negative pressure. In addition, the less scar damaged (non-irradiated) the tissue is, the easier it will be to expand with negative pressure. The following cases serve as extremely diverse examples:

Case 1: Breast augmentation: existing breasts 250 mL size; desired final breast volume: 500 mL. Plan: pre-expansion to desired volume, then graft. Per cent expansion = (500 − 250)/250 = 100%.

Case 2: Reconstruction: patient has mastectomy scar and existing breast skin, subcutaneous fat volume is 50 mL in size; desired volume: 500 mL. Plan: pre-expansion to desired volume, then graft. Per cent expansion = (500 − 50)/50 = 900%.

The mastectomy recipient site has a much more challenging expansion because one is starting with very little parenchyma. We therefore postulate a general guide to the spectrum of serial grafting as it relates to number of required sessions (Table 9.1).

Preferred techniques

Brava®: recipient site preparation

In cases of mastectomy and for augmentation, the Brava® dome is placed for 3–4 weeks and is worn 12

Table 9.1 General guide to the spectrum of serial grafting as it relates to number of required sessions

Type of Intervention	Augmentation	Reconstruction	XRT Reconstruction
Average number of sessions	1	3	5

h daily. For the last 4–5 days prior to fat grafting, the patient is advised to wear the domes 24 h a day. Circumferential pressure at the edges of the domes can create skin sensitivity and this should be explained to patients who should reduce the degree of negative pressure. As previously stated, non-irradiated skin and subcutaneous tissue has greater potential for parenchymal expansion than cases performed in irradiated tissue, and therefore more serial sessions would be required (Figure 9.6).

The location and degree of body fat available is analyzed to evaluate the existence of an adequate amount of donor fat. Because there are so many variables – amount of tumescence, degree of bleeding,

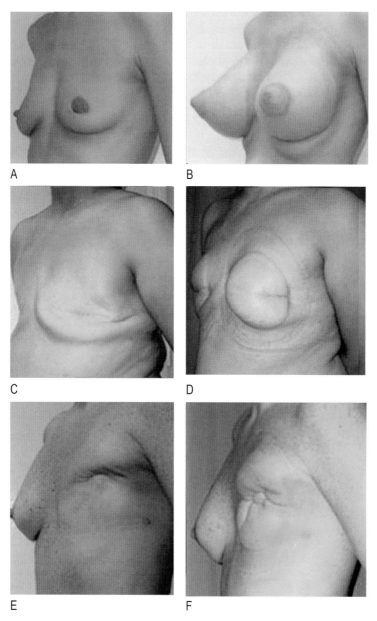

Figure 9.6 Effect of Brava® pre-expansion in three cases: augmentation (A,B), mastectomy (C,D), irradiated mastectomy (E,F) sites with pre-expansion. After 3–4 weeks, note the varying range of expansion possible in each category.

time allowed for tumescent solution to set, it is impossible to formulate a standard ratio of aspirate to actual processed fat by volume. As a conservative rule, four to five times the desired volume of fat needed for grafting should be available to be harvested as aspirate. For example, if reconstruction using 400 mL of fat is planned, the patient should be able to render at least 1600–2000 mL of aspirate to ensure adequate donor material.

Aspirate = 5 × graft; 2000 mL = 5 × 400 mL

Considering the pre-expansion effort the patient must tolerate, it is always better to have more than less fat available.

In the case of augmentation with 300 mL of fat on each side, 3000 mL of aspirate is recommended. Patients with BMIs as low as 23–24 have been successfully treated. Obviously, the lower the BMI, the greater the number of donor sites (abdomen, knees, thighs, etc) that must be entered to harvest adequate amounts of aspirate/fat. It is the surgeon's responsibility to properly select, educate, and support the patient throughout the expansion process to ensure successful results. Patients should spend as much time in office the first time they use their bras to ensure they are properly educated and motivated to use the device.

Lipografting: pre-operative planning

On the day of surgery, patients are photographed and marked as usual for liposuction. Markings are made for injection sites on the breast(s) and lines are made on the breast mound to ensure proper dispersion of the fat grafts. Patients are brought into the operating room still wearing the Brava® bra to maximize expansion closer to the point of injection. Once all the fat is harvested and processed, the Brava® bra is removed, the site is prepped and redraped, and injection takes place.

Harvesting and collection

Fat is harvested using a 12 gauge blunt cannula with multiple side ports. Syringe aspiration is used as opposed to high negative pressure machine techniques. To avoid desiccation, a closed system is employed, transferring the fat from the syringe directly into an empty sterile intravenous bag via an extension tubing setup (Figure 9.7).

Processing

Once an adequate amount of aspirate is harvested, the collected intravenous bags are decanted of unwanted fluid and are placed into a manual centrifuge. This manual centrifuge further separates fluid from the adipocytes without subjecting the cells to excessive handling, desiccation or trauma, as compared to high speed centrifugation in small syringes. Once the fat is properly processed in this manner, the fat is then drawn back into 3 or 5 mL syringes from the intravenous collection bags though intravenous tubing and a non-traumatic, non-clogging valve, and the grafting begins.

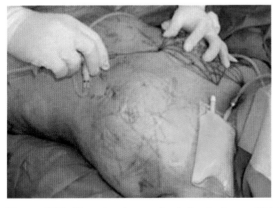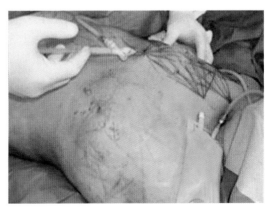

Figure 9.7 Closed system method of collection and fat replantation.

Recipient site techniques: needle band release

Multiple radial 14 g needle puncture wounds are made around the breast mound to maximally disperse the grafted adipocytes and to ensure as many different planes as possible. In many breasts, fibrous ligamenotous tissue or bands distort and restrict the breast mound, such as in constricted inframammary folds or in the case of tuberous or tubular breast deformities. Because expansion of the parenchymal space places these bands under high tension, it facilitates the transaction of these bands using an 18 gauge needle, simply by inserting the needle in the area of the band and through proprioception, 'feeling' the sharp tip of the needle cut the band. In this manner, it is possible to further 'expand' or 'release' these constrictions internally in a manner similar to the external release of a burn scar contracture.

The inframammary fold can be lowered in constricted inframammary folds, and the constricted bases of tubular breasts can be widened in this manner. It is important not to over-release these bands and not to dissect tissue planes, as too large a dead space might ensue. This will reduce the interstices of the tissue and by creating lakes, will reduce the surface to volume characteristics of the recipient site. The idea is to create a three-dimensional mesh pattern expansion, limiting the cuts to small nicks at multiple points in multiple planes avoiding tissue ripping or tears.

Injection technique

Bolus injections are to be condemned as they defeat the purpose of oxygen diffusion and usually result in fat liquefaction and necrosis. The 'mapping' technique previously described involves the use of small (3–5 mL) syringes handheld and connected directly to a 14 g blunt spatulated cannula with a side hole. Through the multiple radial needle insertions around the breast mound, the cannula is advanced in the subcutaneous plane and an exact amount of fat (1–2 mL) is then injected slowly upon withdrawal. The needle is then inserted into another adjacent tunnel and the process is repeated.

Injection into the pre-pectoral fat and the subcutaneous fat is performed in as many different depth planes as the recipient tissue will tolerate. In the case of mastectomy, the first session of grafting will obviously allow fewer planes of grafting and depending upon the pre-operative assessment of the expanded recipient volume, the graft volume during the first session (100–150 mL) should be planned depending upon the amount of expansion and the size of the 'edema' breast created. For subsequent sessions, there are more potential planes, as a thicker interstitial space exists. Generally, the more parenchyma one has to begin with, the larger volumes of fat that can be grafted. For augmentation or in subsequent grafting sessions in reconstruction, 200–300 mL can be planed. For irradiated cases, one should be extremely careful not to over-graft and should expect a minimum of four to five sessions. In no cases of breast augmentation, treating a lumpectomy defect, breast asymmetry or any other cases where any breast tissue remains, is it ever recommended to inject fat directly into the breast parenchymal tissue.

Post-operative management

Patients are instructed to wear the Brava® bra for at least 1 week post grafting. This potentially helps with graft immobilization, potentiates neovascularization, and definitely protects the breast from external pressure or trauma. There is evidence to strongly suggest that wearing Brava® for 10–12 h per day for a few weeks more further stimulates the grafted 'pre-adipocytes' and stem cells and this post operative mechanical stimulation might hold up the operative swelling and gradually induce the formation of fat into these 'edema' interstices similar to the experimental growth chambers of Morrison et al (Hofer et al 2003).

Results

Case 1

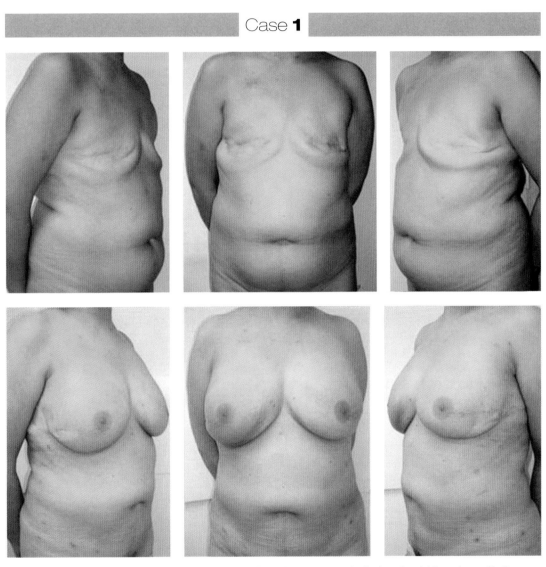

Figure 9.8 Breast reconstruction. This patient had bilateral mastectomy (radical on the right) performed in the distant past. She had refused reconstruction in the past for various personal reasons. She agreed to fat grafting with Brava® pre-expansion and had four serial sessions of Brava® pre-expansion and fat grafting sessions of 150 mL each time.

Case **2**

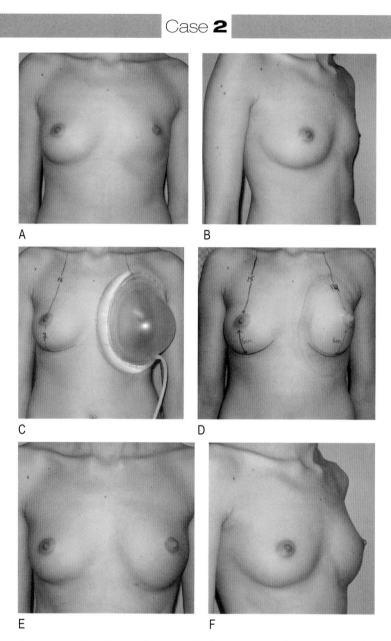

A

B

C

D

E

F

Figure 9.9 Breast asymmetry. This 20-year-old woman had a giant congenital nevus excised as a child and demonstrated hypomastia on the left, documented by MRI. She underwent 3 weeks of Brava® pre-expansions to increase her parenchymal space and to increase the vertical skin envelope deficiency. She underwent a single session with grafting of 300 mL into the left breast. Her post-operative result at 6 months reveals retention of grafted fat volume. (A,B) Patient with severe breast asymmetry and Brava® pre-expansion reconstruction. (C,D) Brava® pre-expansion increases parenchyma and skin envelope. (E,F) Six months after 280 mL of fat transplanted into the left breast.

Case **3**

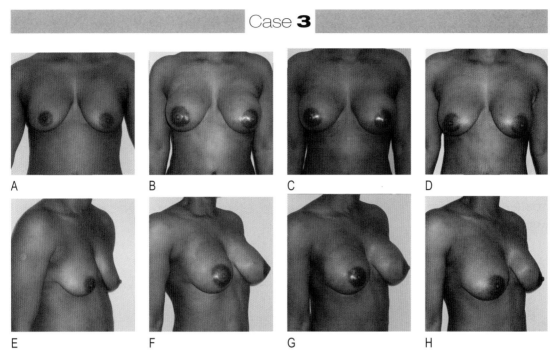

A   B   C   D

E   F   G   H

Figure 9.10   Breast augmentation – ptosis. This 34-year-old woman desired larger breasts after having several children and experiencing some mild deflation and breast ptosis. She did not wish to have breast augmentation with implants. She underwent 3 weeks of Brava® pre-expansions to increase her parenchymal space bilaterally. She underwent a single session with grafting of 300 mL into each breast, with preferential fill to the lower pole to help alleviate the breast ptosis. Her serial photos show some volume decrease but do reveal retention of grafted fat volume at 9 months. (A,B) Before and (C,D) 3 (E,F) 6 and (G,H) 9 months after Brava® pre-expansion augmentation.

Breast reconstruction using three techniques

Table 9.2 helps delineate some of the main differences between currently popular reconstruction options and breast reconstruction using pre-expansion and autologous fat transplantation.

Controversial topics

At the time of this communication, it is still the early days of breast augmentation and reconstruction using fat transplantation. There are more questions than there are answers, and it is easier to ask the question than it is to answer them. The following represent some of the biggest controversies and challenges facing this technique in the near, medium and long-term.

Imaging and detection of breast cancer

In 1987, the American Society of Plastic Surgeon position paper strongly condemned fat grafting to the breast suggesting fat grafting would distort the ability of breast cancer detection. Breast fat grafting has been demonstrated to sometimes result in micro-calcifications. However, following breast fat grafting radiographic findings have been reported to be relatively benign in appearance, and are generally felt to be distinguishable from calcifications of higher grade that are suggestive of malignancy (Missana et al 2007).

Cancer risk

It is well known that one in nine women will experience breast cancer in their lifetime. Although it would

Table 9.2 Main differences between currently popular reconstruction options and breast reconstruction using pre-expansion and autologous fat transplantation

	Tissue expander/implant	TRAM	Brava® fat graft
Pain level	Moderate	High	Low
Number of procedures	2–3	1–2	1–3
General anesthesia	2	2	0–1
Invasiveness/morbidity of the surgery	2–3	4–5	0–1
New scars	0–1	4–5	0–1
Donor site morbidity	NA	High	Bonus-improvement liposuction
Cosmetic result and pt satisfaction with 'feel of reconstructed breast'	2	3–4	4–5
Office visits for expansion	5–7	None	None
Expansion type	Serial–office based	None	Continuous
Recipient site skin	Thinned	NA	Thickened
Hospital days	0–1	3–5	None
Patient compliance	Patient passive	Passive	Compliance is KEY
Reoperation tolerance	Moderately possible	Unlikely	Simple
Cost to system	Moderate	High	Low

take a nearly impossible study size to prove causality or statistical significance, the question has been raised that aromatase, a breakdown product of adipocyte necrosis, might cause breast cancer. The validity of this is unknown. Interestingly, the same study has found that silicone present in breast implants, though now well proven to be non carcinogenic, is a much stronger stimulant of aromatase.

What is known is that surgeons have performed thousands of procedures over the past 20 years in large numbers where some fat invariably survives as a graft and where fat necrosis occurs. Despite thousands of TRAM flaps, with a high degree of fat necrosis in zone II and III, breast liposuctions, mastopexies and breast reductions, there is no evidence, retrospective or prospective, that these procedures are associated with a higher degree of breast cancer (while there are reports of reduced incidence of breast cancer after reduction mammoplasty, a procedure that has a well known 50% incidence of fat necrosis). There is nothing at all in the literature and as experiments

of nature to suggest that fat grafting the breast is carcinogenic.

However, such facts should not be sufficient as to ignore the question of safety. Although there are currently models being developed to evaluate this carcinogenic potential in an animal model, the reality is that the answer in humans will not be available until a few decades follow the widespread use of this technique. Any patients entertaining any breast fat grafting, including reconstruction patients and breast augmentation patients, must be given full informed consent as to the unknown risks of the technique. While many suggest this technique not be performed without the approval of an IRB, the reality is that the technique is already being performed and appears to be safe when well executed. Like everything else in plastic surgery, it is all about adherence to fundamental principles and surgical technique.

We predict a gradual and steady adoption of this technique as safety and good results are reproduced by many independent surgeons, and that such collective data in the literature will eventually help fully delineate the safety issues.

The future

Reconstruction cases

Although it is too early to accurately predict the future of these techniques, there certainly exists the potential for breast reconstruction with natural fat to fill the void for many patients who are otherwise not candidates for autologous flap or implant reconstruction. Lumpectomy patients, patients with co-morbidity, older age, irradiation, and patients averse to implants constitute just some of the many types of orphaned reconstruction cases that may potentially benefit from this technique.

Breast deformities: natural and iatrogenic

In the case of tubular breasts, breast asymmetry, unilateral or bilateral breast agenesis, or Poland's syndrome, fat grafting may also be a useful alternative to achieve a natural result without the long term morbidity of implant reconstructions. The iterative nature of fat grafting, combined with its low morbidity, allows for serial sessions to refine the cosmetic result. In the case of rippling after breast augmentation with saline implants, breast fat grafting may also play a significant role. Rippling is thought to be a direct result of an excessively thin subcutaneous layer, in addition to a potentially under-filled implant. Therefore, pre-expansion with Brava would potentially allow more fat to be inserted with a potentially lower risk of implant damage, as the space would be rendered thicker after pre-expansion.

Breast augmentation

In cases of primary breast augmentation, Brava pre-expansion and fat grafting may play a role as its safety and efficacy is proven in the reconstructive and then in the deformity literature. For patients seeking a cup size increase, as in the multiparous patient with breast deflation who may be entertaining lipo-abdominoplasty, this may be an ideal approach. For the patient who desires a significant breast enlargement and in whom a natural result is not desired, fat grafting is less likely to deliver the desired outcome. In these cases, and in cases where compliance of pre-expansion is in doubt, breast augmentation with implants will always be superior to fat grafting.

Further reading

American Society of Plastic Surgeons. Statistics on breast surgery from American Society of Plastic Surgery: www.plasticsurgery.org/media/statistics/loader.cfm?url=/commonspot/security/getfile.cfm&PageID=29287. 2008.

ASPRS ad-hoc committee on new procedures. Report on autologous fat transplantation, September 30, 1987.

Baker T. Live Presentation on BRAVA, American Society of Aesthetic Plastic Surgery Annual Meeting, April 2006, Orlando, Florida.

Baker T. Live Presentation – Follow up Study on BRAVA, American Society of Aesthetic Plastic Surgery Annual Meeting, April 2008, San Diego, California.

Betti GK. Huixquilucan, Estado de Mexico, 52763 Presentation at the 20th Annual Italian-American Plastic Surgery Meeting, Bologna, Italy, June, 2008.

Billings E, May JW. Historical review and present status of free fat graft autotransplantation in plastic and reconstructive surgery. Plast Reconstr Surg 1989;83:368–381.

Bircoll M. Autologous fat transplantation to the breast. Plast Reconstr Surg 1988;82:361.

Bucky LP, Godek CP. Discussion. The behavior of fat grafts in recipient areas with enhanced vascularity by Baran CN, Celebioglu S, Sensoz O, Ulusoy G, Civelek B Ortak T. Plast Reconstr Surg 2002;109:1652 and unpublished communication.

Coleman, SR, Saboeiro AP. Fat grafting to the breast revisited: safety and efficacy. Plast Reconstr Surg 2007;119:775–785.

Coupdefoudrelingerie.blogspot.com/2008/05/new-bra-statistics-from-consumer.html. Incidence of padded Bra Wearers.

Czerny V. Plastischer Ersatz der Brustdruse durch ein Lipom. Zentralbl Chir 1895;27:72.

Delay, E. Lipomodeling of the reconstructed breast. In: Spear SL (Ed). Surgery of the breast: principles and art. Philadelphia, PA: Lippincott Williams & Wilkins; 2006.

Guyuron B, Majzoub RK. Facial augmentation with core fat graft: a preliminary report. Plast Reconstr Surg 2007;120:295–302.

Hinderer UT, Del Rio J. Erich Lexer's mammaplasty. Aesthetic Plast Surg 1992;16:101.

Hofer SOP, Knight KM, Cooper-White JJ et al. Increasing the volume of vascularized tissue formation in engineered constructs: an experimental study in rats. Plast Reconstr Surg 2003;111:1186–1192.

Illouz YG. Body contouring by lipolysis: A 5-year experience with over 3000 cases. Plast Reconstr Surg 1983;72:591–597.

Kaufman MR, Bradley JP, Dickinson B et al. Autologous fat transfer national consensus survey: trends in techniques for harvest, preparation, and application, and perception of short- and long-term results. Plast Reconstr Surg 2007;119:323–331.

Khouri RK, Schlenz I, Murphy BJ, Baker TJ. Non-surgical breast enlargement using an external soft-tissue expansion system. Plast Reconstr Surg 2000;105:2500–2512.

Kononas TC, Bucky LP, Hurley C, May JW. The fate of suctioned and surgically removed fat after reimplantation for soft-tissue augmentation: a volumetric and histologic study in the rabbit. Plast Reconstr Surg 1993;91(Suppl 5):763S–768S.

Kurita M, Matsumoto D, Shigeura TMS et al. Influences of centrifugation on cells and tissues in liposuction aspirates: optimized centrifugation of lipotransfer and cell isolation. Plast Reconstr Surg 2008:121:1033–1041.

Missana M, Laurent I, Barreau L, Balleyguier C. Autologous fat transfer in reconstructive breast surgery: indications, technique and results. Eur J Surg Oncol 2007;33:685–690.

Morykwas MJ, Argenta LC, Shelton-Brown EI et al. Vacuum assisted closure: a new method for wound control and treatment: animal studies and basic foundation. Ann Plast Surg 1997;38:553–562.

Rigotti G, Marchi A, Galiè M, et al. Clinical treatment of radiotherapy tissue damage by lipoaspirate transplant: a healing process mediated by adipose-derived adult stem cells. Plast Reconstr Surg 2007;119:1409–1422.

Shiffman MA, Mirrafati S. Fat transfer techniques: the effect of harvest and transfer methods on adipocyte viability and review of the literature. Dermatol Surg 2001;27:819–826.

YME National Breast Cancer Organization. Available online at www.yme.org/information/breast_cancer_news/breast_cancer_statistics.php, 2006.

10

Tubular breasts

Liacyr Ribeiro, Affonso J. Accorsi Jr, Roberto B. Rocha

Key points

- Tubular breast is the most severe and most typical form of the so called 'breast base anomalies'.
- Its etiology is an anomaly of the fascia superficialis in the breast.
- It is difficult to treat and has a tendency to recur.
- Its treatment is based in the disruption of the constricting ring that is present in the breast.
- The use of the inferiorly based flap described by the authors allows the disruption of this ring and the redistribution of the breast tissue.

Introduction

Tubular breast is a rare syndrome affecting young women unilaterally or bilaterally. Its real incidence remains unknown. First described in 1976 by Rees and Aston, it received the name of tuberous breast because of its resemblance to a 'tuberous plant root' (Rees 1976). However, its multiplicity of clinical manifestations has led to great confusion among plastic surgeons, mainly in the nomenclature used. Tubular breasts, tuberous breasts, snoopy breasts, domed nipple, herniated areolar complex, constricted breasts, are some of the names used to describe this deformity. Dinner considers it a syndrome rather than a single deformity (Dinner 1998), consisting of: (1) hypertrophy of the nipple/areola complex; (2) pseudoherniation of the breast content into the areola, producing the very typical Snoopy-dog-nose deformity; (3) hypoplasia with commonly related asymmetry with the contralateral side; (4) vertical constriction with the reduced superior inferior diameter; and (5) a constricted transverse base. It is considered the most severe and most typical form of a group of breast anomalies called 'breast base anomalies' and it represents one of the most challenging surgical conditions of the breast because of its tendency to recur.

Etiology

Great controversy exists about its etiology. Recent observations led to the theory of anomalies of the fascia superficialis, in the form of strong adherence between the dermis and the muscular plane or the presence of a constricting fibrous ring as a consequence of a thickening of the superficial fascia (Grolleau et al 1999, Mandrekas et al 2003). In both cases, the result is the impairment of the normal development of the breast, restricting its peripheral expansion, with consequent narrowing of the breast base, and preferential forward development into the areolar area, where the fascia superficialis is absent, giving the breast its tubular appearance and enlarging the areola. Clinical observations favor the presence of the constricting fibrous ring and its disruption is the most important step in the treatment of the disorder (Ribeiro et al 1998, 2002, 2005, Ribeiro & Accorsi 2007).

Classification

The tubular breast is the most typical form of a group of disorders that are characterized by anomalies of the breast base and that generally involve the lower quadrants. Von Heimburg et al classified it in four types: Type I, hypoplasia of the lower medial quadrant; Type II, hypoplasia of the lower medial and lateral quadrants, sufficient skin in the subareolar region; Type III, hypoplasia of the lower medial and lateral quadrants, deficiency of skin in the subareolar; Type IV, severe breast constriction, minimal breast base (von Heimburg et al 1996).

Treatment

Many techniques developed to treat this condition have yielded poor results. Pushing the mammary gland through the pseudohernia and narrowing the areolar diameter, removing a doughnut-shaped piece of skin, will not correct the deformity. Treatment by simply inserting an implant accentuates the deformity, creating a second crease and dropping the entire gland over the implant. As mentioned earlier, to correct the deformity it is necessary to disrupt the constricting ring, which is achieved by the creation of a dermo-adipose-glandular flap inferiorly based, also called inferior pedicle, that was created by the senior author in 1973 (Ribeiro & Baker 1973). Another point is the redistribution of the mammary tissue, to allow the filling of the inferior quadrants and enlarge the base of the breast, which is constricted in the great majority of the cases. The procedure is easily performed and may also include implant placement (Ribeiro et al 2002, 2005, Ribeiro & Accorsi 2007).

Surgical sequence

In cases of severe hypoplasia, breast implants can be used uni- or bilaterally to reach a better result. The surgery, with or without implants, is quite similar, differing only in the inclusion of the silicone implant and the closure of the space in which it was intro-

duced. The surgery is always performed under general anesthesia.

Pre-operative preparation

With the patient in dorsal decubitus and half-seated position, under general anesthesia, the new areola is drawn with a diameter of 4 cm. The external limit of the areola is also drawn, demarcating the excessive areola to be removed. The submammary sulcus is marked, and this represents the inferior limit of dissection of the inferior flap to be created (Figure 10.1). In cases of highly hypoplastic lower quadrant, we discard the actual position of the sulcus and mark it more inferiorly in a new desired position. It is important to mention that asymmetry is frequently present, so the markings are made independently.

Operative techniques

Surgery without breast implants

The circumareolar region is de-epithelialized (Figure 10.2). The inferior based flap is started by dividing the gland in two halves with an incision in the infraareolar region perpendicular to the thoracic wall and reaching the pectoral fascia (Figure 10.3). This creates the superior hemisphere which keeps the nipple–areola complex and the inferior hemisphere from which the inferior flap will be made. The inferior portion of the gland is freed from its skin with the use of scissors limiting the dissection to the sulcus previ-

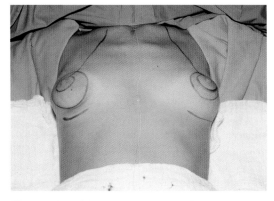

Figure 10.1 Markings. New areola with 4 cm diameter, exceeding halo and a new inframammary fold are drawn.

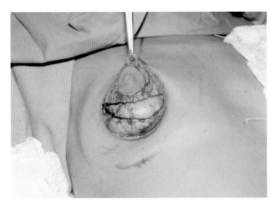

Figure 10.2 Circumareolar region already de-
epithelialized and drawing of the
reference line for gland division into
upper and lower hemispheres.

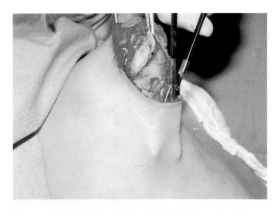

Figure 10.4 Undermining of the inferior pole with
scissors.

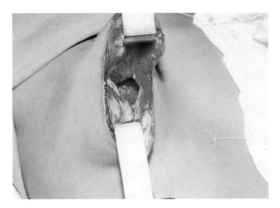

Figure 10.3 Complete breast gland division up to the
muscular plane.

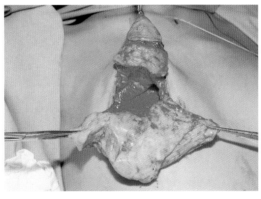

Figure 10.5 Inferior pole completely freed from its
skin.

ously marked (Figure 10.4). The lateral and medial
prolongations of the gland are resected, with care
being taken not to injure the perforating vessels from
the fourth and fifth intercostal vessels (Figure 10.5).
The creation of this flap will lead to the disruption of
the constricting ring which is responsible for the herniation (Figures 10.6, 10.7). Mounting of the breast
begins with the fixation of the inferior flap on the
thoracic wall. Fix the distal end of the flap inferiorly
to its base, bending it over itself, using non-absorbable
sutures (Figures 10.8, 10.9). This maneuver is important to fill the inferior quadrants, which generally are
hypoplastic (Figure 10.10). The upper portion is left
to fall naturally over the inferior flap causing the
mammary base to become enlarged (Figure 10.11).
The breast is closed using a periareolar suture by the

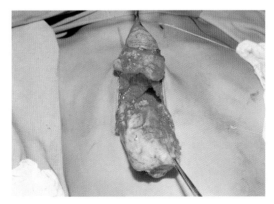

Figure 10.6 Inferior flap created after resection of
the lateral and medial prolongations.

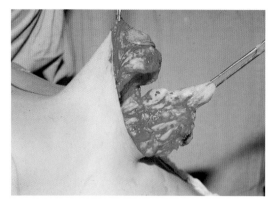

Figure 10.7 Lateral view of the upper pole with the areola and the inferior flap.

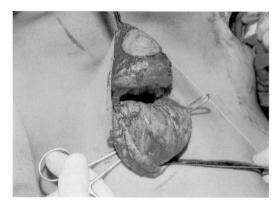

Figure 10.8 Starting the fixation of the flap on the thoracic wall. The flap is bent over itself, inferiorly to its base, so that the inferior quadrants are completed.

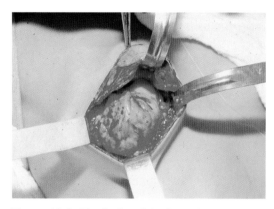

Figure 10.9 The fixation of the flap is done with nonabsorbable sutures.

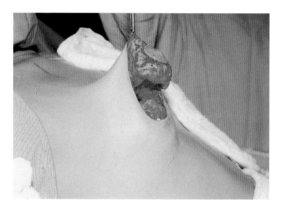

Figure 10.10 Lateral view of the inferior flap in position after being fixed to the thoracic wall. Note the completion of the inferior quadrants.

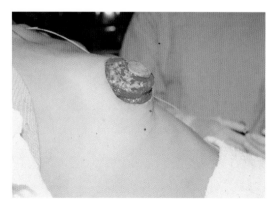

Figure 10.11 The upper hemisphere is left to lie over the inferior flap, promoting an enlargement of the entire breast base.

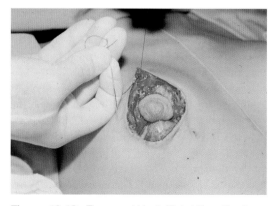

Figure 10.12 The round-block (Peled-Benelli) suture technique.

technique of Peled and Benelli performed with 2-0 nylon (Figures 10.12, 10.13) (Peled et al 1985, Benelli 1991). The areolar suture is done with separate stitches using 6-0 nylon (Figure 10.14). Suction drains are left for 24 hours. Immobilization of the breast with micro-porous tape is important and remains for 7 days (Figure 10.15).

Surgery with breast implants

The surgery is performed in the same way as described above, except that the inclusion of silicone prostheses is done after the fixation of the inferior flap in the thoracic wall. The prosthesis is placed between the superior hemisphere and the inferior flap and left in

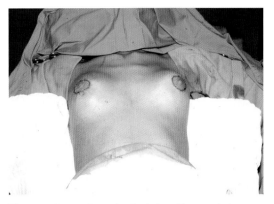

Figure 10.14   Operative final view. The areola is sutured with 6-0 nylon separate stitches.

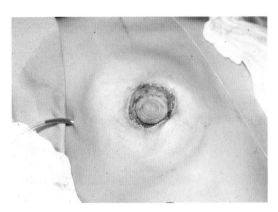

Figure 10.13   The round-block suture completed.

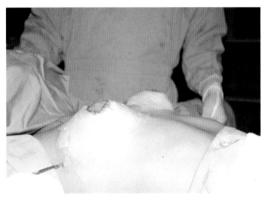

Figure 10.15   Immobilization of the breast with microporous tape. It is left in place for 7 days. Note the suction drain exiting through the axilla.

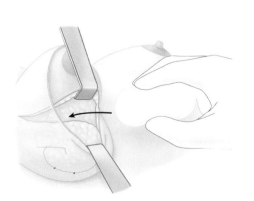

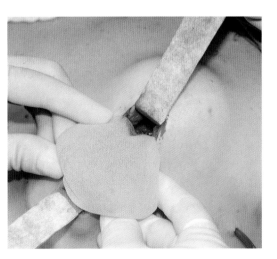

Figure 10.16   The insertion of the implant. The inclusion is made between the superior hemisphere and the inferior flap and left in the existing space between the two.

the existing space between the two (Figures 10.16, 10.17). After the introduction of the implant the space is closed with separate stitches fixing the inferior border of the superior segment to the superior border of the inferior flap (Figure 10.18). The skin is closed in the same way as described above (Figure 10.19).

Pitfalls and how to correct

As asymmetry is present in most cases, great care should be taken in marking the breasts, otherwise asymmetry of the breasts will occur. Hypoplasia of the inferior poles is always present so the actual submammary sulcus is located in a more cranial position. The new sulcus should be marked in a more inferior position so that the distance between the submammary sulcus and the inferior border of the areola is kept at approximately 6-8 cm depending on the breast size. Once one breast is marked, the points are transferred to the opposite breast so that symmetry is preserved.

Another important point is positioning the inferiorly based flap. As previously discussed, it is bent over

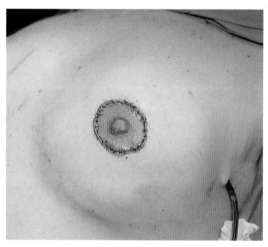

Figure 10.19 End of surgery. The areolar suture is done with separate stitches using 6-0 nylon. The suction drain exits through the axilla.

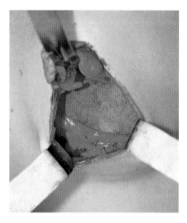

Figure 10.17 The breast implant in place.

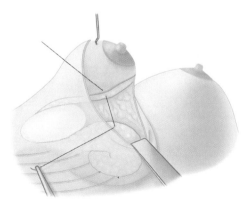 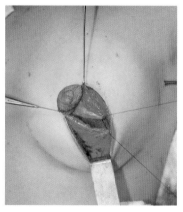

Figure 10.18 After the introduction of the implant the space is closed with separate stitches fixing the inferior border of the superior segment to the superior border of the inferior flap.

itself and fixed in an inferior position so that the inferior quadrants are fulfilled. The important point here is to fix the distal end of the flap to the thoracic fascia at the level of the new submammary sulcus marked on the skin. Failure to do so, with the fixation of the flap superiorly, will result in the maintenance of 'hypoplastic' inferior quadrants. Fixing it too low will result in a breast with the submammary sulcus too low in the thorax.

Post-operative care

The patient remains in hospital until the following morning. At this time the dressings are changed and the suction drains are removed. During the recovery time the patient is advised to limit the movement of the arms. On the seventh post-operative day, the tape immobilization is removed. The removal of the stitches begins on the seventh post-operative day and goes through to the tenth day. The patient is advised to

limit physical activities for 30 days, after which they can resume normal activities.

Conclusion

The abundance of techniques available in the literature for the correction of the tubular breast attests to the great challenge of treating this deformity. The peri-areolar approach with de-epithelialization of the excessive areola and its closure with a round-block suture are common to various techniques. The main feature of our technique, and what separates it from others, is the prevention of recurrence by dividing the gland in half and creating the inferiorly based glandular flap. Both of these maneuvers account for the disruption of the constricting ring. Our technique has successfully corrected this deformity (Figures 10.20, 10.21), which can affect the patients so severely from a psychological standpoint, with pleasing aesthetic results and no recurrence.

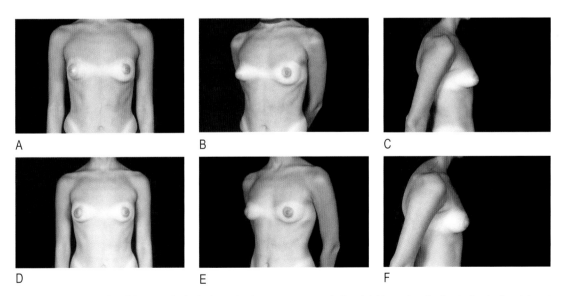

Figure 10.20 (A–C) Mild case of tubular breast where we can see in the right breast reduction in the horizontal and vertical diameters and mild pseudoherniation of the areola. The left breast is normal, except for its small size. (D–F) Correction of the deformity without the use of prostheses. Two years follow-up. The patient wanted small breasts.

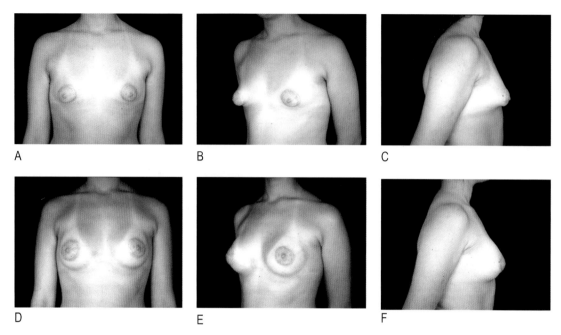

Figure 10.21 (A–C) A case of recurrence after 1 year of surgery. Persistence of the base constriction (fibrous ring) and pseudoherniation of the areola. Note the periareolar scar. Correction with the use of 155 ml round, high profile, prostheses. (D–F) Eighteen months post-operatively.

Further reading

Benelli L. Technique personnelle de plastie mammaire periareolaire: le round block. Cah Chir 1991;77:15.

Dinner MI. Discussion. Tuberous breast: a new approach. Plast Reconstr Surg 1998;101:51.

Grolleau JL, Lanfrey E, Lavigne B et al. Breast base anomalies: treatment strategy for tuberous breasts, minor deformities, and asymmetry. Plast Reconstr Surg 1999;104:2040.

Mandrekas AD, Zambacos GJ, Anastasopoulos A et al. Aesthetic reconstruction of the tuberous breast deformity. Plast Reconstr Surg 2003;112:1099.

Peled IJ, Zagher U, Wexler MR. Purse string suture to reduction and closure of skin defects. Ann Plast Surg 1985;14:465.

Rees TD, Aston SJ. The tuberous breast. Clin Plast Surg 1976;3:339.

Ribeiro L, Baker E. Mastoplastia con pedículo de seguridad. Rev Esp Cir Plast 1973;16:223.

Ribeiro L, Canzi W, Buss A, Jr, Accorsi A, Jr. Tuberous breast: a new approach. Plast Reconstr Surg 1998;101:42.

Ribeiro L, Accorsi A Jr, Buss A, Pessja MCM. Short scar correction of the tuberous breast. Clin Plast Surg 2002;29:423.

Ribeiro L, Accorsi A, Jr, Argencio V. Tuberous breast: a periareolar approach. Aesthetic Surg J 2005;25:398.

Ribeiro L, Accorsi A, Jr. Mama tuberosa. In Rietjens M, Urban CA, eds. Cirurgia da Mama, Estética e Reconstrutora. Rio de Janeiro: Revinter; 2007:191-201.

Von Heimburg HD, Exner K, Kruft S, Lemperle G. The tuberous breast deformity: classification and treatment. Br J Plast Surg 1996;49:339.

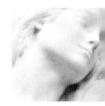

11

Mastopexy: augmentation

G. Patrick Maxwell, Allen Gabriel

Key points

- Goals of mastopexy.
- Breast ptosis etiology.
- Breast ptosis classification.
- Patient evaluation.
- BioDimensional® pre-operative planning.

- Selection of operation.
- Patient marking.
- Operative approach.
- Managing complications.
- Post-operative care.

Mastopexy is one of the most demanding operations in breast surgery and although it may increase the challenge, performing simultaneous breast augmentation can be an effective way of producing an aesthetic breast form. As the breast mound descends on the chest wall, patients will display variability in breast shape, tissue laxity, symmetry, parenchymal distribution, and nipple position. While numerous options exist for restoring a youthful appearing breast, the common goals are to raise the nipple–areola complex, decrease the skin envelope, achieve symmetry, and improve the breast shape, while maintaining or increasing volume. Furthermore, the additional challenge is to provide a correction that will endure the test of time.

Appropriate and thorough pre-operative evaluation will allow the surgeon to select and plan a suitable operation. Choosing the proper technique begins with designing incisions based on scar placement and length. Minimizing scar appearance is fundamental to any operation in plastic surgery. However, scars should not be avoided if they are necessary to provide adequate and durable results. A balance must be accomplished between scar placement and efficacy, as the final result will depend on the harmony of the breast shape and scar appearance.

The terms 'short scar' or 'limited scar' have been used interchangeably and applied to many different techniques. As a result, virtually any procedure that leaves a final scar shorter then the classic inverted-T has been classified as such. Explanation of these terms can be essential when counseling patients who are demanding minimal incision lengths and maximal results. For each patient, the surgeon should develop a strategy for reshaping and positioning the breast parenchyma and also determine the need, if any, for additional soft tissue augmentation with an implant or autologous flap. Breast shaping can be elaborate or

Mastopexy: augmentation

simple and may include combinations of suturing, local flaps, muscle slings, or placement of internal mesh support.

Combining augmentation with mastopexy can be accomplished safely for many patients. Clearly, adding an implant to an already complex operation will increase the number of variables that the surgeon must consider. Many women with ptotic breasts focus more on the loss of upper pole volume that has occurred as their breasts have aged, than on the change in nipple position that has accompanied it. An implant can be a very powerful tool in restoring youthful fullness to the upper pole.

Patient selection

The initial consultation for mastopexy should include a detailed discussion of the patient's goals and expectations and a careful review of medical and psychiatric histories. As with any breast surgery, a personal and family history of breast disease or cancer should be obtained. The surgeon should specifically note a history of any previous breast surgery or radiation therapy. Pre-operative mammography is recommended for any patient with significant risk factors and patients over 35 years of age.

Prior surgical history should include previous augmentation or reduction procedures. When possible, operative notes detailing techniques and implant devices used should be reviewed. Information about past or planned pregnancies and changes in weight and/or brassiere size can also aid in pre-operative assessment. Management of patient expectations is crucial to ensuring satisfaction. The ideal breast aesthetic may vary greatly between patients and surgeons. Every attempt should be made to understand the patient's motivations and anticipated results. Patients who are unrealistic or unwilling to accept the necessary scars should be avoided.

The pre-operative physical examination should include measurements as well as an assessment of tissue qualities and distribution. Significant asymmetries will exist in the majority of patients when carefully examined. It is important to recognize and point out any preexisting asymmetries, spinal curvature, or chest wall deformities as these may be difficult to correct and can become noticeable in the postoperative period. Preoperative photographs with multiple views are obtained on all patients and maintained as part of the office record.

Thorough palpation of the breast and axilla should be performed and documented. Any palpable masses or lymph nodes must be evaluated before proceeding with surgery. Measurements of breast width (BW), breast height (BH), intermammary distance, nipple to suprasternal notch (NSSN), and nipple to inframammary fold (NIMF) should be made and documented. Measurements can aid in planning the operation, recognizing asymmetries, and tracking post-operative results.

The formerly Inamed Corporation has developed the BioDimensional® pre-operative planning system to facilitate planning in augmentation mammoplasty (Table 11.1). The same principles can be applied when preparing for mastopexy or mastopexy augmentation. Essentially, the approach should be to first analyze the existing chest and breast form as described. Following that one should characterize the soft tissue envelope and plan the desired resultant breast form. Once accomplished the surgeon can assimilate the information to select an appropriate implant, if desired, and plan the mastopexy approach.

Indications

Breast ptosis is most often a consequence of aging tissues. Over time, Cooper's ligaments become attenuated and the breast loses its fascial support, frequently with a concurrent decrease in volume. Age-related changes are often hastened or mimicked by weight loss and involutional changes seen with pregnancy/ lactation and menopause. Regardless of the etiology,

Table 11.1 Preoperative planning and dimensional analysis

1. Carefully analyze and measure the dimensions and shape of the existing breast
2. Analyze the character and evaluate the adequacy of the soft tissue envelope
3. Develop an anatomically well-defined goal for the breast shape after mastopexy or mastopexy augmentation
4. Select implant size, shape, height, width & projection to accomplish the individual patient's goals
5. Select surgical approach (incisions) and implant location

Table 11.2 Regnault classification

Grade I	Nipple at the level of the IMF, above the lower contour of the gland
Grade II	Nipple below IMF, above the lower contour of the gland
Grade III	Nipple below IMF and at the lower contour of the gland
Pseudoptosis	Normal nipple position with glandular tissue below the IMF

a useful tool for the surgeon is to classify patients by the degree of ptosis present. The classification system used most frequently was first described by Regnault and grades the breast based on the position of the nipple relative to the inframammary fold (IMF) (Table 11.2). The amount of pre-operative ptosis can be used as a guide to selecting the operation necessary to achieve correction.

Patient marking

Pre-operative markings are made with the patient in an upright position and begin with midline, current IMF, and planned nipple position. Additional marks, determined by the patient's tissue characteristics, are then made as guidelines for resection. Nipple position is established using the current IMF as a guide, by making the mark along the breast meridian while manually palpating the fold. The location of this point is confirmed by checking its distance from the suprasternal notch and mid-clavicle bilaterally. This is usually 20 ± 3 cm from the suprasternal notch. At this point, the surgeon should determine the planned excision pattern and proceed with the appropriate marks. The degree of mastopexy will vary from a periareolar approach to a full inverted-T scar based on the amount of ptosis present. Variations in incision patterns are the same for augmentation mastopexy and mastopexy alone and are gradually increased to accommodate increasing amounts of breast tissue and ptosis.

Minor ptosis is usually addressed with a periareolar approach either concentrically or eccentrically designed. This pattern places the scar at the border of the pigmented areola and the breast skin. A point is first made just superior to the planned nipple position and represents the planned position of the upper areolar border. This should be no more than 3 cm above the transposed inframammary fold mark. The areola to be preserved is outlined using a standard nipple marker at 38–42 mm. The distance from the nipple to the planned position of the upper areolar

border can be used as the radius for designing a concentric pattern. Often it is necessary to adjust this to a more oval shaped or eccentric configuration to correct for asymmetries and variations in tissue distribution.

When addressing moderate ptosis, a vertical excision is marked. This is done by first repeating the initial steps above to determine the position of the new nipple and upper areolar border. The distance from the center of the nipple to the new upper areolar border is then used to set the width of the planned vertical excision. The vertical limbs are drawn connecting to a point 1–2 cm above the IMF. Adjusting the distance between the vertical limbs will accommodate individual tissue characteristics and asymmetries. This is often done when tailor-tacking as described below.

Patients with more severe ptosis usually require greater nipple elevation and a horizontal excision to achieve adequate correction. The horizontal component will vary from a traditional Wise pattern marking to a shorter version that is adapted into the vertical pattern described above. Marking this pattern begins as described as above and places the horizontal scar along the IMF with the T-junction designed to rest along the breast meridian. When planning simultaneous augmentation, these marks are made conservatively to allow for the excess tension that will be created when an implant is placed. This helps to avoid problems with healing at the T-junction. Regardless of the pattern chosen, all marks are customized to the individual patient, carefully measured, and confirmed with tailor-tacking in the operating room before proceeding with excision.

Operative technique

The patient is placed supine on the operating room table with the arms carefully secured at 90 degree angles to the torso. Patient positioning is crucial to permit for upright posture in the operating room as necessary. After induction of general anesthesia the patients are sterilely prepped to allow for complete visualization of the anterior chest and shoulders. When planning a simultaneous augmentation, the author's preference is to divide the operation into two parts. First, a dimensionally based breast augmentation is completed. Then, the patient is placed in the sitting position at 90 degrees, and pre-operative markings are tailor-tacked and adjusted before completing the mastopexy.

Implant selection and placement is judged according to the pre-operative measurements. Decisions on implant size, shape, surface texture, and filling material are made based on the soft tissue components present. Selection of an implant with enhanced projection can offer the mechanical advantage of raising the position of the nipple–areola complex. In patients with minor amounts of ptosis, this approach can sometimes alleviate the need for a mastopexy. Likewise, it may in a sense 'down stage' a patient from one degree of ptosis to the next. Therefore, a patient who would need a circumvertical scar to achieve an adequate result may only need a periareolar tightening once the implant is in place. Our preference is to use an anatomic, form-stable cohesive gel implant with enhanced projection for optimal results.

Once a device is selected, the surgeon must determine the implant's location. Patients with a superior pole pinch test result of 2 cm or greater can be considered for subglandular or subfascial implant placement. The subfascial plane may offer additional soft tissue coverage and support. Thinner patients will be at risk for implant palpability and visibility and may also risk blood supply to the nipple–areola complex when concurrent mastopexy is performed. For these patients, a subpectoral dissection is planned. During submuscular implant placement, our preference is to release the inferior portion of the pectoralis major muscle leaving the implant in a partial subpectoral position.

At this point, the pre-operative markings are confirmed with tailor-tacking in the sitting position before proceeding with mastopexy. When using the periareolar approach, the outer and inner circumferences are incised and the intervening skin is de-epithelialized. Often the dermis is then incised at the periphery to create a ledge for closure. When no glandular resection or undermining is performed, nipple vascularity is maintained via perforating vessels. If the vascularity is potentially compromised, care is taken to preserve the subdermal plexus during de-epthelialization and

dermal incisions are avoided. Closure is secured with a non-absorbable Gore-Tex® suture on a straight needle using a 'pin-wheel' or 'wagon-wheel' technique. When correctly placed, this suture controls the areolar diameter, helps to prevent areolar widening, and reduces periareolar wrinkling and pleats by evenly distributing tissues. A running subcuticular 5-0 Monocryl® is then placed superficially with care not to disrupt the previous suture.

Patients with moderate degrees of ptosis will often require a vertical component to the scar with or without a short horizontal excision. The vertical component can be part of the pre-operative design or added intraoperatively to distribute excess tissue encountered with the periareolar excision. In either situation, the inferior extent of the resection is kept at least 1–2 cm above the location of the IMF. As above, the preoperative markings are used as a guide and are confirmed and adjusted before making incisions. Tightening of the lower pole helps redistribute fullness superiorly to a more desired location improving breast shape and projection. This may be helpful when correcting glandular or pseudoptosis as well and in this instance can sometimes be done without a periareolar scar. In addition, if the breast appears flattened or the lower pole prominent after the periareolar excision, vertical skin plication can offer correction. In cases where a vertical excision can be easily predicted, access for implant placement in any plane can be gained through the center of the vertical incision.

Severe ptosis is corrected with an inverted-T excision varying the length of the horizontal scar to accommodate the soft tissue needs. As this often requires greater degrees of nipple elevation, consideration is given to maintaining vascularity on a dermoglandular pedicle. Our preference is to use a superiomedial pedicle as this offers ease of nipple elevation and flexibility for implant placement. However, other pedicles could be safely employed. Skin patterns are conservatively designed when an implant is anticipated.

Closure

After implant insertion and tailor-tacking, flaps are raised and the breast mound is reshaped and secured over the implant. Periareolar closure is performed as described above and a layered closure of the vertical and horizontal limbs follows. Drains are considered when more extensive dissection has been completed.

Operative steps

- BioDimensional® approach.
- Plan and carry out two operations at once.
- Sit patient up 90 degrees and tailor tack.
- Non-absorbable 'pin-wheel' closure.
- Maintain nipple vascularity.

Case **1**

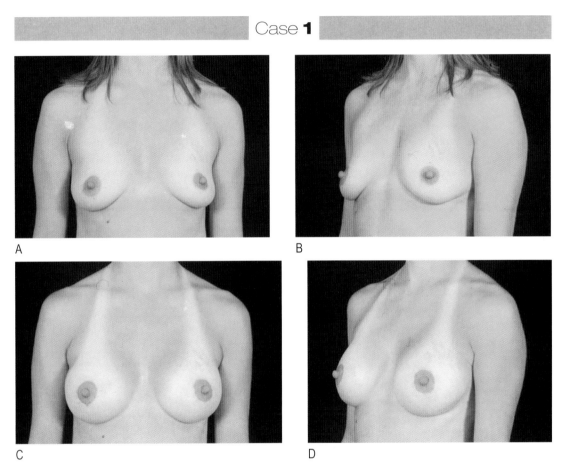

A

B

C

D

Figure 11.1 A 32-year-old woman with pseudoptosis to first degree ptosis treated with subpectoral placement of a 280 mL silicone gel implant with a periareolar purse string mastopexy. (A) Pre-operative frontal view. (B) Post-operative frontal view. (C) Pre-operative lateral view. (D) Post-operative lateral view.

Case **2**

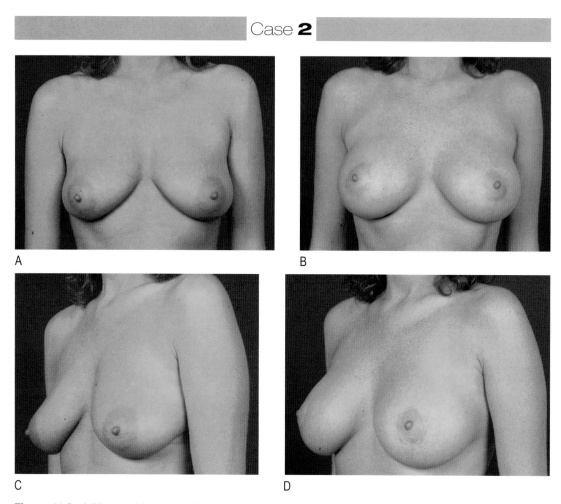

A

B

C

D

Figure 11.2 A 30-year-old woman with first to second degree ptosis treated with subfacial placement of 250 mL silicone gel implants with periareolar purse string mastopexy. (A) Pre-operative frontal view. (B) Post-operative frontal view. (C) Pre-operative lateral view. (D) Post-operative lateral view.

Case **3**

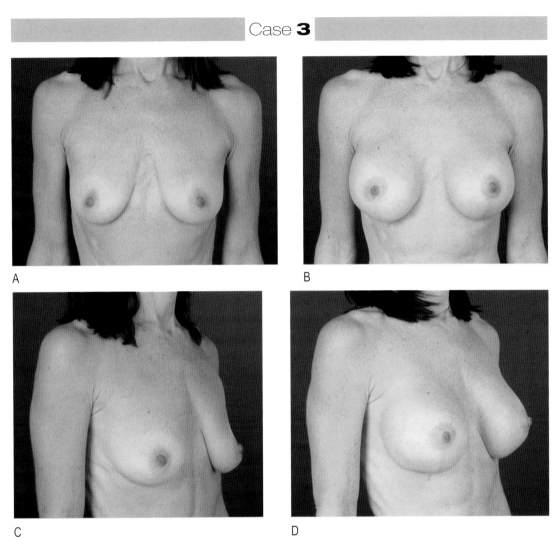

A

B

C

D

Figure 11.3 A 40-year-old woman with second to third degree ptosis treated with subpectoral placement of 375 mL 410 form stable silicone gel anatomical breast implants and a periareolar purse string mastopexy with vertical and transverse skin excision. (A) Pre-operative frontal view. (B) Post-operative frontal view. (C) Pre-operative lateral view. (D) Post-operative lateral view.

Mastopexy: augmentation

Case **4**

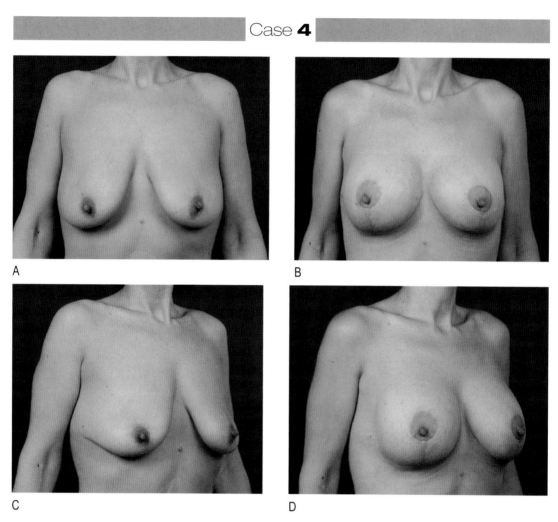

A

B

C

D

Figure 11.4 A 45-year-old woman with second to third degree mammary ptosis treated with subpectoral 350 mL silicone gel breast implants and periareolar purse string plus wise pattern type skin excision. (A) Pre-operative frontal view. (B) Post-operative frontal view. (C) Pre-operative lateral view. (D) Post-operative lateral view.

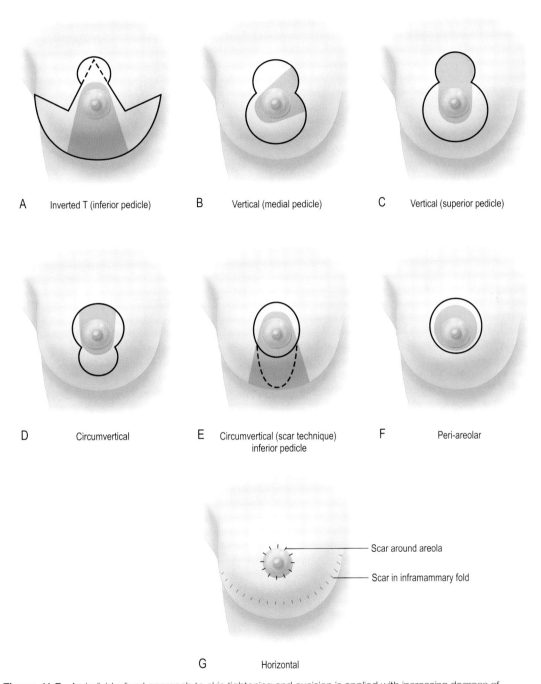

A   Inverted T (inferior pedicle)

B   Vertical (medial pedicle)

C   Vertical (superior pedicle)

D   Circumvertical

E   Circumvertical (scar technique) inferior pedicle

F   Peri-areolar

Scar around areola

Scar in inframammary fold

G   Horizontal

Figure 11.5 An individualized approach to skin tightening and excision is applied with increasing degrees of mammary ptosis. Thus lesser degrees of ptosis require no or little skin excision whereas increasing degrees require the most skin tightening or excision. (A) Periareolar approach with internal rearrangement or insertion of implant. (B) Periareolar excision. (C) Circumareolar with vertical excision. (D) Circumareolar plus 'J' excision, which, with increasing ptosis, turns into a wider 'J' or 'B' excision. (E) Circumareolar with vertical and small transverse excision. (F) Wise pattern-type excision. With all these skin patterns an implant may be inserted, internal tissue rearrangement performed, or simply skin tightening.

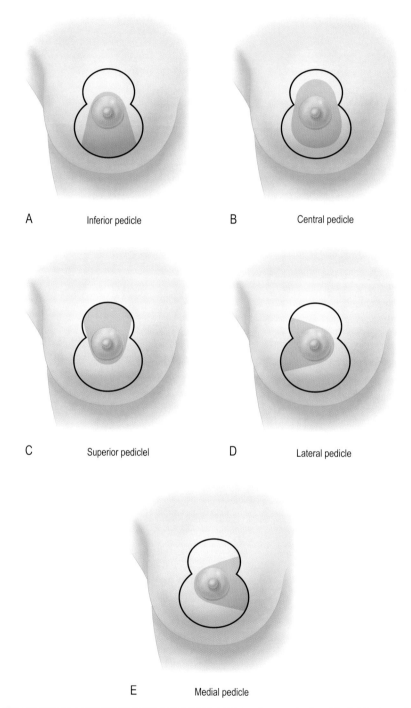

A   Inferior pedicle   B   Central pedicle

C   Superior pediclel   D   Lateral pedicle

E   Medial pedicle

Figure 11.6 The addition of a periareolar purse string gives enhanced power to the skin tightening adjustments and uplifts the lower skin excess, so that all vertical to 'T' type scars are minimized with the addition of the purse string. (A) Periareolar purse string mastopexy. (B) Extended periareolar purse string mastopexy. (C) Circumvertical periareolar mastopexy. (D) 'J' to 'B' excison plus periareolar purse string mastopexy. (E) Transverse 'T' excision plus periareolar purse string mastopexy. (F) Wise type pattern plus periareolar purse string mastopexy.

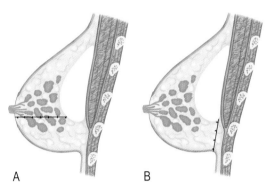

Figure 11.7 In performing the 'two operations in one' augment mastopexy, the implant is inserted via a periareolar (A) or inframammary (B) approach. It is placed in its desired respective pocket (subpectoral, subfascial or subglandular), and the parenchyma is sutured off securing the implant in its proper position.

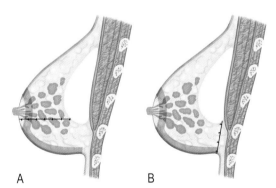

Figure 11.8 For more excessive degrees of ptosis, the second stage of the 'two operations in one' includes a circumvertical or circumvertical plus transverse skin excision component, performed over the implant secured in its deep pocket.

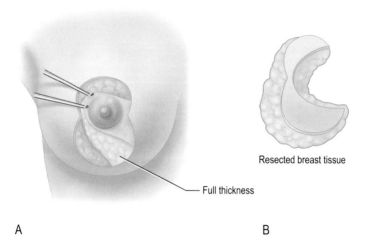

Resected breast tissue

Full thickness

A

B

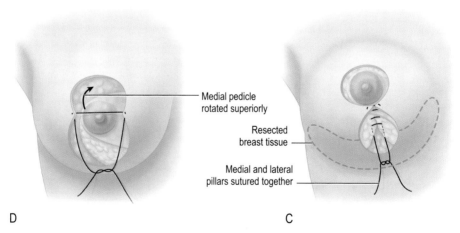

Medial pedicle
rotated superiorly

Resected
breast tissue

Medial and lateral
pillars sutured together

D

C

Figure 11.9   Once the implant is secured, the second step of the 'two operations in one' is performed. Here a periareolar purse string mastopexy is applied to the soft tissue envelope over the implant secured in its pocket.

Pitfalls and how to correct

Complications can be subdivided temporally and by relation to breast implantation. Patient education and photo documentation cannot be overemphasized. When combining mastopexy with augmentation, complications inherent and unique to the implant device must be anticipated and explained to the patient. Specifically, this would include capsular contracture and implant rupture or deflation.

In the perioperative period, hematomas and infections can be encountered. Careful pre-operative counseling regarding cessation of any prescription or over-the-counter herbs or medications that may impair clotting or platelet function is essential. Immediate evacuation of any recognized hematoma is recommended in order to avoid possible late sequelae. Infections can range from superficial cellulitis to purulent periprosthetic collections. Prophylaxis is administered prior to induction of anesthesia with a single dose of intravenous antibiotics and is continued with an oral regimen for three post-operative days. Alterations in nipple sensation can be transient or permanent and are often a major source of concern for the patient. Careful attention is directed during implant placement to avoid overdissection or transection of the lateral intercostal cutaneous nerves.

Errors in nipple placement can be difficult to correct especially when the nipple position is too high on the breast mound. This is best treated by avoiding the problem with careful measurements. Placing the implant first and then tailor-tacking the mastopexy design into place before re-measuring and assessing the patient in an upright position is crucial to avoiding this problem. Nipple–areola necrosis is avoided by maintaining blood supply via glandular perforators or a dermoglandular pedicle. Caution should be exercised when a subglandular plane is dissected or in patients with diabetes, collagen vascular disease, or a smoking history.

Asymmetries can often be corrected at the time of operation but may persist or become more noticeable in the recovery period. Again, photo documentation and patient education are paramount to ensuring satisfaction. Minor asymmetries that persist can be addressed in a second stage that should be delayed at least 6 months. It is our preference to perform mastopexy augmentation as a single stage rather than with two separate operations even though this may increase the need for minor revisions. These revisions are often much less invasive and are regularly performed with local anesthesia in the office setting when necessary.

Late consequences include recurrent ptosis and scar widening or hypertrophy. Problems with areolar spreading have been largely addressed with the use of permanent sutures and the 'pin-wheel' technique. We avoid horizontal scars on the medial and lateral aspects of the chest wall when possible. If scar hypertrophy is encountered, this is usually addressed with local steroid injections. Recurrent ptosis is an unfortunate consequence of poor tissue quality and lack of fascial support. There are many different maneuvers designed to minimize this, as described above, but none can stop the effects of gravity on aging tissues.

Post-operative care

The vast majority of these procedures are performed in the outpatient setting. Wounds are dressed with Steri-Strips and a supportive gauze dressing. Patients are allowed to shower on post-operative day 2. After 3–5 days, the patients are seen in the office for their first follow up visit. At that time, patients with smooth implant devices are instructed in implant mobility exercises. Patients felt to be at risk for superior implant displacement are managed with an elastic band across the superior pole providing gentle downward pressure. Upper body and vigorous exercise is restricted for 2–4 weeks. Regular follow up appointments are scheduled at 1 month, 3 months and 1 year. All patients are photographed in the post-operative period.

Conclusion

Mastopexy and mastopexy augmentation present a unique challenge to the plastic surgeon. Emphasis should be placed on thorough preoperative evaluation combined with a biodimensional approach. Performing the operation in two parts in the same setting will allow for safe, predictable outcomes.

Further reading

Benelli L. A new periareolar mammaplasty: the 'round block' technique. Aesthetic Plast Surg 1990;14:93–100.

Benelli LC. Mastopexy and reduction: The 'round block'. In: Spear SL (Ed). Surgery of the Breast: Principles and Art 2nd edn. Philadelphia, PA: Lippincott Williams & Wilkins; 2006: 977–990.

Goes JC, Landecker A, Lyra EC et al. The application of mesh support in periareolar breast surgery: clinical and mammographic evaluation. Aesth Plast Surg 2004;28:268–274.

Graf R, Biggs TM. Mastopexy with a pectoralis muscle loop. In: Spear SL (Ed). Surgery of the Breast: Principles and Art, 2nd edn. Philadelphia, PA: Lippincott Williams & Wilkins; 2006: 1008–1020.

Graf RM, Bernardes A, Auersvald A, Damasio RCC. Subfascial endoscopic transaxillary augmentation mammoplasty. Aesth Plast Surg 2000;24:216–220.

Graf RM, Bernardes A, Rippel R et al. Subfascial breast implant: a new procedure. Plast Reconstr Surg 2003;111:904–908.

Hammond DC. The SPAIR mammaplasty. Clin Plast Surg 2002;29:411–421.

Hammond DC. Augmentation mastopexy: General considerations. In: Spear SL (Ed). Surgery of the breast: Principles and Art, 2nd edn. Philadelphia, PA: Lippincott Williams & Wilkins; 2006: 1403–1416.

Hammond DC. Reduction mammaplasty and mastopexy: General considerations. In: Spear SL (Ed). Surgery of the Breast: Principles and Art, 2nd edn. Philadelphia, PA: Lippincott Williams & Wilkins; 2006: 971–976.

Regnault B. Breast ptosis. Definition and treatment. Clin Plast Surg 1976;3:193–203.

Regnault P, Rolin DK, Breast ptosis. In: Regnault P (Ed) Aesthetic Plastic Surgery. Boston, MA: Little, Brown & Co.; 1984: 539–558.

Rohrich RJ, Beran SJ, Restifo RJ, Copit SE. Aesthetic management of the breast following explantation: evaluation and mastopexy options. Plast Reconstr Surg 1998;101:827–837.

Rohrich RJ, Hartley W, Brown S. Incidence of breast and chest wall asymmetry in breast augmentation: a retrospective analysis of 100 patients. Plast Reconstr Surg 2003;111:1513–1519.

Rohrich, RJ, Thornton JF, Jakubietz RG et al. The limited scar mastopexy: Current concepts and approaches to correct breast ptosis. Plast Reconstr Surg 2004;114:1622–1630.

Spear SL, Kassan M, Little JW. Guidelines in concentric mastopexy. Plast Reconstr Surg 1990;85:961–966.

Spear SL, Giese SY, Ducic I. Concentric mastopexy revisited. Plast Reconstr Surg 2001;107:1294–1299.

Whidden PG. The tailor-tack mastopexy. Plast Reconstr Surg 1978;62:347–354.

Periareolar/vertical/ small horizontal scars

James C. Grotting, Phillip L. Lackey

Key points

- Reduction of scar burden and concealing of scars by placement in inconspicuous areas improves aesthetic outcomes in breast surgery.

- Periareolar incisions concealed in the breast skin–areola interface, while aesthetically advantageous, provide only limited access for breast reshaping or nipple repositioning. Correction of only mild ptosis and reductions <500 g are possible under the best of circumstances.

- Vertical scar breast techniques are well suited for reductions of <1500 g and correction of moderate breast ptosis.

- The extent to which pleasing aesthetic results can be achieved by periareolar and vertical scar breast techniques is heavily influenced by the quality of the breast gland and skin with more youthful breast and skin allowing for best results.

- Scar burden and visibility contribute only in part to overall aesthetic results in breast surgery. Breast shape, symmetry, and proportion to body habitus are equally important and efforts to limit scars may adversely affect the capacity to achieve other aesthetic goals.

Patient selection

Aesthetic results of periareolar or vertical scar breast techniques are heavily dependent on the quality of the breast gland and skin. Periareolar techniques are almost exclusively limited to younger patients with good skin thickness and elasticity. Firmer breasts with preserved integrity of Cooper's ligaments are also desirable, especially if any amount of breast reshaping or reduction is to be performed. If significant atrophy of the breast gland is present an implant may be needed to fill the skin envelope before using a periareolar technique to reposition the nipple. Generally, correction of mild ptosis and reductions of up to 500 g of breast tissue are possible with a periareolar approach.

Vertical scar techniques are more versatile than periareolar techniques. Reductions of up 1500 g and correction of moderate ptosis are possible. These techniques allow for more extensive breast parenchymal rearrangement and hence even fatty breast can be supported by columns and pillars of repositioned breast gland. Youthful breast skin and gland is still desirable but not as limiting as in the periareolar approach. A firmer breast will hold shape better and hence give longer lasting results while more elastic skin will have a lessened tendency to form widened scars (which because of its location over the anterior breast is already prominent). As in the periareolar technique, an implant may be used if additional volume is required at the time of vertical scar mastopexy.

Periareolar operative techniques

Concentric mastopexy without parenchyma reshaping

In women with good skin thickness and elasticity, nipple ptosis is often mild. Unless there is an accompanying significant degree of glandular ptosis or breast atrophy, periareolar skin excision alone can effectively recentralize the areola over the breast mound. The nipple can be repositioned up to 3 cm without undue tension. In women with mild ptosis and glandular atrophy, placing an implant in the same setting fills the skin envelope providing additional lift.

Pre-operative preparation

In the standing position, the superior areola position is determined by measurement from the sternal notch 19–22 cm along the breast meridian. This point is marked for each breast and symmetry is confirmed by measurement from the sternum to the marked position. Differences in symmetry can be 'split' between the breasts with final adjustments of position based on the centering of the nipple over the breast mound.

Based on the new areola position, a circular line of excision is marked. The diameter of the proposed line of excision ($D_{outside}$) based on the areolar diameter ($D_{original}$) and any amount of planned areolar reduction (D_{inside}) is constructed as defined by Spears (Figure 12.1). The final diameter of the closure can be predicted (Figure 12.1 Rule #3) for each breast and adjustments made to account for any asymmetry between the breasts.

Technique

Intraoperatively with the patient supine, the areola is distended and marked with an areolar sizer. The skin between the outer and inner circular marks is infil-

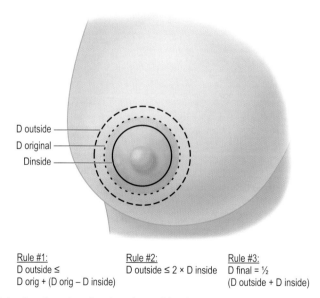

D outside
D original
D inside

Rule #1:
D outside ≤
D orig + (D orig − D inside)

Rule #2:
D outside ≤ 2 × D inside

Rule #3:
D final = ½
(D outside + D inside)

Figure 12.1 Determining the diameter of periareolar excision in concentric mastopexy. (Modified from Spear SL, Giese SY, Ducie I. Concentric mastopexy revisited. Plast Reconstr Surg 2001; 107:1294.)

trated using 0.5% lidocaine with 1:200 000 epinephrine and de-epithelialized. The caudal edge of exposed
dermis is then incised at its outer border from 2 o'clock
to 10 o'clock and elevated off the breast. This creates
a dermal flap which reduces tension on the skin
closure and may be folded underneath the areola to
maintain projection.

Closure

A deep dermal permanent suture (4-0 gore-tex or
mersilene) is placed in a running purse-string fashion
along the breast skin edge and cinched to the final
areolar diameter. Half-buried horizontal mattress 4-0
nylon sutures with the knot over the areolar skin are
then placed tacking the areola to the breast skin. A
running subcuticular 4-0 monocryl or PDS suture provides final skin closure.

Operative steps

- Infiltrate dermis between periareolar marks with local
  anesthetic containing epinephrine and
  de-epithelialize.
- Incise inferior border of de-epithelialized flap and tuck
  under areola.
- Cinch the breast skin down around the areola using
  a permanent suture run in the dermis as a purse-
  string cerclage.
- Approximate the areola and breast skin with half-
  buried mattress sutures and a running absorbable
  subcuticular suture.

The Benelli periareolar technique

The Benelli periareloar technique extends the periareolar approach to the breast to include a limited
reduction of the breast gland. Removal of central and
inferior glandular tissue followed by 'reconization'
parenchymal rearrangement is accomplished through
a periareolar incision. A decreased base diameter of
the breast results and pushes the areola superiorly
supported by breast parenchyma. This technique is
limited to <500 g of glandular excision although a
1200 g excision has been reported with good results.

Pre-operative preparation

Pre-operative marks are made with the patient standing. The midline and the estimated meridian of the
reshaped breast are marked. The estimated meridian

intersects the clavicle 6 cm from the midline. The level
of the inframammary fold is projected to the anterior
breast with finger tips and the superior border of the
new areolar position (point A) is marked 2 cm superior along the meridian. The future inferior border of
the areola (point B) is marked with the patient supine
5–12 cm superior to the inframammary fold. The
anticipated volume reduction and skin excision must
be considered when identifying this point as a larger
final volume of the breast will dictate a longer length.
The medial and lateral limits of the proposed skin
excision (points C and D respectively) are then placed
equidistant from the meridian at a level between A
and B with point C 8–12 cm lateral to the midline at
the level of the sternum. Points A through D are then
connected forming an ellipse. Point S is marked at the
midpoint of the inframammary fold (Figure 12.2).
The opposite breast is marked in a similar fashion,
insuring symmetry by the sternal notch to areola
distance and distance from the midline along the

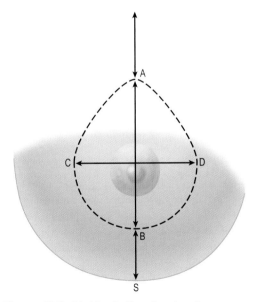

Figure 12.2   Marking for Benelli periareolar
mammaplasty. Point A marks the new
superior areolar position. Point B is the
inferior extent of excision. Points C and
D mark the medial and lateral limits of
excision. Point C lies 9–12 cm from
midline. Point S marks the midline of
the inframammary fold.

sternum to areola. Simulation of the final closure from points A to B and points C to D is performed to ensure there is no excess tension.

Technique

A wetting solution of 1000 mL saline mixed with 0.25 mg epinephrine and 20 mL of 2% lidocaine is infiltrated subcutaneously 3 cm outside the periareolar marks and into the prepectoral space. The areola is distended and marked under tension with a sizer. The skin between the sized areola and the marked ellipse is de-epithelialized. The de-epithelialized dermis is incised 1 cm from its outer border between the 2 o'clock and 10 o'clock positions. Subcutaneous dissection extending out from the incised ellipse follows over the upper outer, inferior, and medial breast being mindful to conserve adequate flap thickness to ensure blood supply (Figure 12.3A). Over the upper outer quadrant of the breast, dissection is more superficial to preserve extensions of the lateral thoracic artery.

Glandular resection follows, beginning with a semicircular incision through the gland some 3 cm from the inferior areolar edge. The incision is carried deep to the level of the prepectoral space. The inferior gland is incised vertically beyond the breast meridian to the level of the fascia creating four flaps: (1) a superior dermatoglandular flap carrying the areola; (2) a glandular medial flap; (3) a glandular lateral flap; and (4) a detached skin flap (Figure 12.3B). The glandular flaps are trimmed being cautious of reduction along the distal ends of the flaps which will reduce their length. If the breast requires no reduction or parenchymal rearrangement, no trimming is performed.

Closure

The breast is reassembled beginning with suture elevation of the superior dermatoglandular flap high on the chest wall to the pectoralis fascia (Figure 12.4A). Trimmed medial and lateral flaps are then folded over one another with the medial flap rotated first and sutured to the pectoralis fascia. The lateral flap is folded over the medial flap and sutured in place forming a 'cone' of glandular tissue (Figure 12.4B,C). If no trimming of the medial and lateral flaps was performed, the edges of the flaps can be simply plicated and invaginated to cone the breast shape.

Additional coning of the breast is accomplished with 'full-breast lacing'. Large-bite inverted sutures of braided 2-0 polyester are placed across the inferior

gland as retention sutures. The sutures are tied under minimal tension and help maintain shape, particularly when the gland is fatty and less firm (Figure 12.5). The deep dermal areolar undersurface is then suspended from the dermis of the superior border of the de-epithelialized ellipse with a suture passed through a small incision made at the 12 o'clock position (Figure 12.6A). The incision allows for the knot to be buried as the suture supports the areola without tension on the skin. A running intradermal permanent suture on a straight needle is then passed along the outer perimeter of the de-epithelialized ellipse through the 12 o'clock dermal incision. The suture is cinched down to the diameter of the areolar template and tied (Figure 12.6B). Diametrical transareolar U-stitches are then placed, anchored into the dermis of the breast skin edges, to help prevent areolar protrusion and better define the circular shape of the areola (Figure 12.6C). A 4-0 vicryl intradermal suture is run around the areola for final skin closure.

Operative steps

- Infiltrate subcutaneous and prepectoral spaces with dilute local anesthetic containing epinephrine 3 cm outside the planned area of excision.
- De-epithelialize periareolar skin between marks and then incise the de-epithelialized flap 1 cm from its outer edge between 2 and 10 o'clock.
- Undermine the skin over the upper outer, inferior and medial breast and then incise the inferior breast gland horizontally then vertically down to chest wall fascia to create four flaps.
- Suture the superior flap carrying the areola high on the chest wall to fascia.
- Trim excess gland tissue from medial and lateral gland flaps if needed and then secure the flaps over one another in a 'criss-cross' fashion giving addition support with placement of retention sutures.
- Cinch the periareolar breast skin down around the areola with a purse-string suture cerclage placed intradermally with the knot buried. Place additional transareolar 'U' stitches to support the areola and close skin with running subcuticular suture.

Góes periareolar technique with mesh support

The Góes periareolar technique supports the areola on a central dermatoglandular column created by

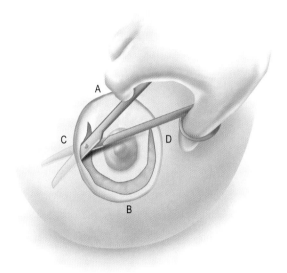

A

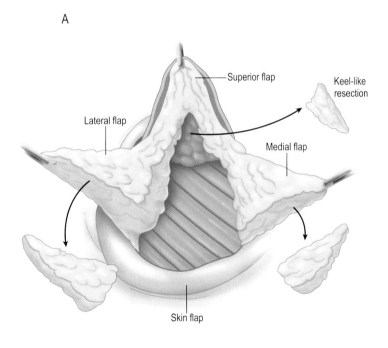

B

Figure 12.3 Benelli periareolar mammaplasty: (a) Skin undermining through incision in the de-epithelialized periareolar flap. (b) Creation of four flaps following glandular excisions which will be rearranged. (Modified from Benelli LC. Periareolar Benelli mastopexy and reduction: the 'round block'. In: Spear SL (Ed). Surgery of the Breast: Principles and Art, 2nd edn, Vol II Philadelphia, PA: Lippincott Williams & Wilkins; 2006: 70)

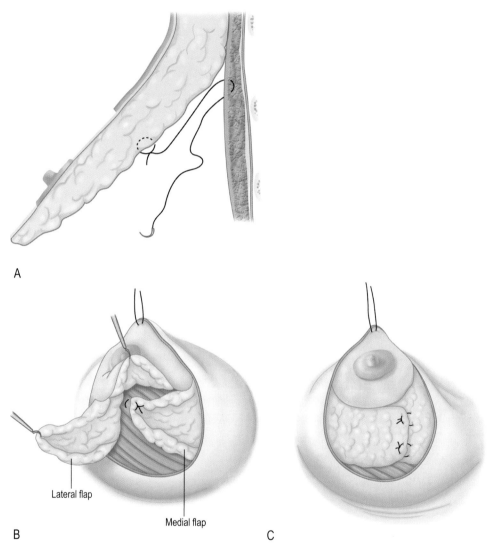

A

B

C

Lateral flap

Medial flap

Figure 12.4 Reassembly of the breast flaps in Benelli periareolar mammaplasty. (A) The superior flap carrying the areola is sutured from its undersurface high on the chest wall. (B) The medial breast flap is rotated laterally under the areola and sutured to the chest wall. (C) The lateral flap 'criss-crossed' over the medial flap and secured with sutures. (Modified from Benelli LC. Periareolar Benelli mastopexy and reduction: the 'round block'. In: Spear SL (Ed). Surgery of the Breast: Principles and Art, 2nd edn, Vol II. Philadelphia, PA: Lippincott Williams & Wilkins 2006: 70)

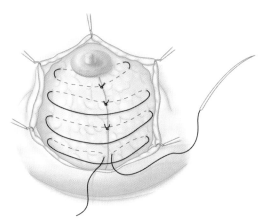

Figure 12.5 Benelli periareolar mammaplasty 'full breast lacing'. Inverted transverse 2-0 Mersilene® sutures are placed to cone and support the breast and tied under minimal tension. The first suture is placed transareolarily and helps control the nipple-areolar anterior projection. (Modified from Benelli LC. Periareolar Benelli mastopexy and reduction: the 'round block'. In: Spear SL (Ed). Surgery of the Breast: Principles and Art, 2nd edn. Vol II. Philadelphia, PA: Lippincott Williams & Wilkins; 2006: 70)

excision of parenchyma superiorly and inferiorly. A mixed vicryl and polypropylene (Vipro II™) mesh is also placed which acts as an 'internal brassiere' providing long-term shape to the breast. Initially the mesh is palpable but softens over time as it is incorporated. The mesh does not interfere with mammography. Again, the degree of gland reduction is generally limited to <500 g and is best suited for younger patients with good skin quality.

Pre-operative preparations

Four cardinal points are marked with the patient standing: the superior border of the new areola (point A) is marked 19–22 cm from the sternal notch; the new inferior border of the areola (point B) is marked 5–12 cm from the inframammary fold; the medial margin of excision (point C) lies 9 cm lateral of midline; and the lateral margin of resection (point D) lies 12 cm medial to the anterior axillary line. The four points are joined as an ellipse defining the limits of skin de-epithelialization (Figure 12.7).

Technique

The areola is distended and marked under tension using a sizer. The skin between the areola and the pre-operative marks is de-epithelialized after intradermal injection of a local anesthetic containing epinephrine. The outer perimeter is incised circumferentially and skin over the superior breast is undermined with progressive flap thickening down to the chest wall. Once the chest wall is encountered, undermining continues superiorly for another 5 cm over the pectoralis fascia. Turning inferiorly the dissection continues subglandular, preserving vascular perforators, until approximately one-third of the central gland has been freed. Skin over the inferior breast is then undermined forming a thin skin flap that extends down to the inframammary fold (Figure 12.8A). Wedges of excess breast tissue in the superior and inferior poles are then excised. Tissue at the base of the gland is not included in the excision in order to maintain gland attachments to the chest wall (Figure 12.8B).

Closure

The opposing edges of excised breast gland are closed with absorbable suture. The de-epithelialized dermis of the periareolar flap is then stretched over the gland and sutured superiorly to breast connective tissue and inferiorly to pectoralis fascia. Vipro II™ mesh is inserted between the breast skin and breast mound, encasing the glandular breast. The mesh is secured to the underlying breast and pectoralis fascia creating an 'internal brassiere' (Figure 12.9). A closed suction drain is placed and the breast skin is redraped over the mesh and the stretched periareolar flap dermis. A 2-0 mersilene suture on a straight needle is run in the deep dermis of the breast skin perimeter, cinched to the final areolar diameter, and tied. A continuous 4-0 monocryl periareolar subcuticular suture is then run for final skin closure (Figure 12.10).

Operative steps

- Infiltrate dermis between periareolar marks with local anesthetic containing epinephrine and de-epithelialize.
- Incise outer perimeter of de-epithelialized flap circumferentially, undermine skin superiorly and inferiorly, and separate the superior third of the central breast gland off the chest fascia.

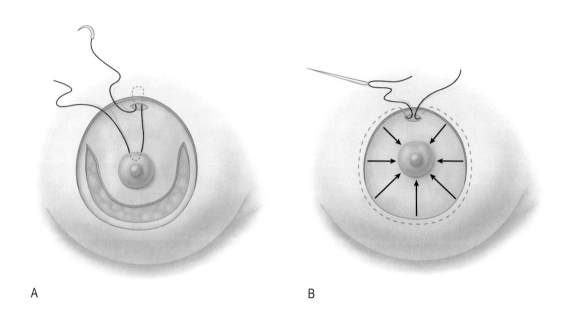

A   B

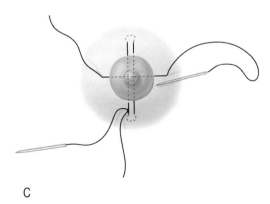

C

Figure 12.6 Closure of the periareolar incisions in Benelli periareolar mammaplasty. (A) Though a small 12 o'clock incision in the areolar flap, the areolar dermis undersurface is suture suspended from the breast skin to relieve tension. (B) A permanent suture on a straight needle is passed through the same incision as a purse-string cerclage 'round-block' in the breast skin dermis and cinched down. (C) Transareolar sutures passed through breast skin and areolar dermis to diametrically opposed poles further shape and secure the areolar shape. (Modified from Benelli LC. Periareolar Benelli mastopexy and reduction: the 'round block'. In: Spear SL (Ed). Surgery of the Breast: Principles and Art, 2nd edn, Vol II. Philadelphia, PA: Lippincott Williams & Wilkins; 2006: 70)

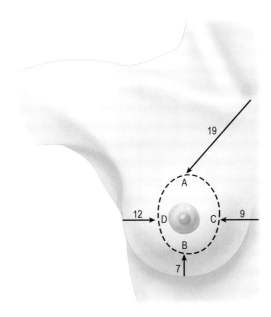

Figure 12.7 Cardinal marks of the Góes periareolar mammaplasty with mesh support. (Modified from Góes JCS: Periareolar mammaplasty: Double-skin technique with application of mesh support. In: Spear SL (Ed). Surgery of the Breast: Principles and Art, 2nd edition, Vol II. Philadelphia, PA: Lippincott Williams & Wilkins; 2006: 71)

- Excise superior and inferior wedges of breast tissue and suture close opposing edges of excised breast gland.
- Support the breast gland by suturing the circumferentially distended dermis of the periareolar flap and a circumferentially placed piece of Vipro II™ mesh to the breast and chest wall.
- Cinch the breast skin to the final areolar diameter with a running purse-string cerclage placed intradermally and close the skin with a running subcuticular suture.

Pitfalls and complications of periareolar breast techniques

Precise placement and closure of the periareolar incision at the skin–areola interface is essential to achieving scar camouflage. Scar widening may occur, especially where there is excess tension on the wound closure. Sources of excess wound tension include excess skin excision, excess breast mass, or the weight of a breast implant. Placement of the purse-string cerclage in the breast skin dermis helps minimize tension on the areolar closure. Alternately, the dermis of the breast skin and the areola can be secured to one another using a 4-0 gore-tex suture placed in a 'spokes on a wheel' interlocking fashion as described by Hammond (Figure 12.11). This maneuver distributes tension between the dermis of the areola and the breast skin to resist widening (Figure 12.12).

Prominence or exposure of the permanent cerclage suture requires removal. This may be performed in the office setting under local anesthesia. Key to prevention of this complication is the placement the suture in the deep dermis. The knot securing the periareolar cerclage should always be placed at the same position in every instance to allow easy identification of the ends of the suture for removal if necessary.

The areolar skin is heavily colonized with bacteria as is true for other skin areas of apocrine glands (axilla and circumanal regions). Good hygiene and post-operative antibiotics are imperative as even sub-clinical infection may contribute to poor scarring. When mesh support is used, it may be difficult to distinguish infection from the normal inflammatory process that accompanies mesh incorporation. Generally, however, the mesh is completely incorporated by 2 months post-operatively. Development of seroma beyond this point in time is highly suggestive of infection and requires removal of all mesh material.

There is a tendency toward a flattening of the areolar complex giving a 'pancake' appearance with periareolar techniques. Supporting the areolar flap with additional tissue as described for the various techniques helps to prevent this. However, the patient must be informed pre-operatively of the possibility of areolar flattening and be willing to accept a potentially less than perfect breast shape in order to have a minimal periareolar scar.

Post-operative care following periareolar breast surgery

A supportive, semi-occlusive adhesive dressing is placed over the entire breast, except the nipple, post-operatively. Either Tegaderm™ or a thin polyurethane foam tape may be used. This dressing is maintained for 2 weeks. A supportive bra which lifts but does not compress the breast is worn day and night for 2 months. Half-buried sutures over the areola if used

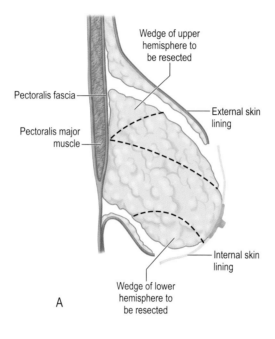

Wedge of upper
hemisphere to
be resected

Pectoralis fascia

External skin
lining

Pectoralis major
muscle

Internal skin
lining

Wedge of lower
hemisphere to
be resected

A

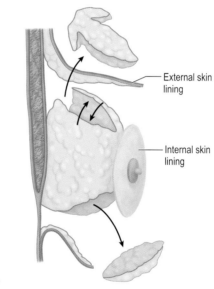

External skin
lining

Internal skin
lining

B

Figure 12.8 Góes periareolar mammaplasty with mesh support. (A) Superior skin is undermined to the chest wall with progressive flap thickness. At the chest wall the dissection is carried another 5 cm superiorly. The upper third of the central breast mound is also dissected off the chest wall. Inferiorly, skin is undermined off the breast down to the inframammary fold. (B) Wedge excisions of superior and inferior poles of the central breast mound are performed being careful to preserve remaining breast attachments to the chest wall. (Modified from Góes JCS: Periareolar mammaplasty: Double-skin technique with application of mesh support. In: Spear SL (Ed). Surgery of the Breast: Principles and Art, 2nd edition, Vol II. Philadelphia, PA: Lippincott Williams & Wilkins; 2006: 71)

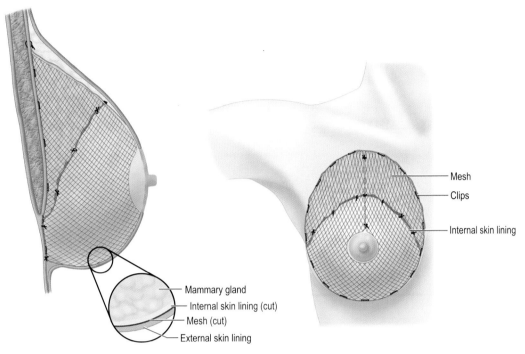

Figure 12.9   Góes periareolar mammaplasty with mesh support. The de-epithelialized dermis of the areolar flap is distended over the breast and sutured to the breast and chest wall. The Vipro II™ mesh is placed over the entire breast mound and secured to the breast and chest wall circumferentially as an 'internal brassiere'. (Modified from Góes JCS: Periareolar mammaplasty: Double-skin technique with application of mesh support. In: Spear SL (Ed). Surgery of the Breast: Principles and Art, 2nd edn, Vol II. Philadelphia, PA: Lippincott Williams & Wilkins; 2006: 71)

should be removed after 1 week. Once the incision is uncovered, twice daily cleaning with peroxide should be performed until all scabs have been removed. Drains are removed as soon as possible, usually by the second post-operative day. If mesh was placed, Góes recommends keeping the drains for 5 days post-operatively.

Vertical scar operative techniques

A reduction up to 1500 g and correction of moderate ptosis is possible using various vertical scar breast techniques. Most techniques incorporate a superior or superomedial based dermatoglandular flap to carry the areola. Central to all vertical scar techniques is the elimination or reduction of the horizontal scar component integral to the 'inverted-T'. Vertical scar techniques advance excess skin into the periareolar skin excision. The amount of excess that can be advanced and removed however is limited. Generally, if >1000 g

of reduction is performed or if the inframammary fold to areola distance is >15 cm a horizontal excision will be needed.

Senior author's preferred vertical scar operative technique

Pre-operative preparation

With the patient standing the inframammary fold, midline, and breast meridian marked. The superior border of the new areola is marked 2 cm above the level of the projection of the inframammary fold on the anterior breast (Figure 12.13A). The breast is distracted superomedially and a perpendicular to the inframammary fold is marked in line with the midpoint of the inframammary fold. The breast is then

Periareolar/vertical/small horizontal scars

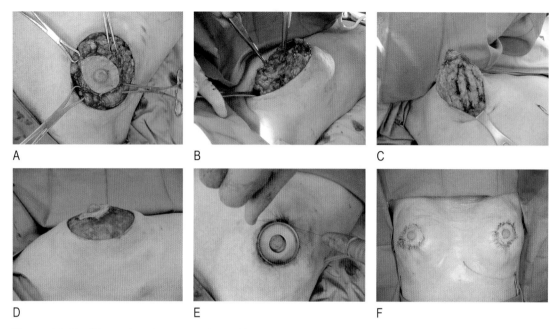

Figure 12.10 Góes periareolar mammaplasty with mesh support: intraoperative technique. (A) The areola is carried on a central dermatoglandular flap. (B) After skin undermining a superior wedge of central breast gland is excised and closed. (C) Similarly an inferior wedge of central breast is marked and excised and closed. (D) The de-epithelialized central flap is secured over the breast gland and Vipro II™ mesh is placed, encasing the reshaped breast. (E) The skin is redraped and the periareolar incision cinched with a permanent purse-string cerclage down to the desired areolar diameter. (F) Final skin closure is made and the breast dressed with a semi-occlusive adhesive dressing.

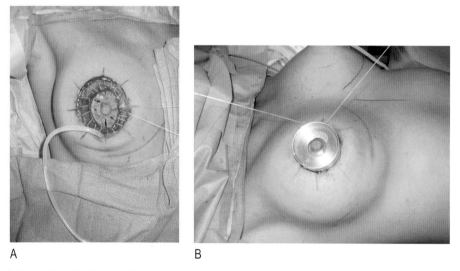

Figure 12.11 Periareolar closure using gore-tex suture placed between the areola and the breast skin as described by Hammond. (A) Suture is passed in a 'spokes-on-wheel' fashion circumferentially. (B) Suture is cinched down to the planned areolar size and tied.

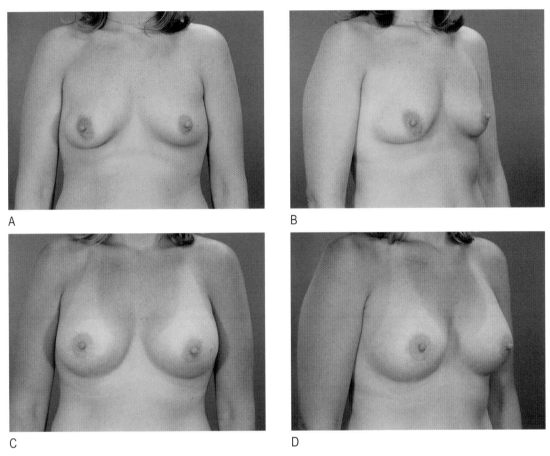

Figure 12.12 Concentric periareolar mastopexy with implant augmentation. (A,B) Pre-operative photographs showing mild post-partum atrophy with mild ptosis of the right breast and areolar asymmetry. (C,D) Six month post-operative photographs.

distracted superolaterally and a perpendicular to the inframammary fold is marked in line with the mid-point of the inframammary fold (Figure 12.13B). These lines mark the lateral and medial extent of breast excision. The force of displacement applied during these maneuvers approximates final wound tension and the direction of the applied force gives a simulation of the final breast shape. If a small reduction is to be performed or an implant is to be placed, a lesser degree of distracting force should be applied than if a large reduction is planned.

The superior extent of breast excision is marked along the medial and lateral lines. These marks are joined with the superior areola mark as a semicircular perimeter that defines the future periareolar closure. The semicircular perimeter should measure 12–16 cm

to ensure proper tension at closure. The semicircular perimeter is completed inferiorly as a concave line placed 3–4 cm away from the nipple. This marks the lower border of a superior based flap that will carry the areola. If excess folding of the superior flap is anticipated with nipple transposition a superomedial flap is preferred and marks are adjusted accordingly.

The inferior extent of breast excision is marked as a concave arc between the medial and lateral lines of incision 2–3 cm above the inframammary fold. Convex lines extending medially and laterally are marked out from this level down to the inframammary fold identifying areas of inferior breast gland that will be removed. Mirrored markings are made on the opposite breast and symmetry of the markings confirmed by measurements from the sternal notch and

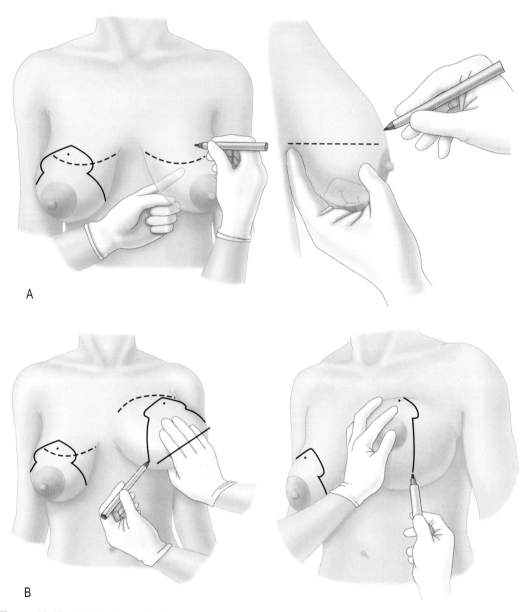

Figure 12.13   Markings for vertical scar mammaplasty. (A) The new superior border of the areola is marked 2 cm above the projection through the breast of a finger placed at the inframammary fold. (B) Lateral and medial lines of excision are marked inline with the midline of the inframammary fold with the breast distracted as shown.

the midline. Differences in measurements are adjusted for taking note of volume or shape discrepancies between the breasts. Centralization of the new areola position over the final breast shape is of primary importance and should serve as a guide in making any adjustments of the final marks (Figure 12.14).

Technique

The areola is distended and marked under tension with a sizer. The skin between periareolar marks is injected intradermally with 0.5% lidocaine with 1:200 000 epinephrine and de-epithelialized. Additional subcutaneous and intraglandular injection of anesthetic is made along medial and lateral lines of excision and over the marked inferior skin flap. Using a spinal needle, anesthetic is also infiltrated into the prepectoral space. The marked inferior arc between the medial and lateral lines of excision above the inframammary fold is incised through the skin. The lower skin flap is distended away from the chest wall with skin hooks and undermined off the breast gland down to the level of the inframammary fold. At the level of the inframammary fold the dissection turns directly

down on to the chest wall fascia such that no lowering of the fold occurs. Undermining extends out medially and laterally over the entire area of planned inferior gland removal.

The breast gland is mobilized off the chest wall by subglandular dissection. The pocket formed is packed with a sponge (Figure 12.15A). The breast gland is then distracted superomedially such that lateral extent of excision is brought in line with the midpoint of the inframammary fold. Incision is performed along the marked extent of the lateral line of excision through the gland down to the level of the sponge packing. The incision plane is beveled as needed to excise either more or less of the central gland. The medial line of excision is incised in a similar fashion but with the breast distracted superolaterally (Figure 12.15B).

The free inferior border of the incised gland is then grasped with skin clamps and distracted caudally. The inferior border of the de-epithelialized periareolar flap is then incised for a depth of at least 2 cm. Beyond 2 cm the plane of incision can be beveled under the flap carrying the areola to thin it if needed. The completed incision frees the central breast specimen, which is passed off the field (Figure 12.15C). The areola is then stapled to its new superior position. Dermis under the staple is then grasped with a skin clamp and the areola distracted off the chest wall. A ruler is placed perpendicular to the chest wall at the medial free skin edge of the flap carrying the areola. A distance of 6–7 cm from the medial skin edge is marked perpendicular to the ruler along the medial breast gland pillar up to the skin markings over the lower skin flap. The ruler is then placed laterally in the same manner. A 6–7 cm

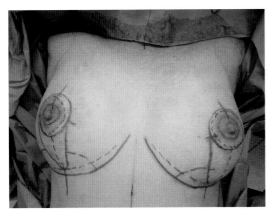

Figure 12.14 Senior author's markings for vertical mastopexy with small reduction. The area between the sized areola and the periareolar marks (solid ellipse) is de-epithelialized. The 'v' area is excised as a keel. The convex arcs extending medially and laterally mark areas of inferior breast gland that will be removed.

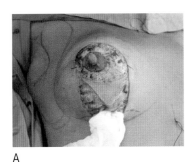
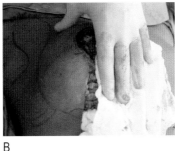
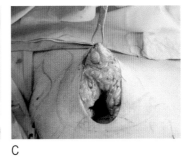

A
B
C

Figure 12.15 (A) The periareolar flap is de-epithelialized and the inferior breast skin undermined. The skin over the area of central gland excision is scored. The breast gland is freed from the chest wall forming a subglandular pocket which is packed with a sponge. (B) The medial and lateral extents of the central gland excision are made with the breast distracted to the midline. (C) The superior attachments of the central gland to the periareolar flap are incised, completing its excision.

perpendicular level is now marked along the lateral breast gland pillar. These marks define excess breast gland which is excised from the lateral and medial flaps (Figure 12.16).

Closure

With the areolar flap still distracted off the chest wall a 2-0 vicryl suture is placed between the undersurface of the areolar flap and the pectoralis fascia suspending the flap high on the chest wall. Medial and lateral flaps are approximated superiorly with a deep dermal 2-0 vicryl suture such that the flaps join at the 6 o'clock periareolar position. (Figure 12.17A) Several interrupted 2-0 vicryl sutures are then placed between the undersurfaces of the medial and lateral flaps narrowing the breast base (Figure 12.17B). The lateral and medial flaps are then secured to one another with deep dermal 2-0 Vicryl sutures. The skin clamp is released and the areola is allowed to relax back on the chest wall. A 15 French closed suction drain is placed. A 2-0 vicryl suture is then placed in the lateral breast gland and secured to the fascia over the midline of the inferior chest wall, rounding the shape of the lateral breast.

A temporary staple closure of the skin is performed. If skin at the inferior portion of the vertical closure is of such excess that it cannot be gathered and closed without dog-earing, the redundant skin can be excised as a short horizontal extension (Figure 12.17C). Final skin closure of the vertical limb and any horizontal extension is accomplished in layers of interrupted intradermal 3-0 PDS sutures followed by a running subcuticular suture. The periareolar skin is closed with half-buried 4-0 nylon sutures placed with the knot

oriented over the areola followed by a running subcuticular 4-0 PDS (Figure 12.17D). A mirror procedure is performed on the adjacent breast and symmetry of the nipple position and breast shape checked with the patient raised upright. Final shaping and symmetry is aided by selective liposuction; particularly over the axillary tail.

Operative steps

- Infiltrate dermis between periareolar marks with local anesthetic containing epinephrine and de-epithelialize.
- Incise skin along inferior extent of planned breast excision and undermine skin along lower skin flap down to the inframammary fold.
- Free the breast gland from the chest wall by subglandular dissection.
- Incise along medial and lateral lines of excision with the breast distracted.
- Incise along the inferior border of the areolar flap to free the central breast specimen.
- Staple the areola to its new superior position, hold the areolar flap up off the chest wall, and suture the undersurface of the flap high on the chest wall.
- Mark and excise portions of inferior glandular tissue that must be removed to preserve 6–7 cm of breast projection.
- Suture approximate medial and lateral pillars of breast gland and deep dermis, temporarily close skin with staples.
- Mark redundant skin in the vertical closure for excision horizontally along the inframammary fold, excise away redundant skin, and make final skin closure.

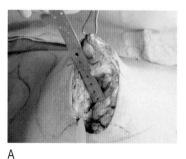 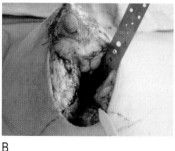 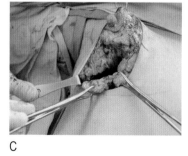

A B C

Figure 12.16 (A) The aerola is held off the chest wall and the medial and lateral flaps marked such that 6–7 cm of areolar projection will be maintained. (B) Excess inferior gland is then distracted with clamps from the medial and lateral gland and excised.

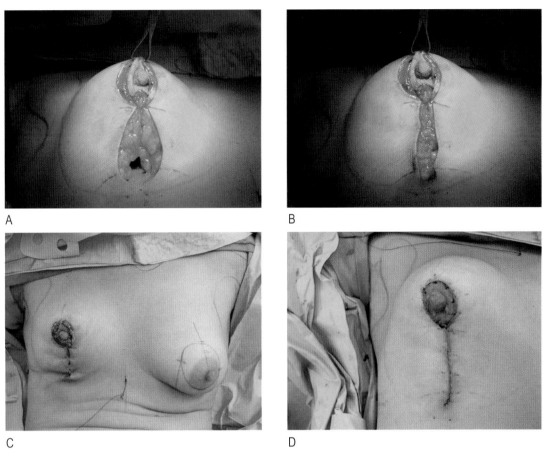

A   B

C   D

Figure 12.17   (A) With the areola held in a position of projection off the chest wall, the medial and lateral flaps are sutured together superiorly with a deep dermal suture at the 6 o'clock periareolar position. (B) The medial and lateral flaps are further secured to one another with sutures passed between the flap undersurfaces and deep dermis. (C) A temporary staple closure is made and the patient placed upright. Redundant skin at the base of the vertical closure as shown is marked for excision as a small horizontal extension. (D) Final closure of the vertical and periareolar skin is made. Note the periareolar half-buried nylon sutures placed with their knots of over the areolar skin.

Post-operative care

Sheets of Tegaderm are placed over the entire breast, except the nipple, without tension. This dressing will remain in place for 2 weeks. A supportive bra which lifts the breast is worn day and night for the next 6 weeks. Drains are removed the first day post-operatively. Periareolar permanent sutures are removed after 1 week and perioperative antibiotics are continued for 7 days.

Pitfalls and complications in vertical scar breast surgery

The initial appearance of the breast post-operatively is that of an 'upside-down' breast with exaggerated upper-pole fullness. Patients must be counseled pre-operatively that this shape is expected and that the final breast shape will not be apparent for 3 months. (Figure 12.18). The nipple position may appear asymmetric as the breast shape evolves during this period. Again, this is to be expected and usually resolves without the need for revision.

Minor wound complications occur as with other breast techniques and perioperative antibiotics are recommended. In larger breasts, extensive wound dehiscence around the periareolar closure may occur. This can be allowed to heal by secondary intention and revised at a later date if necessary. Fat necrosis resulting in palpable firm masses can be observed

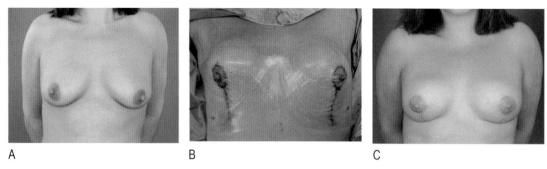

A   B   C

Figure 12.18 Evolution of breast shape following vertical mammaplasty of patient depicted in previous photos Intraoperatively: (A) Pre-operative photo. (B) Immediate postoperative photo showing exaggerated fullness in upper pole giving an 'upside-down' appearance of the breast. (C) Three month post-operative photo with resolution of 'upside-down' appearance.

even years after surgery and can cause extreme patient anxiety. These areas should be excised and any suspicion of malignancy should prompt pathologic examination.

Seroma along the undermined lower skin flap prevents the skin from retracting as it heals and should be drained. Repeated aspiration is commonly required. If retraction of the lower skin flap does not progress, a fold is created along the inframammary fold which will require excision.

Conclusion

Aesthetic techniques in breast surgery continue to evolve. Efforts to minimize and conceal scars must be balanced against the limitations that minimal incisions impose on the ability to reshape the breast. Periareolar approaches allow correction of only mild degrees of ptosis and small reductions. Vertical scar techniques are suitable to accomplish moderate breast reductions and lifts.

Further reading

Benelli L. A new periareolar mammaplasty: The 'round block' technique. Aesthet Plast Surg 1990;14:93.

Benelli LC. Periareolar Benelli mastopexy and reduction: The 'round block'. In: Spear SL (Ed). Surgery of the Breast: Principles and Art, 2nd edn, Vol II. Philadelphia: Lippincott Williams & Wilkins; 2006: 70.

Berthe JV, Massaut, J, Greuse M et al. The vertical mammaplasty: A reappraisal of the technique and its complications. Plast Reconstr Surg 2003;111:2192.

Boehm K, Nahai F. Vertical reduction: Techniques. In: Mathes SJ (Ed). Plastic surgery, 2nd edn, Vol 6. Philadelphia: Saunders-Elsevier; 2006: 136.

Chiari A Jr, Grotting JC, Seidel SP. The L short-scar mammaplasty. In: Spear SL (Ed). Surgery of the Breast: Principles and Art, 2nd edn, Vol II. Philadelphia: Lippincott Williams & Wilkins; 2006: 83.

Davison SP, Mesbahi AL, Ducie I et al. The versatility of the superomedial pedicle with various skin reduction patterns. Plast Reconstr Surg 2007;120:1466.

Góes JCS. Periareolar mastopexy: Double-skin technique. In: Hinderer UT (Ed). Plastic Surgery, Vol II. New York: Elsevier; 1992: 575.

Góes JCS. Periareolar mammaplasty: Double-skin technique with application of mesh support. In: Spear SL (Ed). Surgery of the Breast: Principles and Art, 2nd edn, Vol II. Philadelphia: Lippincott Williams & Wilkins; 2006: 71.

Grotting JC, Chen SM. Control and precision in mastopexy. In: Nahai F (Ed). The Art of Aesthetic Surgery: Principles and Techniques, Vol III. St Louis: Quality Medical; 2005: 51.

Grotting JC, Marx AP, Chen SM. Mastopexy. In: Mathes SJ (Ed). Plastic Surgery 2nd edn, Vol 6. Philadelphia, Saunders-Elsevier; 2006: 120.

Gruber RP, Jones HW Jr. The 'donut' mastopexy: Indications and complications. Plast Reconstr Surg 1980;65:34.

Hall-Findlay EJ. A simplified vertical reduction mammaplasty: Shortening the learning curve. Plast Reconstr Surg 1999;104:748.

Hammond D. Short scar periareolar inferior pedicle reduction (SPAIR) mammaplasty. Plast Reconstr Surg 1999;103:890.

Hammond D, Khutaila DK, Kim J. The interlocking gore-tex suture for control of areolar diameter and shape. Plast Reconstr Surg 2007;119:804.

Hidalgo DA. Vertical mammaplasty. Plast Reconstr Surg 2005;113:1179.

Lassus C. Breast reduction: evolution of a technique. A single vertical scar. Aesthet Plast Surg 1987;11:107.

Lassus C. A 30-year experience with vertical mammaplasty. Plast Reconstr Surg 1996;97:373.

Lassus C. Vertical scar breast reduction and mastopexy without undermining. In: Spear SL (Ed). Surgery of the Breast: Principles and Art, 2nd edn, Vol II. Philadelphia, Lippincott Williams & Wilkins; 2006: 73.

Lejour M. Vertical mammaplasty and liposuction of the breast. Plast Reconstr Surg 1994;94:100.

Lejour M. Vertical mammaplasty: Early complications after 250 personal consecutive cases. Plast Reconstr Surg 1999;104:764.

Lejour M. Vertical mammaplasty: Update and appraisal of late results. Plast Reconstr Surg 1999;104:771.

Rohrich RJ, Thorton JF, Jakubietz RG et al. The Limited Scar Mastopexy: Current concepts and approaches to correct breast ptosis. Plast Reconstr Surg 2004;114:1622.

Spear SL, Kassan M, Little J. Guildlines in concentric mastopexy. Plast Reconstr Surg 1990;85:961.

Spear SL, Giese SY, Ducie I. Concentric mastopexy revisited. Plast Reconstr Surg 2001;107:1294.

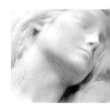

13

The circumvertical breast reduction technique

A. Aldo Mottura

Key points

- For the last 10 years, vertical reduction mammaplasties have become a modern trend in breast reductions. Some surgeons, however, are reluctant to adopt them because they consider that the procedure is neither easy to learn nor is it easy to obtain a nice, shaped projected breast. Additionally, the results can not be observed at the end of the surgery. The circumvertical technique is easy to learn. The parenchyma removal and its remodeling is the same as in the w-pattern techniques and a round-shaped breast is observed at the end of the surgery.

- In the circumvertical technique, the skin is de-epithelialized as in circumareolar plus vertical techniques. The inferior half of the breast skin is undermined and separated from the pectoralis fascia.

- The parenchyma removal follows the w-pattern. Pillars are firmly sutured in two to three layers or imbricated to build a round-conic projected breast whose inferior edge is sutured to the pectoralis facia.

- The areola is transposed without any pedicle. The areola is sutured using the cinching running suture.

- At the end of the surgery a nice, round-shaped breast is observed with a harmonious distribution of the wrinkles around the areola. The vertical scar never crosses the submammary fold.

- Most of the inferior breast skin resected in the inverted T technique will retract in the circumvertical technique and will become part of the chest wall.

13 The circumvertical breast reduction technique

Patient selection

This technique is indicated when there is an acceptable volume of good skin quality, when the amount to be removed is less than 1000 g and when the areola elevation is no more than 10 cm. During the surgery I follow the penciled line and the estimation of the glandular removal I planned before surgery. This is especially important when there are asymmetries. As there is a great variety of breast hypertrophies, before surgery, I also plan from which part of the breast I have to remove more tissue and, when there are difficult asymmetries, I draw a draft of the future areas to be removed as a surgical guide.

Indications

I use the periareolar technique in minor hypertrophies. The circumvertical is a technique which should only be used in moderate or big hypertrophies but good results are not obtained in gigantomasties, where the vertical scar usually trespasses the submammary fold (SMF) or the vertical has to be transformed into an inverted T technique. When the patient has firm skin, the skin is marked and then resected in a conservative way, because during and after surgery, it will retract.

Operative technique

Pre-operative preparation

With the patient in a standing position I evaluate what her size preference is and if she wishes to have projected breasts or small flat ones. I then have an idea of what volume I have to remove and from what area of the breast. This is marked on the breast skin. I also study the areolar position and the natural asymmetries of each patient.

First, I mark the submammary fold. The vertical lines passing through the nipple go to the external notch if I wish to move the areola superiomedially but to the mid-clavicular line if I wish to move the areola superiorly. I then move the areola to the position I think it should be placed, that is, its projection above the future submammary fold, and I mark the superior areola position on the vertical line. According to what I think will be the periareolar skin resection, I mark 5–6 cm on each side of the nipple. This can be 4–7 cm

if I wish to move a lateralized areola more medially. From the superior mark to the lateral ones, I then mark a semi-circumference and from there I drop two vertical lines converging 2–4 cm above the SMF. I draw the same mark on the contra-lateral side or I can make different marks if the breast is bigger, smaller or more ptotic.

Technique

Before beginning the surgery, each breast is thoroughly infiltrated with 250–300 mL of anesthetic solution at the submammary, prepectoralis layer, at the subcutaneous inferior half of the breast skin and under the areola. The anesthetic solution is prepared with 25 mL 2% lidocaine, 25 mL 0.5% bupivacaine, 1 mL 1:1000 epinephrine diluted in 450–550 mL of Ringer's lactate solution. Once the whole periareolar skin is de-epithelialized, the skin is undermined at the inferior half of the breast medially and laterally, leaving 1 cm thick subcutaneous tissue to preserve its blood supply (Figure 13.1). The inferior half of the breast is also detached from the pectoralis major muscle up to the fourth intercostal space, where the perforant of the fourth intercostal nerve usually emerges (Figure 13.2). In this way, the dissected breast comes out and, holding up the breast with a hook, I mark a w-pattern resection (Figure 13.3), that is at the inferior quadrant and at the inferior part of the medial and lateral quadrants, marking 10 cm distance of what will be the future areola–SMF distance (Figure 13.4).

After the resection, the lateral and medial glandular edges are sutured medially in two to three layers using

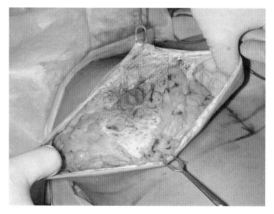

Figure 13.1 The inferior half of the skin breast is medially and laterally undermined.

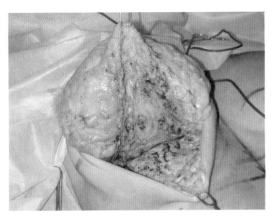

Figure 13.2 The breast is dissected from the pectoralis fascia until the fourth intercostal space.

a 3-0 vicryl suture. In case I want a central projection of the breast, both pillars can be imbricated. To have a more projected breast, two to three stitches are placed at the base of the cone in order to keep the pillars together (Figure 13.5). Once I have obtained a conic shaped breast, the inferior edge of the parenchyma is fixed to the pectoralis facia where it now sits using 5–7 3-0 vicryl separate stitches placed all along what will be the future SMF (Figure 13.6) At this time, some de-fatting can be performed in order to create a more even and round breast shape. I then move the areola to the superior border of the skin and I fix it with two to three subdermal 3-0 vicryl sutures (Figure 13.7). To finish the surgery, a stitch is placed

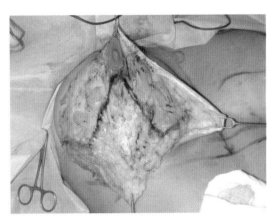

Figure 13.3 The W pattern to be resected is marked on the parenchyma.

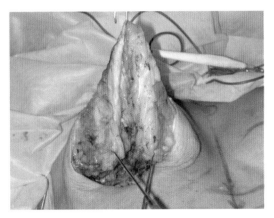

Figure 13.5 Once the parenchyma has been resected the pillars are approximated to be sutured.

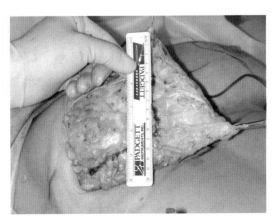

Figure 13.4 A 10 cm mark is placed on the vertical limb of the W pattern.

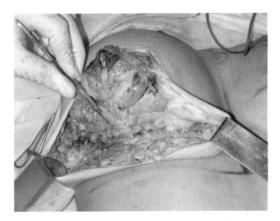

Figure 13.6 The inferior parenchyma edge is sutured to the pectoralis fascia to avoid future breast rotation and to form the new SMF.

The circumvertical breast reduction technique

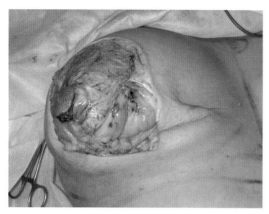

Figure 13.7 Pillars have been sutured. The low position of the areola can be observed.

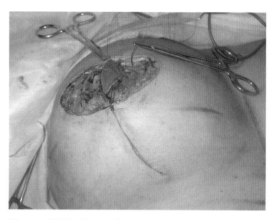

Figure 13.9 The vertical wound already sutured.

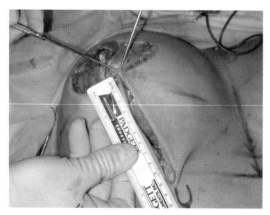

Figure 13.8 The areola is sutured to the superor skin markings. Ten cm from the inferior skin angle, a stitch devides the wound in two parts, the periareolar and the vertical parts.

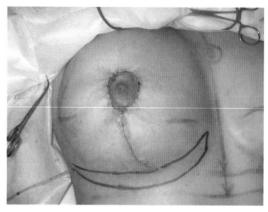

Figure 13.10 The areola sutured. A round shaped breast can be observed, with a harmonious distribution of the wrinkles and the vertical not crossing the new SMF.

at 8–10 cm from the inferior part of the skin angle, dividing the wound in two figures: the superior round periareolar and the inferior vertical ellipse (Figure 13.8).

Closure

The inferior wound is sutured in a vertical fashion with a 3-0 vicryl subdermal running suture (Figure 13.9). The periareolar skin is sutured to the areolar border with another subdermal cinching running suture. This running suture takes big 10–20 horizontal bites at the skin dermis and 2–3 mm vertical bites at the areola dermis. In this way, after three passes the

thread is strongly pulled and the skin gathers toward the areola. I then continue the suturing all along the areola to have a harmonious distribution of the wrinkles all along the areola and no spaces are left. To finish the surgery, all the wounds are closed with intradermal 5-0 vicryl suture (Figure 13.10). Aspiration drains are placed laterally and a paper tape fixes the wounds. To keep the flap attached to the parenchyma, I use strong aspirative drainage. When the inferior part of the breast is removed, the skin that previously covered the breast will now attach to the thoracic wall. As the pleats are harmoniously distributed at the periareolar and vertical wounds and the undermined skin retracts during surgery, an acceptable result can

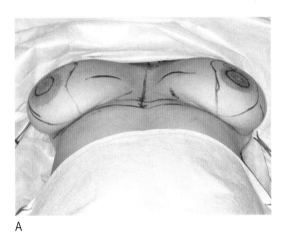
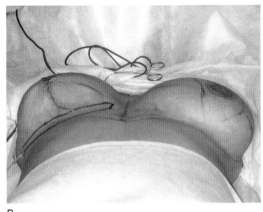

A

B

Figure 13.11 (A) The breast before surgery. (B) The right surgery is already finished.

be observed when the surgery is finished (Figure 13.11).

Operative steps

- Profuse infiltration with anesthetic solution is used with lidocaine–bupivacaine–epinephrine.
- The skin is de-epithelialized within the circumvertical markings (Figure 13.12).
- The inferior half of the breast skin is undermined and the parenchyma is separated from the pectoralis fascia.
- Following the w-wise pattern, the parenchyma is removed (Figure 13.13).
- Pillars are sutured. The base of the cone can be sutured (Figure 13.14).
- The areola is transposed without a pedicle.
- The wound is divided into vertical and round wounds (Figure 13.15).
- Once the skin is gathered to the areola, all the undermined inferior skin breast ascends as does the vertical wound and in this way avoids crossing the SMF (Figure 13.16).
- The vertical is sutured in two to three layers. The periareolar follows the cinching running suture.

Results

I began performing the Circumvertical Technique and have experienced breast reductions over 300 g since 1992. However, where prospective reductions

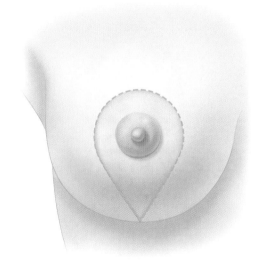

Figure 13.12 The skin undermined within the circumvertical markings.

are around 200 g, I use periareolar techniques and where reductions are between 200 g and 1000 g, the circumvertical technique is used. Where reductions are over 1000 g. I prefer the inverted T technique. I have used the circumvertical technique removing more the 1200 g but even when the scars are vertical, the results are suboptimal. The ideal breast (from a young

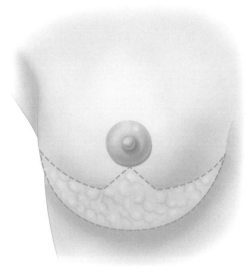

Figure 13.13 The parenchyma to be removed is marked following the w pattern.

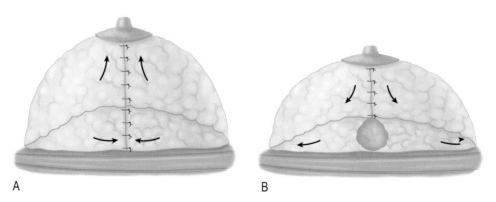

A   B

Figure 13.14 (A) If the base of the cone is sutured, the breast can be projected. (B) In case it is not sutured, the breast can remain flat.

woman) is a round firm breast with minor ptosis and the least ideal, a flat hanging breast with a poor skin quality.

The main complication I have encountered is skin sloughing at the periareolar–vertical junction, but as I am removing a very limited amount of skin and I am not compressing the flaps, this problem is very rarely observed. Hematomas are present in 4% of cases and as I wash out all the wounds with cefuroxone before suturing. I have no incidents of infection to report. As no pedicle is used and the blood supply of the areola is preserved, no areolar necrosis has been found.

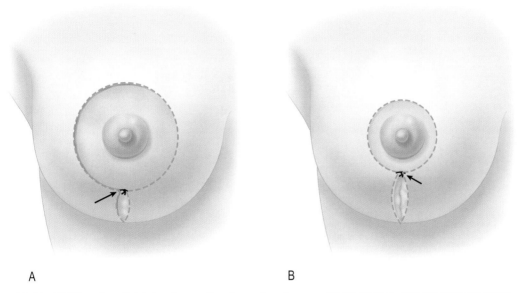

A   B

Figure 13.15 (A) When the stitch is in a low position the periareolar wound is big and the vertical is short. (B) When the stitch is high, the periareolar wound is smaller and the vertical longer.

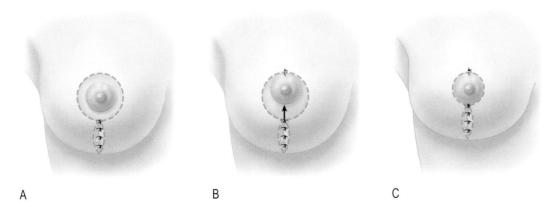

A   B   C

Figure 13.16 When the areola is sutured, the skin moves upward towards the areola and the vertical wound ascends.

The circumvertical breast reduction technique

Case **1**

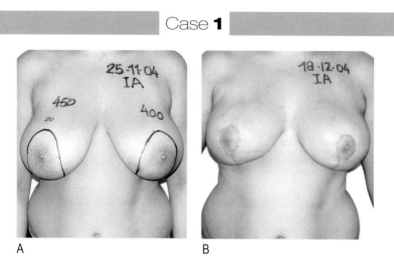

A B

Figure 13.17 A 25-year-old woman presented requesting a breast reduction for large, heavy breasts. The breasts were symmetrical and a circumvertical breast reduction was planned with a reduction estimated at 400 g on each side and an areola elevation of 6 cm. The wound healed uneventfully and periareolar wrinkles were hardly visible, as shown in the 4-week post-operative picture. (A) A moderate breast hypertrophy. (B) Four weeks post-op. A nice breast shape with a harmonious distribution of the periareolar wrinkles can be observed.

Case **2**

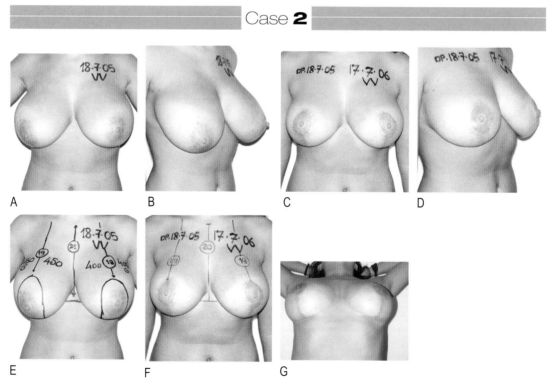

A B C D

E F G

Figure 13.18 A 20-year-old woman consulted for a reduction of her large breasts. The right breast was approximately 50 g bigger with moderate ptosis. The areola had to be elevated 5 cm. It was planned to remove 450 g on the right side and 400 g on the left side. Wound healing was uneventful. (A,B) Moderate breast hypertrophy. (C,D) One year post-op. (E,F) Pre- and post- markings. (G) The vertical scar does not cross the submammary fold.

Case **3**

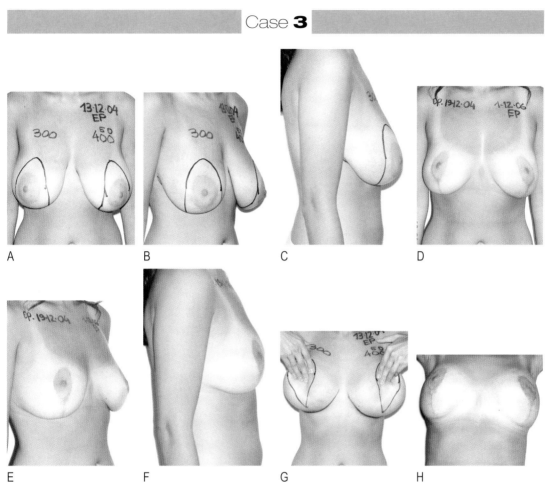

A B C D

E F G H

Figure 13.19 A 25-year-old woman requested a breast lift and reduction. She had lax skin, marked ptosis for the elevation of the areola 6 cm and removal 400 g of the left and 300 g of the right side was planned. Wound healing resulted in a small 1 cm wound dehiscence at the junction of the periareolar and vertical wound at the right side, the weakest point of the sutures. This was resolved using medical treatments. (A–C) Moderate hypertrophy with marked ptosis. Poor skin quality. (D–F) Two years post-op. (G) Circumvertical pre-op. markings. (H)The vertical scars not crossing the SMF.

Case **4**

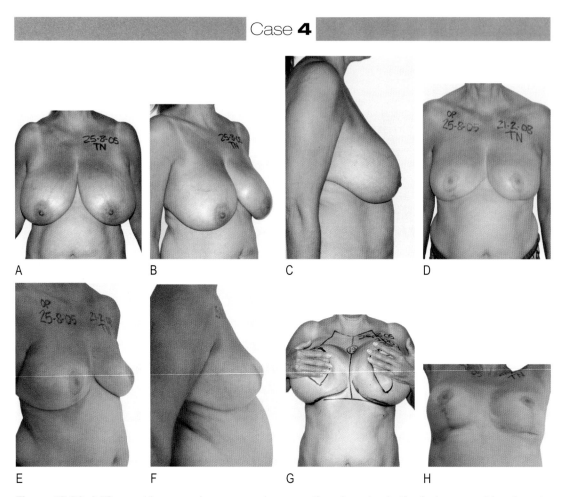

A   B   C   D

E   F   G   H

Figure 13.20 A 50-year-old woman who was a smoker requesting a breast reduction for large, pendulous breasts. Her breasts were big, with marked ptosis and poor skin quality. She was under mycosis treatment for her breast skin for 2 months prior to consultation. A circumvertical technique was planned with a resection of 700 g on each side and an areola elevation of 7 cm. Post-operatively, she developed wound healing problems in both breasts at the vertical wounds which needed to be re-sutured under local anesthesia. Small retraction at the submammary fold is the consequence of too much defatting of this area, (A-C) Moderate hypertrophy with marked ptosis and poor skin quality. (D–F) post-op. (G) The inferior part of the marking finishes 4 cms above the SMD. (H) The vertical scar finishing at the SMF, but some retraction of the SMF skin is observed as a consequence of too much defatting.

Case 5

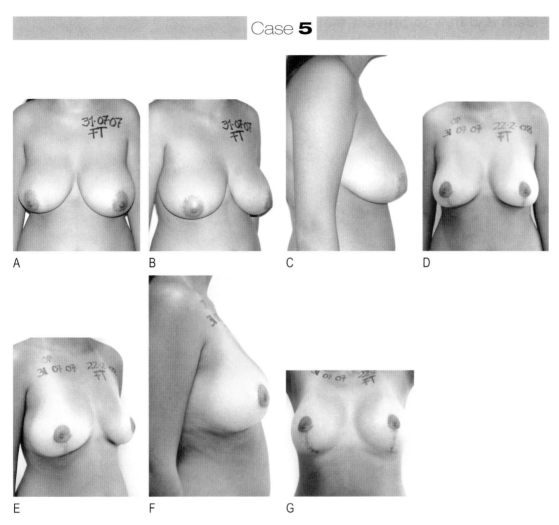

A   B   C   D

E   F   G

Figure 13.21   A woman with moderate breast ptosis and asymmetric hypertrophy presented for a breast reduction. The skin quality was acceptable. I removed 250 g on the left side and 350 g on the right side. Wound healing was uneventful and results are shown at 5 month follow-up. (A–C) Moderate hypertrophy and ptosis. (D–F) Five months post-op follow-up. (G) The vertical scar not crossing the SMF.

The circumvertical breast reduction technique

Pitfalls and how to prevent them

- To prevent a bloody surgery, profuse infiltration is suggested.
- Using bupivacaine in the infiltration, there are 2–4 h of post-operative pain relief.
- Avoids too large skin resection, so the skin tension and the possibility of wound dehiscence diminish.
- Avoid thin skin undermining. To preserve an optimal blood supply, I suggest dissecting 10 mm or even thicker skin flaps.
- To avoid a flat breast, the pillars have to be sutured in two to three layers and also at the base of the breast.
- Suturing the inferior parenchyma edge to the pectoralis fascia, a clear SMF is defined and the gland is fixed to the muscle, thus avoiding the possible bottoming out of the breast.
- Moving the areola without a pedicle upwards avoids lactation, blood supply and sensation problems.
- The suture that divides the wound can be regulated during surgery. If it is placed in a higher position, the periareolar diameter will be reduced and the vertical one enlarged. However, if it is placed in a lower position, the periareolar diameter becomes bigger and the vertical wound is shortened. This possibility of variations is important to consider when a harmonic distribution of the wrinkles has to be determined.
- Suturing the areola with the cinching running suture makes a more harmonious distribution of the wrinkles.

- When the glandular removal is at the inferior part of the breast and the areola is transposed upwards without a pedicle, the normal anatomy remains almost unaltered, an important factor to control the breast with mammograms over the years.
- Leaving aspirative drainage and soft tapes on the skin flaps avoids skin necrosis at the vertical wounds.
- Liposuction is not used to reduce the volume because a firm conic breast can be better reshaped with scalpel and sutures.
- The inferior part of the skin that attached to the breast will now be attached to the chest wall. This skin was routinely removed with the inverted T technique, which is the main difference between the techniques.

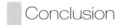

Conclusion

Once the breast is removed, using the circumvertical reduction mastoplasty, there is a conic breast reshaping, a new SMF is defined and the parenchyma is fixed to the pectoral fascia. Most of the skin is gathered around the areola, there is a harmonic distribution of the pleats all along the wounds and the vertical wound never crosses the submammary fold. Furthermore, without any pedicle for areola transposition, its blood supply and breast feeding function remain unaltered. An important difference from the vertical techniques is that a nice result can be observed at the end of the surgery.

Further reading

Benelli L. A new periareolar mammaplasty: The 'round block' technique. Aesth Plast Surg 1990;14:93–100.

Graft R. Breast shape: a technique for better upper pole fullness. Aesthet Plast Surg 2000;24:348.

Hall FE. A simplified vertical reduction mammaplasty: shortening the learning curve. Plast Reconst Surg 1999;104:748.

Hammond D. The SPAIR mammaplasty. Clin Plast Surg; 2002;29:411–421.

Lassus C. Breast reduction: evolution of a technique: a single vertical scar. Aesth Plast Surg 1987; 11:107–112.

Lassus C. Update on vertical mammaplasty. Plast Reconstr Surg 1999;104:7.

Lejour M. Suction mammaplasty. Correspondence. Plast Reconstr Surg 1992;89:1.

Lejour M. Vertical mammaplasty and liposuction of the breast. Plast Reconstr Surg 1994;94:1.

Menke H, Restel B, Olbrisch RR. Vertical scar reduction mammaplasty as a standard procedure – Experiences in the introduction and validation of a modified reduction technique. Eur J Plast Surg 1999;22:74–79.

Mottura AA. Mastoplastia reductiva con anestesia local. Rev Argent Mastol 1990;9:56–61.

Mottura AA. Zirkumverticale Mammareduktionplastik. In: Lemperle G (Ed). Aesthetische Chirurgie. Ecomed, Grand Werk; 1998, pp 1–5.

Mottura AA. Circumvertical reduction mastoplasty. Aesthet Surg J 2000;20:199–204.

14

Vertical breast reduction

Elizabeth J. Hall-Findlay

Key points

- The pedicle, the skin resection pattern and the parenchymal resection pattern should all be treated as separate entities.

- The Wise pattern (not just the keyhole opening) is an excellent pattern for what parenchyma should be left behind.

- The resection is in the shape of a vertical ellipse rather than the horizontal ellipse that is common with an inferior pedicle inverted T pattern. The vertical wedge excision results in coning of the breast with good projection and an absence of

medial and lateral dog-ears. There are, however, two vertical dog-ears, one into the areola and one inferiorly.

- The excess parenchyma should be excised by direct excision and then tailored out by liposuction.

- Neither the pillars nor the skin should be closed under tension.

- Under-resection will result in bottoming out over time.

Introduction

Vertical breast reduction is not just one procedure. There are many breast reduction techniques which fit into the category of 'short scar' or 'vertical' approaches. The word 'vertical' applies only to the fact that there is a vertical scar (as well as a scar around the areola) but little or no inframammary scar. It is important to separate the concepts of the skin resection pattern (which results in a vertical scar), the pedicle design, and the parenchymal resection. Different pedicles can be adapted to different skin resection patterns.

The pedicle will dictate the parenchymal resection to some degree but there are still multiple possible variations.

This chapter will describe the medial pedicle design with a vertical skin resection pattern and an inferior parenchymal resection pattern. An inferior pedicle will dictate a superior resection and a more difficult skin closure. The technique described here can easily incorporate a superior, a lateral or a medial pedicle. The medial pedicle is chosen because it has a reliable blood supply, it has good sensation and it is easy to inset. The fact that the inferior border of the medial pedicle becomes the medial pillar allows the surgeon to give the patient an immediate good shape with an elegant lower pole.

Patient selection

The best patients for a vertical type approach using a medial pedicle are those with good skin quality and who require a small to medium breast reduction (up to 1000 g). The same technique can be used with larger breast reductions but the skin resection pattern may need to be altered to include a 'J', and 'L' or a 'T' extension along the inframammary fold. The surgeon's threshold for conversion will occur earlier in patients (such as massive weight loss) with poor skin quality.

There are very few patients where a superomedial or medial pedicle cannot be used. A truly supero-medial pedicle is more likely to include the strong descending artery from the second interspace, but it may be more difficult to inset than a purely medial pedicle. The advantage to persisting with a medially or superomedially based pedicle even in very large breast reductions is that the heavy inferior breast tissue is removed (thereby defying gravity) and the superior breast tissue remains still attached to the chest wall and the superior skin. Extremely large patients could be warned that the surgeon may need to convert to free nipple grafts intraoperatively but this would only rarely happen.

Patients and surgeons need to understand that the breast cannot be elevated on the chest wall. Some patients are 'high-breasted' and some are 'low-breasted'. Some patients will have a narrow vertical breast footprint and some will have a very long vertical breast footprint. The upper breast border cannot be changed with sutures but the inframammary fold can be elevated slightly. Much of plastic surgery is about managing patient expectations and a patient who understands that her brassiere band or underwire will remain at the same level will be more appreciative of the final result.

There are very few flaps that have been able to increase upper pole fullness long-term. Only implants and fat injections seem successful at elevating the upper breast border and increasing upper pole fullness and unfortunately many of the procedures that remove tissue in the upper pole create an actual loss in upper pole fullness. I tried suturing breast tissue up higher onto the chest wall in 77 patients (43 with PDS and 34 with braided polyester) and in not one of the patients who returned for follow-up did the improvement in upper pole fullness last for more than a few months. The medial pedicle vertical breast reduction, however, does maintain upper pole fullness. It is important for surgeons to realize that pushing tissue into the upper pole will only end up with bottoming-out and a poor result.

Indications

Surgeons and patients (and only some insurance carriers) are well aware that breast reduction surgery of any type will improve upper back and neck pain, shoulder grooving, skin rashes, posture, exercise tolerance and self-esteem. The medial pedicle vertical breast reduction is a good choice for patients who want to preserve sensation and the possible ability to breastfeed. The statistics for breastfeeding after medial pedicle reduction are about the same as for other full thickness pedicles such as the inferior pedicle (about 60%). About 85% of patients recover normal to near-normal sensation with this technique. This is comparable to most of the other pedicle techniques.

There is no question that patients who are overweight will not get as good a cosmetic improvement as those patients who are closer to their ideal body weight. The obese patient is more prone to complications. These patients tend to believe that they will lose weight after the surgery but it has been my experience that if they have not changed their lifestyle prior to surgery they are unlikely to change it after surgery.

Operative technique

Pre-operative preparation

It is important to note and explain to the patient about the breast footprint and whether they are 'high-breasted' or 'low-breasted' (Figure 14.1). They also need to be aware of how much upper pole fullness they have (or not) and that this upper slope will not change. They also need to be aware that there will still be some breast skin resting on the chest wall after surgery. They often bring in photos of women where the nipple sits well above the inframammary fold but they need to realize that the nipple will be lower with an inferior curve to the lower pole of the breast. The nipple will still sit about one-third to one-half up the breast mound, but the breast mound shape will be

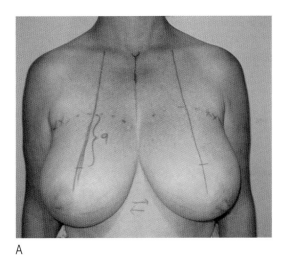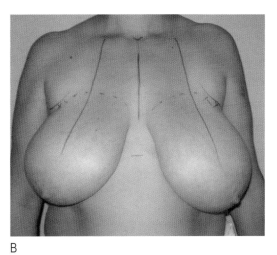

A   B

Figure 14.1 (A) This patient is 'high breasted' with her breasts high on the chest wall. She has a long vertical breast footprint with a high upper breast border and a low inframammary fold. (B) This patient is 'low breasted' with her breasts lower on the chest wall. She has a lower upper breast border but a high inframammary fold. She has a narrow vertical breast footprint.

slightly lower than that achieved in many breast augmentation patients.

Markings

Upper breast border

The upper breast border sits just above the pre-axillary indentation and it is usually just above any striae that may be present (Figure 14.2). This border is marked to give the surgeon an idea of where the nipple should be – usually about 9–11 cm below this border.

Inframammary fold

The inframammary fold is often a good guide for the new nipple position but it can be misleading in patients with either a very long or very short vertical breast footprint. The upper breast border is actually a better guide.

Breast meridian

The breast meridian should be drawn where it is desired, not where it is. The surgeon should ignore the current nipple position and draw the breast meridian where it should be. This will usually be about 10 cm from the midline at the medial extent of the inframammary fold. The medial pedicle vertical breast reduction is more effective than an inverted T inferior

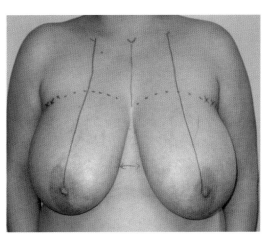

Figure 14.2 It is important to mark the upper breast border just anterior to the pre-axillary depression (marked with x's). It is shown as a dotted line. The inframammary fold is marked between the breasts. The new breast meridian is drawn where it should be, ignoring the nipple position.

pedicle technique at reducing the lateral breast fullness so the meridian can be drawn a bit more medially. It is, however, better to have the new nipple position marked too far laterally than too far medially (the same rule applies to making it lower rather than higher).

New nipple position

The new nipple position should be at the intersection of the mark made on the breast meridian which will be about 10 cm below the upper breast border (Figure 14.3). This will often be (except in about 15% of patients) about the level of the inframammary fold. The nipple is best placed lower in patients who have poor upper pole fullness and the surgeon needs to be aware that the nipple will appear to be higher because of the increased projection that is achieved with this technique. In asymmetry cases the new nipple position should be placed slightly lower on the larger breast to accommodate for the skin stretch in the larger breast and the fact that closure of a wider ellipse will push the superior end of the ellipse higher.

Upper areolar border

The upper border of the areola is then marked about 2 cm above the new nipple position (Figures 14.4, 14.5). The areola is designed to be about 4–5 cm in diameter and 2 cm works well as a standard measurement.

Areolar design

The areola is designed so that it ends up as a circle when it is closed (Figure 14.6). It does not need to be 'mosque' shaped. A good template is a large paper clip

made into a circle and then opened out. A large paper clip is 16 cm in length and 16 cm is the circumference around a 5 cm diameter areola. The original Wise pattern had a 14 cm diameter areola which matches a 4.5 cm diameter areola.

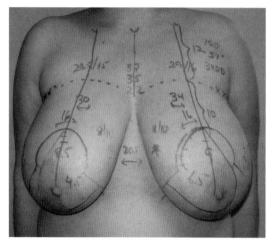

Figure 14.4 The areola is marked 2 cm above the new nipple position. The areola is marked 16 cm in circumference (which matches a 5 cm diameter areola). The medial pedicle is marked with the base half way into the areolar opening with a base of about 8 cm. The rest of the numbers are for statistical study only and are not necessary for the design.

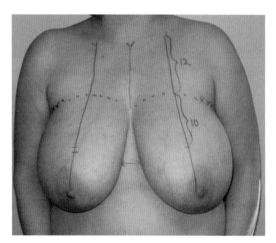

Figure 14.3 The new nipple position is marked about 10 cm below the upper breast border. In this patient it is somewhat higher than the inframammary fold level.

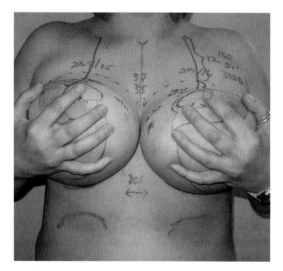

Figure 14.5 The skin resection pattern follows the standard Wise pattern but instead of extending laterally and medially the two limbs are joined together about 2–4 cm above the inframammary fold.

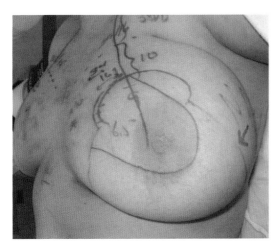

Figure 14.6 The skin resection pattern and the medial pedicle are shown. The red arrows mark the arteries that can be determined by Doppler examination. The descending branch of the artery from the second interspace usually enters the areolar opening just medial to the breast meridian and it is about 1 cm deep to the skin surface. The superficial branch of the lateral thoracic artery is also marked. The deep perforators and the medial supply are too deep to be heard with a Doppler.

Skin resection pattern

The vertical limbs of the usual keyhole opening are then drawn and instead of extending them laterally and medially for the standard anchor pattern, they are then circled around and joined together about 2–4 cm above the inframammary fold. It is important to draw this as a 'snowman' and curve the lower end of the incision as a 'U' and not as a 'V' or otherwise too much skin will be left behind. The surgeon can pinch the skin to make sure that the closure will not be under tension (the skin does not act as a brassiere but instead adapts to the breast shape).

Medial pedicle

The pedicle is then designed with about half of the base in the areolar opening and about half below. The base of the pedicle is usually about 6–10 cm. The medial pedicle base rotates so that the inferior border of the medial pedicle will become the medial pillar. The medial pedicle also allows for easy access to the excess lateral breast tissue. If the pedicle is very long it might be prudent to try to include the descending branch of the artery from the second interspace (from the internal mammary artery) which usually enters the areolar opening about the level of the breast meridian. Including this artery can make the pedicle more difficult to inset than a purely medial pedicle. The artery can be found by Doppler because it is usually no more than 1 cm deep to the skin surface. It is also prudent to include one of the veins that can be seen through the skin. The superficial venous system is separate from the arteries and the veins can be found just beneath the dermis and they can be seen to be draining medially and superiorly. The pedicle should be designed so that a cuff of dermis is left around the areola.

Liposuction areas

The areas to be suctioned are marked. This includes the area along the inframammary fold below the Wise pattern, the pre-axillary area and the lateral chest wall fullness.

Operative technique

Infiltration

Xylocaine with epinephrine is infiltrated into the areas to be liposuctioned only. The incision lines are not infiltrated because the needles can damage the superficial veins. Tumescent type infiltration is used in these areas when the patient is overweight (Figures 14.7, 14.8).

Creation of the pedicle

The pedicle is de-epithelialized and then cut straight down to chest wall as a full thickness pedicle. The arterial supply is deep at the sternal border medially and progresses superficially and a dermal pedicle at the level of the areola should have good blood supply but a full thickness pedicle is more likely to maintain innervation and preserve breast feeding potential. Most of the blood vessels will be encountered in the first couple of centimeters deep to the surface. Either cutting cautery or a scalpel can be used. If the assistant puts too much traction on the pedicle it can be inadvertently undermined.

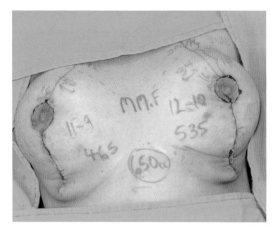

Figure 14.7 The patient shown in these figures had 465 g removed from the right breast and 535 g removed from the left breast. Another 650 mL of fat was removed with liposuction. Note that the vertical incisions are not shortened and that the pucker is left uncorrected.

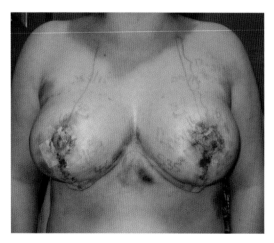

Figure 14.8 The same patient is shown the morning of the first post-operative day.

Parenchymal resection

The parenchyma is then resected en bloc by beveling out laterally, medially and inferiorly. Tissue is left over the pectoralis fascia to preserve innervation and to prevent excessive bleeding. The artery and its venae comitantes to the inferior pedicle will be encountered about 4–6 cm above the inframammary fold just medial to the breast meridian. It is important to seek this out and make sure that hemostasis is secured. The superficial branch of the lateral thoracic artery will also be encountered a couple of centimeters deep to the skin surface on the lateral aspect but often more caudal than what would normally be incorporated into a lateral pedicle.

It is difficult with this technique to remove enough breast tissue – the best place to resect more is laterally. A lateral pillar which is about 2 cm thick should be left attached to the skin. Tissue deep to this and inferior to the pillar (leaving the pillar length about 5–7 cm) can be excised. It is usually quite fibrous and not amenable to removal by liposuction. Extra tissue is removed down to the inframammary fold and medially making sure to remove tissue in the ghost areas (as described by Carolyn Kerrigan) which are the areas below the Wise pattern. As Louis Benelli has said, the Wise pattern (Figure 14.9A,B) is a good geometric design for the breast tissue but not for the skin. These inferior flaps will need to be thin but must still maintain some fat on the undersurface to prevent scar contracture.

Liposuction

The dermis is closed first so that the areas to be suctioned can be better visualized. The dermal closure makes it easier to perform the liposuction because of the resistance created. All the fibrous tissue below the Wise pattern will need to be directly excised and liposuction can be used for peripheral tailoring.

 Closure

Pillar closure

The base of the areola is closed first with an interrupted 3-0 monocryl suture (Figure 14.10). This allows for assessment of the resection and for pillar orientation. The pedicle is then easily inset by rotating it into position. If there is any resistance tissue deep to the surface can be removed superiorly and medially because the blood supply is superficial. The inferior border of the medial pedicle becomes the medial pillar. The pillars follow the Wise pattern and are about 5–7 cm in length. Pillar closure starts inferiorly (it helps to pull up on the areola to keep the pillars in good position). The lower border of the pillars is not at the inframammary fold or even at the lower aspect of the skin, but about half way up the skin opening.

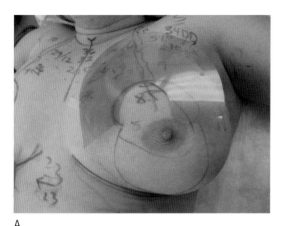
A

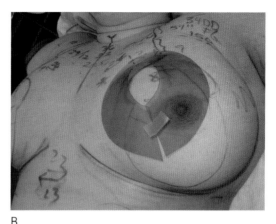
B

Figure 14.9 (A) The Wise pattern is not just the keyhole opening but a design created from a brassiere pattern. The Wise pattern is a good pattern for the parenchyma that is left behind. (B) When the Wise pattern is closed (and the pillars brought together) the breast achieves a good shape and good projection.

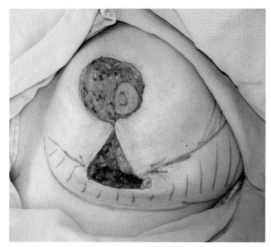

Figure 14.10 The base of the areolar opening is closed. The inferior border of the medial pedicle becomes the medial pillar and the whole base of the pedicle rotates. This gives an elegant curve to the lower pole of the breast. The bases of the pillars are brought together with about 3 sutures and the closure starts about half way up the skin opening. The parenchyma below the Wise pattern is marked by cross hatching and this is the area that needs to be resected (and tailored out by liposuction peripherally). The skin will then adapt to the new breast design rather than the other way around.

The surgeon should keep the Wise pattern in mind when assessing the parenchymal shape. The pillars are closed with about three interrupted 3-0 monocryl sutures place about 1–2 cm deep to the skin surface. The sutures do not need to be deep and constricting but should just grasp some fibrous tissue to allow fibrous tissue to heal to fibrous tissue. Neither the pillars nor the breast tissue need to be sutured up to the chest wall.

Deep dermal closure

The dermis is closed with only enough sutures to allow dermal to dermal apposition (Figure 14.11). Too many sutures will cause constriction of the blood supply to the wound margins. Interrupted buried 3-0 monocryl sutures are used. The dermis does not need to be sutured up to breast tissue. Liposuction is performed after deep dermal closure. Four deep interrupted sutures are placed around the areola.

Skin closure

3-0 monocryl is also used for the subcuticular closure. The original vertical designs attempted to shorten this vertical length but that only resulted in wound healing problems. It is important not to gather the vertical incision. I measured this distance before surgery, before closure and at each follow-up visit and the incision just lengthened. Surgeons have trouble

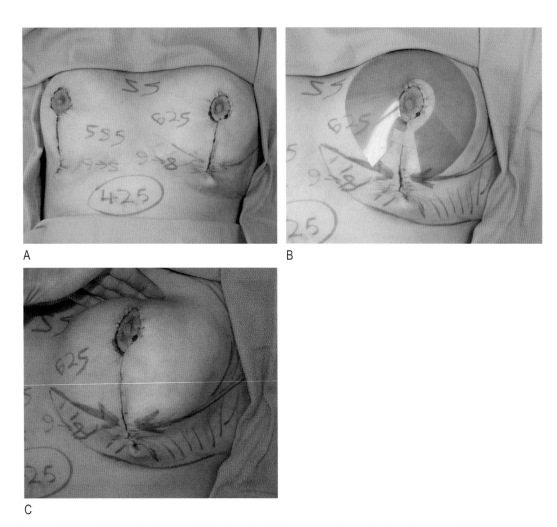

A

B

C

Figure 14.11   (A) The patient shown in this figure had 585 g removed from the right breast and 625 g removed from the left breast. Another 425 mL of fat was removed by liposuction. The pucker is not sutured down or corrected. The vertical incision is not shortened or pleated. (B) The Wise pattern over the breast at the end of the procedure shows how good a design it is for determining what to remove and what to leave in a medial pedicle vertical breast reduction. (C) This maneuver shows that the breast descends back to its normal position and the pucker tucks in.

understanding that a long vertical incision is actually quite acceptable. A good shape can be achieved with 9–11 cm scar length below the areola in a large 'C' cup shape. The gathered or pleated incision looks better at the end of the procedure but it actually delays resolution. The pucker will tuck in quite quickly in the weeks after surgery. The pucker does not need to be sutured down to chest wall because the actual location may be difficult to determine. The areola is also closed with a subcuticular 3-0 monocryl suture.

Post-operative care

Drains are only rarely used. Drains do not prevent or treat a hematoma. The incisions are covered with paper tape. Patients shower the next day and just pat the tape dry. The tape provides a good bandage and it stays in place for 3–4 weeks. When the tape comes off the incisions are nicely approximated. Brassieres are used only to hold gauze in place. It would be good to apply pressure to the lateral chest wall area where liposuction was performed, but excess pressure could cause problems with the nipple–areola complex.

Operative steps

- Marking in the standing position including new nipple position.
- Infiltration only in the areas to be suctioned avoiding damage to the veins.
- Creation of a full thickness medially based pedicle.
- Resection of parenchyma by beveling out laterally, medially and inferiorly.
- Extra resection can be performed laterally deep to the lateral skin flap.

- Inferior border of the medial pedicle becomes the medial pillar.
- Pillar closure starting about half way up the skin opening.
- Deep dermal closure with not too many sutures.
- Liposuction beyond the direct excision areas to leave a Wise pattern behind.
- Subcuticular closure without gathering.
- No drains.
- Paper tape for 3–4 weeks and brassiere only to hold bandages in place.

Results

Case **1**

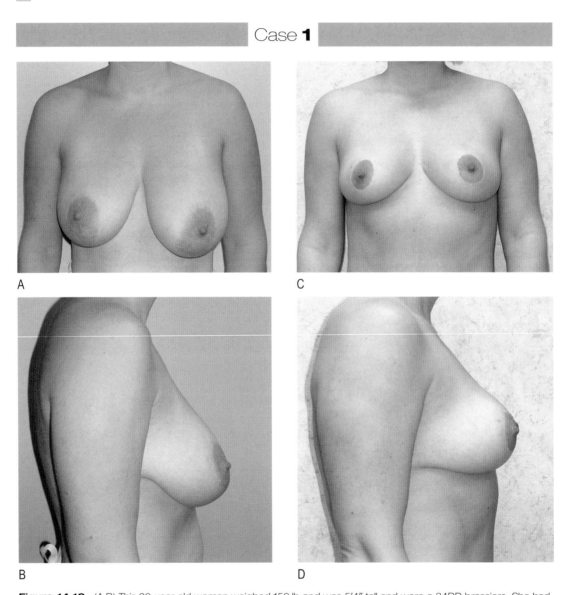

A

C

B

D

Figure 14.12 (A,B) This 30-year-old woman weighed 150 lb and was 5′4″ tall and wore a 34DD brassiere. She had 250 g removed from the right breast and 400 g from the left breast. The liposuction amount was 150 mL. The slight asymmetry shows that it is important to place the new nipple position slightly lower on the larger side (which was not done in this case). She reported a complete return of nipple sensation. (C,D) The follow-up photos are shown at 18 months after surgery.

Case 2

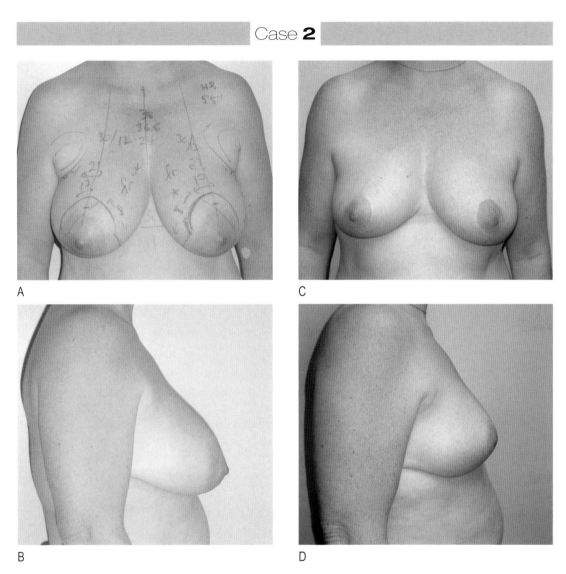

A

B

C

D

Figure 14.13 (A,B) This 50-year-old woman weighed 180 lb, was 5'5" tall and wore a 38D brassiere. She had 410 g removed from the right breast and 440 g removed from the left breast. She also had 575 mL of fat removed by liposuction. She reported a complete return of nipple sensation. (C,D) The follow-up photos are shown at 4 years after surgery.

Case **3**

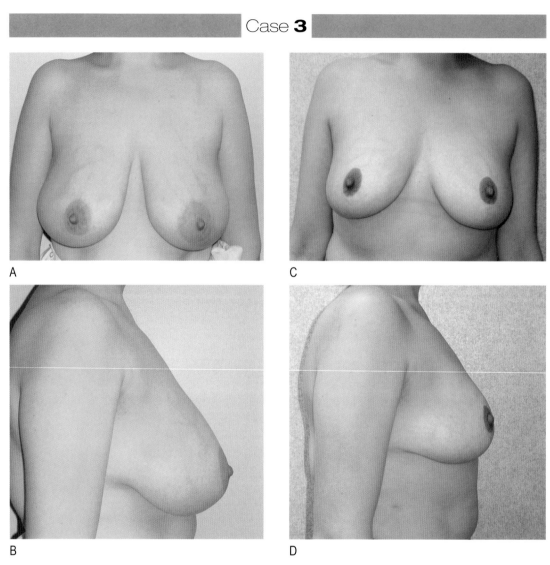

A   C
B   D

Figure 14.14   (A,B) This 36-year-old woman weighed 160 lb and was 5′9½″ tall and wore a 38DD brassiere. She had 600 g removed from the right breast and 550 g removed from the left breast. She had 475 mL of fat removed by liposuction. She reported a complete return of nipple sensation. (C,D) The follow-up photos are shown at 3½ years after surgery.

Pitfalls

The main pitfall with this vertical approach is that sometimes the pucker at the inferior end of the vertical incision may need to be excised under local anaesthesia in the office. Most puckers disappear and it is important to warn the patients that this can take a full year although it usually settles in the first few weeks or months. The key to correcting the pucker is to understand that it is usually a problem of excess subcutaneous tissue rather than a problem of excess skin.

Surgeons will try to avoid the pucker by carrying the skin excision down to the inframammary fold but this will only result in a scar that ends up on the chest wall. It is important to leave at least 2–4 cm of skin above the inframammary fold. It is also important to excess the skin inferiorly as a 'U' rather than a 'V' otherwise there will be too much skin left behind as well as excess subcutaneous tissue. The pucker often results because the inframammary fold rises. Purposely elevating the fold by excision of fold fibers can give a better shape to the breast but it can increase the revision rate. When a pucker does need correction the best method is to excise a small amount of skin in a vertical direction (not horizontal unless the scar is below the fold) and then excise the fat out laterally and medially.

Case **4**

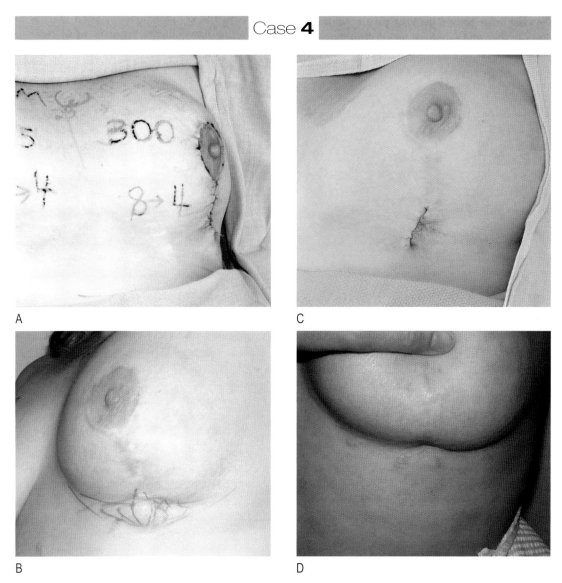

A

B

C

D

Figure 14.15 (A,B) This patient had a pucker after removal of 300 g from the left breast. The pucker was corrected with a vertical skin excision and the fat was excised laterally and medially. (C,D) The correction is shown a few weeks later.

The second major pitfall is to close the skin under tension. Surgeons are so comfortable with the inverted T inferior pedicle technique and using the skin as a brassiere that they find it hard to leave the skin loose. Unfortunately the inverted T methods have more wound healing problems than the vertical techniques because the skin is closed under tension. It is also important for surgeons to realize that the best final breast shape is to leave behind a Wise pattern of parenchyma without closing the pillars under tension. It is better to close the parenchyma loosely and excise all the extra tissue beyond the Wise pattern (with both direct excision and peripheral liposuction).

Post-operative care

Patients are allowed to resume activities fairly quickly and they are instructed to use their discomfort level as their guide. They will usually return to work in 2–3 weeks. They will usually wear the post-operative brassiere for about 2 weeks day and night but mostly to give them a sense of support. There will be some bruising from the liposuction and patients need to realize that there will be some hardening especially in the lateral chest wall during resolution.

A patient with a hematoma will probably need to be taken back to the operating room. Seromas, on the other hand, do occur but do not usually need to be treated. They can be aspirated but they will drain out and disappear without intervention. If nipple congestion is seen the treatment would be to relieve the pressure - either by removing sutures or taking the patient back to the operating room. If necrosis is evident after the first 24 h it is probably best to allow the necrosis to demarcate without intervention.

Conclusion

The medial pedicle vertical breast reduction gives excellent short-term and long-term results. The shape is good 'on the table' and it resolves quickly. A pucker will need to be corrected in about 5% of cases but this revision rate is no different from other procedures in plastic surgery. It is actually easier to correct this inferior pucker than it is to correct the medial and lateral pucker that can result after an inverted T approach. The key to achieving a good result is to remove the heavy inferior breast tissue in order to defy gravity. The breast tissue is left in the brassiere design shape reported by Robert Wise in 1956. All the tissue beyond the Wise pattern is removed by direct excision and then tailored out peripherally with liposuction.

It is important for surgeons to understand that a good breast shape after reduction or mastopexy has a longer inferior pole than what is usually sought after breast augmentation. The breast shape curves down below the inframammary fold rather than immediately curving upwards. The breast augmentation shape and the breast reduction shape are both good shapes but they are different. The nipple in both cases is 'centralized' on the breast mound but the breast mound is completely above the fold in many augmentations but closer to the level of the inframammary fold in many reductions. The surgeon also needs to understand the concept of, and the variations of, the breast footprint so that patients can understand that they may be either 'high-breasted' or 'low-breasted'. A pre-operatively informed patient is the surgeon's best ally.

Further reading

Arie G. Una nueva tecnica de mastoplastia. Rev Iber Latino Am Cir Plast 1957;3:28.

Asplund O, Davies DM. Vertical scar breast reduction with medial flap or glandular transposition of the nipple-areola. Br J Plast Surg 1996;49:507–514.

Benelli L, A new periareolar mammaplasty: The 'round block' technique. Aesth Plast Surg 1990;14:93.

Courtiss EH, Goldwyn, RM, Reduction mammaplasty by the inferior pedicle technique. An alternative to free nipple and areola grafting for severe macromastia or extreme ptosis. Plast Reconstr Surg 1977;59:500.

Cruz-Korchin N, Korchin L. Breast-feeding after vertical mammaplasty with medial pedicle. Plast Reconstr Surg 2004;114:890–894.

Hall-Findlay EJ. A simplified vertical reduction mammaplasty: shortening the learning curve. Plast Reconstr Surg 1999;104:748.

Hall-Findlay EJ. Vertical breast reduction with a medially based pedicle. Operative strategies. Aesth Surg J 2002;22:185–195.

Hammond, DC. Short scar periareolar inferior pedicle reduction (SPAIR) mammaplasty. Plast Reconstr Surg 1999;103:890.

Lassus C. A technique for breast reduction. Int Surg 1970;53:69.

Lejour M, Abboud M, Declety A, Kertesz P. Reduction des cicatrices de plastie mammaire: de l'ancre courte a la verticale. Ann Chir Plast Esthet 1990;35:369.

McKissock PK, Reduction mammaplasty with a vertical dermal flap. Plast Reconstr Surg 1972;49:245–252.

Marchac D, de Olarte G. Reduction mammaplasty and correction of ptosis with a short inframammary scar. Plast Reconstr Surg 1982; 69:45–55.

Mottura A, Circumvertical Reduction Mammaplasty. Aesthetic Surg J 2000;20:199–204.

Peixoto G, Reduction mammaplasty: a personal technique. Plast Reconstr Surg 1980;65:217.

Skoog T. A technique of breast reduction - transposition of the nipple on a cutaneous vascular pedicle. Acta Chir Scand 1963;126:453–465.

Spear SL, Howard MA. Evolution of the vertical reduction mammaplasty. Plast Reconstr Surg 2003;112:855–868.

Strombeck JO. Mammaplasty: report of a new technique based on the two-pedicle procedure. Br J Plast Surg 1960;13:79–90.

Wise RJ. A preliminary report on a method of planning the mammaplasty. Plast Reconstr Surg 1956;17:367.

Wuringer E, Refinement of the central pedicle breast reduction by application of the ligamentous suspension. Plast Reconstr Surg 1999;103:1400.

Vertical mammaplasty

Ruth M. Graf, André R.D. Tolazzi, Maria Cecília C. Ono

Key points

- Vertical mammaplasty causes fewer scars, narrows the wide breast, reduces the bottoming out phenomenon, improves projection, and offers better long-term shape when compared with the inverted T techniques.

- It can be performed in patients with several degrees of breast hypertrophy and ptosis, but the best results have been achieved in mild and moderate cases. Parenchyma resection follows the vertical principle, which narrows the base, increasing breast projection and avoiding the flat and broad shape. Periareolar skin compensation reduces the length of the vertical scar, avoiding its elongation across the inframammary crease.

- In order to obtain a better long-term outcome, it is mandatory to redefine breast shape with internal tissue, not with skin sutures, therefore avoiding exaggerated scar tension.

- Better and long-term breast shape can be achieved using the chest wall based flap under a sling of major pectoralis muscle, together with liposuction to the lateral breast area.

Introduction

Breast reduction and mastopexy remains one of the most challenging operations in plastic surgery. Since the surgeon is usually faced with hypertrophic and/or ptotic breast tissue that requires a well-planned and careful approach, many believe that perfection is hard to achieve. The fact that many different options exist does not necessarily make this problem any easier. The goal of mammaplasty /mastopexy is to provide long-lasting results, reducing the breast size, improving upper pole fullness, repositioning the nipple–areola complex and tightening the skin brassiere.

Currently, aesthetic breast surgery not only reduces breast size, but also restores a firm and youthful look to the breast. This is not possible without placing incisions on the breast. However, in some cases, hypertrophic scarring may also jeopardize the final appearance. Thus, minimizing the extent of scarring remains a key point when modifying existing techniques and introducing innovative procedures. The so-called 'short scar or limited scar mammaplasty' has evolved out of the necessity to reduce the length of the incisions, as patients are highly concerned with the aesthetic outcome and often request the shortest scar possible. Trading a ptotic breast for a visibly scarred breast with a chance of recurrent ptosis is a poor choice. The term 'short scar mammaplasty' is not limited to one specific technique but is used to describe techniques that minimize the extent of scarring. There are basically four different scarring patterns, with some variations to each one (periareolar, vertical, L-shape and inverted T short scars). Usually, a number of different techniques exist for each pattern (Rohrich et al 2004).

Vertical mammaplasty is an appealing technique because it promises fewer scars, narrowing of the wide breast, reducing the bottoming out phenomenon, improved projection, and stable long-term shape when compared with the inverted-T techniques (Hidalgo 2005). Several authors have reported vertical techniques that are conceptually similar but vary in some details. Issues that differ among previous descriptions include the role of liposuction (integral or incidental), pedicle design (superior or medial), and whether or not to undermine the lower pole skin, imbricate the lower pole, or elevate the parenchyma by suture to the pectoralis major muscle (Hall-Findlay 1999, 2002, Lassus 1970, 1987, 1996, Lejour & Abboud 1990, Lejour 1994a, b). Vertical mammaplasty is quite different from inverted T techniques in both design, execution, immediate and long-term results (Balch 1981, Bostwick 1983, Courtiss & Goldwyn 1977, Finger et al 1989, Hester et al 1985, Hugo & McClellan 1979, Labandter et al 1982, McKissock 1972, Orlando & Guthrie 1975, Pitanguy 1967, Robbins 1977, Robbins & Hoffman 1992). It is inherently more intuitive and requires a certain amount of experience before a surgeon becomes proficient. Parenchyma resection follows the vertical principle, which narrows the base, increasing breast projection and avoiding the flat and broad shape. Immediate postoperative result quite frequently is not optimal due to pleating of the skin in order to avoid extending the scar, which is presumed to 'settle out' favorably over time. The vertical component of the scar is longer than in inverted T techniques, because less pronounced parenchyma descent is expected, causing minimal elongation of the vertical scar.

Dartigues was the first author to describe a vertical scar technique used for mastopexy (Dartigues 1925). In 1957, Arie described a technique for reduction mammaplasty finishing with a vertical scar which did not gain popularity because the vertical scar often crossed the inframammary crease and extended onto the chest wall, leaving an unsightly scar (Arie 1957). It was only in 1969 that Lassus renewed interest in vertical scar breast reduction by developing a technique using a superior dermoglandular pedicle for

transposition of the nipple–areola complex; a central excision en bloc of skin, fat, and gland; no undermining and finishing with a vertical scar (Lassus 1969, 1970). In 1994, Lejour described a modification of Lassus's technique, beginning the breast reduction with liposuction to eliminate fat contributing to breast volume (Lejour 1994a, b). The skin surrounding the excised area was undermined and the superior dermoglandular pedicle was sutured to the pectoralis fascia, joint pillars to improve breast shape, and suturing the skin of the vertical wound above the inframammary crease.

Lassus's and Lejour's techniques demonstrated positive outcomes when applied not only in mild and moderate cases of breast hypertrophy, but in severe cases as well. Hammond adds the vertical component intraoperatively in his short scar periareolar inferior pedicle reduction mammaplasty/mastopexy, initially using a periareolar incision and then working redundant skin to the lower portion of the areola where it can be excised in a vertical fashion (Hammond 1999). Graf & Biggs (2002) described an interesting concept to increase longevity and especially enhance upper-pole fullness of the breast. They use a chest wall based flap passed under and held by a pectoralis muscle sling (Graf & Biggs 2002).

Recently, working with the philosophy of the periareolar technique associated with the vertical scar technique, it has been possible to reduce scar length, thus avoiding its elongation across the inframammary crease by compensating for skin excess around the areola. It was observed that in every single technique performed, the breast shape after descent resulted in loss of upper pole fullness. Some authors used the inferior portion of breast tissue to fill in the upper pole or the areola to achieve a better breast shape. In addition to scar evolution, since 1994 we have been using a sling of major pectoralis muscle to allow long-term maintenance of upper pole volume (Ribeiro 1975, de Auraújo Cerqueira 1998). In order to obtain a better long-term outcome, it is mandatory to redefine breast shape with internal tissue, not with skin sutures, therefore avoiding exaggerated scar tension. It has been observed that passing the chest wall based flap under a sling of pectoralis major muscle permits a longer definition of the breast shape and upper pole fullness. Liposuction on the lateral breast area helps to better define the lateral fold.

Therefore, Ribeiro's technique was then utilized, which is an inferior pedicle flap (Ribeiro 1975), modified by Daniel, who associated a bipedicled flap of major pectoralis muscle to keep Ribeiro's flap in a higher position (Daniel 1995). The approach was switched from inferior pedicle flaps to flaps based only on the thoracic wall vasculature, completely detached from the surrounding structures, keeping the overlying dermis to give better support and shape to the flap, fixating it to pectoralis fascia. The association of vertical mammaplasty principles with chest wall based flap held by a bipedicle pectoralis muscle flap has improved long-term results.

The upper pole of the breast remains with a good volume and the vertical scar is placed above or at the level of the new inframammary crease with a minimal breast descent. This technique is indicated either in patients who need only a mastopexy and reduction, no breast tissue or for breast reductions where excessive breast tissue is resected from the columns or base of the breast, after the thoracic wall flap is built and fixed. With this technique we realized that less breast tissue is resected compared with the other techniques without the thoracic flap. In large hypertrophies or severe ptosis, the 'D' point should be marked higher to the 'M' point, by up to 4 cm. This maneuver is done to leave skin and subcutaneous tissue of the lower breast pole as part of the thoracic wall, with a higher new inframammary crease, decreasing skin compensation in the vertical scar.

The redundant skin in the vertical can be compensated with a subcuticular suture that shortens this scar. During the first 2 months of the post-operative period there is flattening of the wrinkles with no need to remove skin horizontally in the inferior portion of this scar, as suggested by Marchac (Marchac & Olarte 1982). A periareolar round block suture is done with the purpose of reducing even more the length of vertical scar by compensating skin excess around the areola. Taking larger suture bites in the outer skin circle in order to compensate the skin around the areolar.

The goals of a vertical scar technique associated with chest wall based flap and bipedicled major pectoralis muscle flap are: maintain the breast upper pole fullness with the patient in a standing position, providing a better aesthetic outcome in the long-term follow-up; avoid vertical scar crossing the new inframammary crease; project the nipple–

areolar complex even using the periareolar round block suture.

Personal technique

Preoperative preparation

Usually every patient is being followed annually by a mastologist. If not, the patient is referred for a specialized breast evaluation prior to the operation. Preoperative mammograms and, when necessary, a breast ultrasound is routinely ordered. Smokers are requested to stop smoking at least 1 month before and for 2 weeks after surgery. On the day before the operation, skin is marked and an antiseptic soap is prescribed.

Markings

The same skin markings can be used to perform either breast reduction or mastopexy, with the only difference being during surgery where tissue removal is performed where indicated. A line from the sternal notch to the xiphoid process is drawn (midline). The meridian line is drawn from the midclavicle to the NAC, crossing the inframammary crease ('M' point), which is 12 cm or more from the midline. The 'A' point is marked 18–20 cm from the clavicle or 20–22 cm from the sternal notch. With a horizontal maneuver, the breast is moved medially and laterally and two points ('B' and 'C') are marked, using the vertical line inferior to the areola as a reference, which demonstrates the skin in excess. Using these three points as a reference, a curved line is drawn around the areola in an oval shape, similar to the periareolar technique. The medial portion of this line is, on average, 9 cm from the midline, and the lateral portion is, on average, 12 cm from the anterior axillary line. Point 'D' is marked, 2–4 cm above point 'M'. Points 'BD' and 'CD' are joined together in a curved line of approximately 5–7 cm (Figures 15.1, 15.2).

Surgical technique

Surgery begins with de-epithelialization of the area previously described keeping the subdermal plexus intact. Dermis is incised along the marked lines, up to 1.5–2 cm superior to points 'B' and 'C' sparing the upper portion of the areola, which is the pedicle for the NAC (Figure 15.3). Dermis is also incised

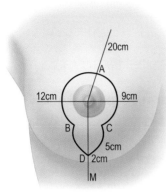

Figure 15.1 Basic markings of vertical technique. A point, 20 cm from the clavicle; B and C points, pinching maneuver; D point, 2 cm above the inframammary crease.

horizontally 1 cm inferior to the areola and subcutaneous tissue is incised perpendicular to the plane of the thoracic wall, reaching the pectoral fascia at the level of the fourth intercostal space.

The incision is then made obliquely in the upper portion of the flap, leaving enough breast tissue on either side (future breast pillars) (Figure 15.4). Breast tissue is undermined to the level of the second intercostal space, at the level of the pectoralis major fascia. The lower portion of the flap is dissected carefully down to the original inframammary crease leaving a 0.5–1 cm mastectomy flap, widening its base until the chest wall flap is formed, which will be based on the arteries of the fourth and fifth intercostal spaces, with approximately the following dimensions: 6–8 cm of width and 4 cm of thickness (Figure 15.5). A 2 cm wide bipedicled flap of pectoralis major muscle is dis-

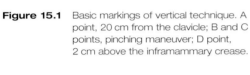

Figure 15.2 Skin demarcation before surgery.

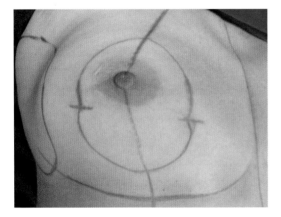

Figure 15 3 Deepithelization and dermal incision following demarcation, up to 2 cm above B and C points.

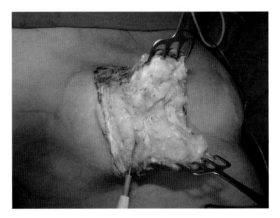

Figure 15.4 Undermining of chest wall based flap, lateral view.

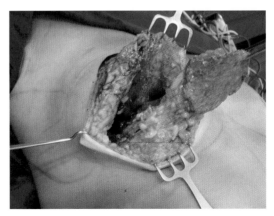

Figure 15.5 Chest wall based flap.

sected just superior to the base of the chest wall flap, using only 50% of the muscle thickness, long enough to accommodate the chest wall based flap with no compression at all (Figures 15.6, 15.7). The usual length of the muscle sling is 8–10 cm. After the flap is passed under the muscle sling (Figure 15.8), the donor area of the muscle is sutured with two separated sutures (2-0 nylon) followed by fixation of the thoracic flap to pectoralis fascia using a continuous suture of 2-0 nylon, beginning laterally, reaching the second intercostal space and finishing medially. The size of this flap is similar to a 100–200 g implant, so it gives volume to the upper pole of the breast. At this stage, breast tissue is excised as needed as a wedge from the lateral area and also from the superior flap of the breast maintaining the perforating vessels to the gland in order to avoid necrosis of the nipple–areola complex, to achieve the desired breast size and shape

(Figure 15.9). It is important to preserve enough tissue in the medial column to avoid flattening of the medial breast. The upper part of the breast is sutured to pectoralis fascia at the second intercostal space, bringing together the medial and lateral pillars to improve breast shape (Figure 15.10).

The medial and lateral pillars are sutured in an inferior to superior fashion using 2-0 nylon sutures (Figure 15.11). Deep dermis is sutured placing together points 'B' and 'C' as the first suture (Figure 15.12), and then the vertical segment (Figure 15.13). A round block suture is made in order to compensate the skin around the areola. Another option, which is our preferred method, consists of distributing and suturing the outer deep dermis of the periareolar skin to the areolar deep tissue, (Figures 15.14–15.16). Point 'D' is fixed to the deep plane so that the vertical suture is

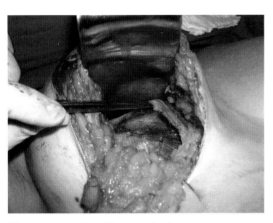

Figure 15.6 Bipedicle muscular flap.

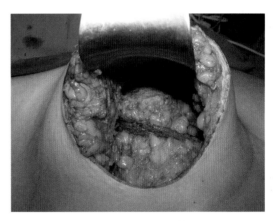

Figure 15.8 Passage of chest wall based flap under the bipedicle muscular flap.

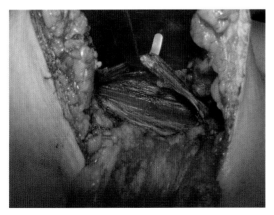

Figure 15.7 Muscular flap elevated.

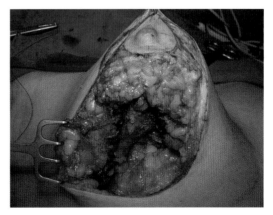

Figure 15.9 Glandular resection.

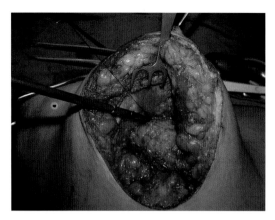

Figure 15.10 Cranial fixation of chest wall based flap.

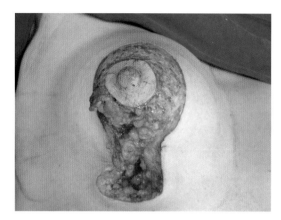

Figure 15.11 Aspect of the breast after breast column suture.

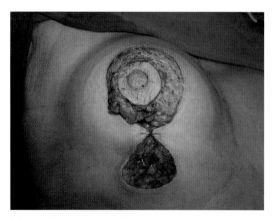

Figure 15.12 Suture of B and C points.

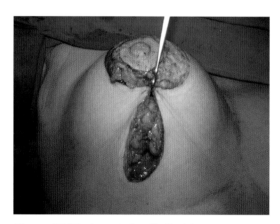

Figure 15.13 Aspect of vertical incision.

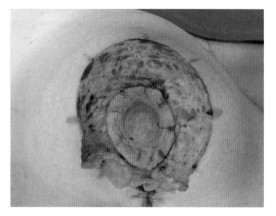

Figure 15.14 Schematic view of the areola suture.

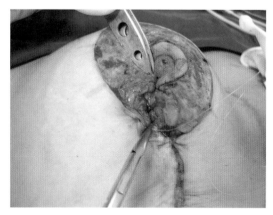

Figure 15.15 Suture of the nipple–areola complex and dermis.

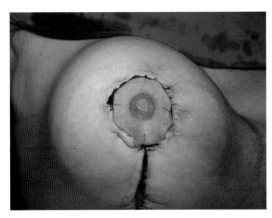

Figure 15.16   Aspect of the areola after dermal suture.

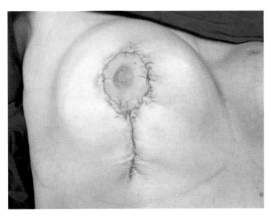

Figure 15.17   Final skin closure with shortening of vertical incision and round block suture around the areola.

kept at the same level as the new inframammary crease. A subcuticular suture with 4-0 monocryl is made in the vertical scar to shorten it (Figure 15.17). No suction drainage is used.

Post-operative care

A compressive bra is used for 1 to 3 months to support the breast during healing time. Lymphatic massages for the breast and arms are recommended from the third day through the fourth post-operative week. Antibiotic ointment is used over the wounds during the first week to maintain humidity and improve cell migration. To prevent wide scars, sterile strips are rou-

tinely used and silicone gel or sheets can be used to avoid hypertrophic scars. Walking start in the first post-operative day and physical activities can be started after 3 weeks.

Operative steps

- Skin is marked with the patient in the upright position. Moving the breast mound medially and laterally, two vertical lines are drawn to guide the area of skin resection. Point A (supra-areolar), B and C (infra-areolar), and D (end of the vertical markings) are marked.
- The entire marked area is de-epithelialized. Dermis is incised, sparing the superior portion of the periareolar marking, which will be the NAC pedicle.
- About 1 cm below the NAC, the dermolipoglandular flap is dissected, keeping a wide base attached to the chest wall. The remaining hypertrophic breast tissue is excised.
- A 2 cm wide bipedicled flap of pectoralis major muscle is dissected just superior to the base of the mammary flap, using only 50% of the muscle thickness.
- The mammary flap is passed under the muscle sling and sutured superiorly to the pectoralis fascia. Medial and lateral breast pillars are sutured together.
- Periareolar skin is compensated using a round block suture. The skin of the vertical incision is sutured aiming to shorten it and to avoid the point D ending below the new inframammary crease.

Complications

The most common complication related to the thoracic wall flap is fat necrosis in the distal portion of this flap, which can be dealt with by surgical revision to remove this tissue. Seroma or hematoma is avoided with careful hemostasis during the surgery. Another complication seen is wound healing problems in the vertical scar due to the wrinkles related to the shrinking of the scar. Post-operative mammograms have clearly shown the whole breast parenchyma and the mammary flap passed under the pectoralis muscle sling. Occasionally, the flap presents some changes in density compared to the surrounding breast parenchyma. Calcifications in the flap are uncommonly seen, and probably result from insufficient blood supply.

Vertical mammaplasty

Results

The vertical technique can be performed in patients with several degrees of breast hypertrophy and ptosis, but the best results, as with any other technique, have been achieved in those patients with mild and moderate breast ptosis, Good results can also be accomplished in large hypertrophies, especially in patients with good skin quality. In the case of severe breast ptosis, point 'D' must be marked at a greater distance to the 'M' point, up to 4 cm, leaving skin and subcutaneous tissue of the lower pole of the breast as part of the chest wall, therefore elevating the infra-mammary crease and also decreasing skin compensation of the vertical scar. Throughout the first 2 months of the post-operative period, it has been noticed that there is a settlement of the vertical scar, with no need for scar revision (horizontal scar) in the majority of patients.

Case 1

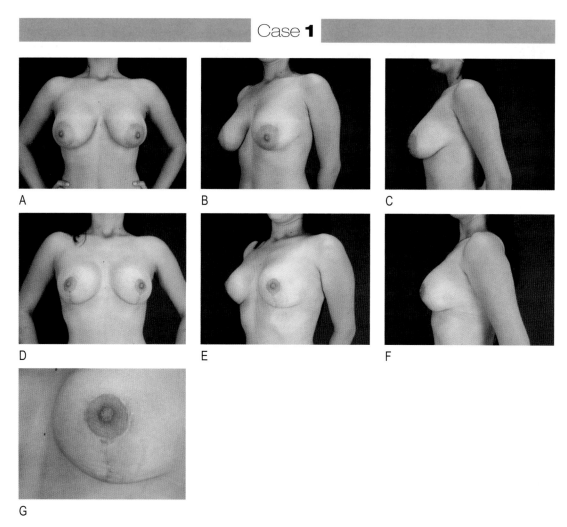

A

B

C

D

E

F

G

Figure 15.18 A 24-year-old woman with breast hypertrophy. (A–C) Pre-operative. (D–F) One year following vertical breast reduction using the chest wall based flap and the pectoralis loop. (G) Close-up of scar one year post-operatively.

Case **2**

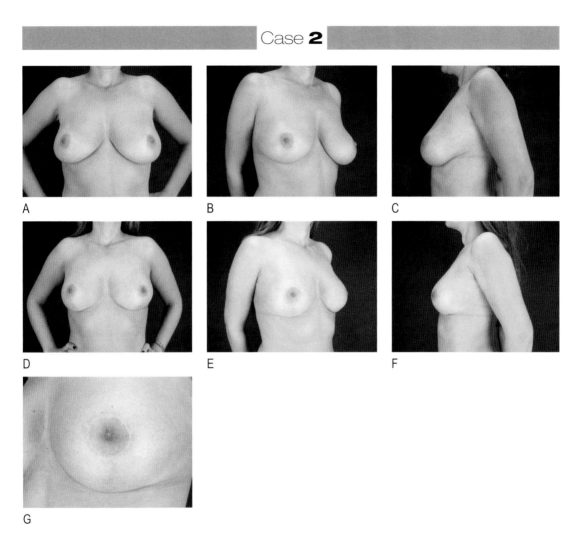

A

B

C

D

E

F

G

Figure 15.19 A 28-year-old woman with breast hypertrophy. (A–C) Pre-operative. (D–F) Two years following vertical breast reduction using the chest wall based flap and the pectoralis loop. (G) Close-up of the vertical scar, 2-years post-operatively.

Vertical mammaplasty

Case **3**

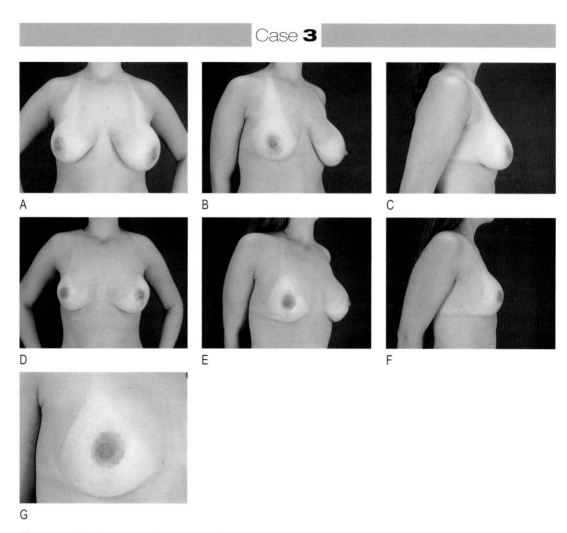

A   B   C

D   E   F

G

Figure 15.20 A 19-year-old woman with breast hypertrophy and asymmetry. (A–C) Pre-operative. (D–F) Four years following vertical breast reduction using the chest wall based flap and the pectoralis loop. (G) Close-up of the vertical scar, 4-years post-operatively.

Conclusion

Vertical mammaplasty is conceptually different from classical inverted T techniques, and offers several advantages that should be considered when choosing the best technique for each patient. Its design produces fewer scars, avoiding unaesthetic scars from the infra-mammary crease incision. Parenchyma resection follows the vertical principle, which narrows the base, increasing breast projection and avoiding the flat and broad shape. The chest wall based flap fills the upper pole of the breast, and, held by a sling of pectoralis major muscle, promotes longer maintenance of breast shape.

Further reading

Arie G. Una nueva tecnica de mastoplastia. Rev Latinoam Cir Plast 1957;3:23.

Balch CR. The central mound technique for reduction mammaplasty. Plast Reconstr Surg 1981;67:305–311.

Bostwick J. Breast reduction. In: Aesthetic and Reconstructive Breast Surgery. St Louis, MO: Mosby, 1983.

Courtiss EH, Goldwyn RM. Reduction mammaplasty by inferior pedicle technique. Plast Reconstr Surg 1977;59:500–507.

Daniel MJB. Mammaplasty with pectoral muscle flap. Presented at 64th American Annual Scientific Meeting, Montreal, 1995.

Dartigues L. Traitement chirurgical du prolapsus mammaire. Arch Franco Belg Chir 1925;28:13.

De Auraújo Cerqueira A. Mammoplasty: breast fixation with dermoglandular mono upper pedicle under the pectoralis muscle. Aesth Plast Surg 1998;22:276–283.

Finger RE, Vasquez B, Drew GS, Given KS. Superomedial pedicle technique of reduction mammaplasty. Plast Reconstr Surg 1989;83: 471–480.

Graf R, Biggs TM. In search of better shape in mastopexy and reduction mammaplasty. Plast Reconstr Surg 2002;110:309–317.

Hall-Findlay EJ. A simplified vertical reduction mammaplasty: Shortening the learning curve. Plast Reconstr Surg 1999;104:748–759.

Hall-Findlay E. Vertical breast reduction with a medially based pedicle. Aesth Surg J, 2002;22:185.

Hammond D. Short scar periareolar inferior pedicle reduction (SPAIR) mammaplasty. Plast Reconstr Surg 1999;103:890–901.

Hester TR, Jr, Bostwick J, Miller L, Cunningham SJ. Breast reduction utilizing the maximally vascularized central breast pedicle. Plast Reconstr Surg 1985;76:890–900.

Hidalgo DA. Vertical mammaplasty. Plast Reconstr Surg 2005;115:1179–1197.

Hugo NE, McClellan RM. Reduction mammaplasty with a single superiorly based pedicle. Plast Reconstr Surg 1979;63:230–234.

Labandter HP, Dowden RV, Dinner MI. The inferior segment technique for breast reduction. Ann Plast Surg 1982;8:493–503.

Lassus C. Possibilités et limites de la chirurgie plastique de la silhouette féminine. Hopital 1969;801:575.

Lassus C. A technique for breast reduction. Int Surg 1970;53:69–72.

Lassus C. Breast reduction: Evolution of a technique: a single vertical scar. Aesth Plast Surg 1987;11:107–112.

Lassus C. A 30-year experience with vertical mammaplasty. Plast Reconstr Surg 1996; 97:373–380.

Lejour M, Abboud M. Vertical mammaplasty without inframammary scar and with breast liposuction. Perspect Plast Surg 1990;4:67.

Lejour M. Vertical mammaplasty and liposuction of the breast. Plast Reconstr Surg 1994a;94:100–114.

Lejour M. Vertical mammaplasty and liposuction of the breast. St Louis, MO: Quality Medical, 1994b.

McKissock PK. Reduction mammaplasty with a vertical dermal flap. Plast Reconstr Surg 1972;49:245–252.

Marchac D, Olarte G. Reduction mammaplasty and correction of ptosis with a short scar. Plast Reconstr Surg 1982;69:45–55.

Orlando JC, Guthrie RH. The superiomedial dermal pedicle for nipple transposition. Br J Plast Surg 1975;28:42–45.

Pitanguy I. Surgical treatment of breast hypertrophy. Br J Plast Surg 1967;20:78–85.

Ribeiro L. A new technique for reduction mammaplasty. Plast Reconstr Surg 1975;55:330-334.

Robbins TH. A reduction mammaplasty with the areola-nipple based on an inferior dermal pedicle. Plast Reconstr Surg 1977;59:64–67.

Robbins LB, Hoffman DK. The superior dermoglandular pedicle approach to breast reduction. Ann Plast Surg 1992;29:211–216.

Rohrich RJ, Thornton J, Jakubietz RG et al. The limited scar mastopexy: current concepts and approaches to correct breast ptosis. Plast Reconstr Surg 2004;114:1622–1630.

No vertical scar breast reduction/ mastopexy

Donald H. Lalonde, Janice F. Lalonde

Key points

- Where does the no vertical scar technique fit in the armamentarium of reduction/mastopexy techniques relative to the vertical scar and the T scar techniques?

- The ideal patient for the no vertical scar technique has a lot of ptosis with at least 5 cm between the areola and the new areolar site.

- The main advantages of the no vertical scar technique are a nice periareolar scar with the only other scar hidden in the inframammary fold. There is no vertical scar on the visible breast mound.

- The main disadvantages of the no vertical scar technique are the same as those of the T scar: medial and lateral dog ears as well as a possible boxy shape problem if attention is not given to detail.

- Intraoperative breast sizers are useful to ensure that remaining breast tissue is of equal volume on both sides before the skin is closed.

Patient selection

The no vertical scar reduction/mastopexy is essentially the same reliable operation as the T scar inferior pedicle reduction except that it has one less scar; the vertical scar (Figures 16.1–16.3). The most common cause of patient dissatisfaction after breast reduction is the scar (Celebiler et al 2005). We believe that many patients can achieve a good breast shape with a modification of the T scar operation which deletes the verti-cal scar. If we can achieve good shape with one less scar than is achieved with a T scar reduction, then why not do it? The most important factor in patient selection for the no vertical scar technique is that the ideal patient is one who has 5 cm or more skin between the areola and the new areolar site (Figure 16.4). In other words, this is a good technique for a patient who has a lot of ptosis and excess skin.

Most surgeons would be reluctant to perform a breast reduction on a patient with a BMI of 45. With

No vertical scar breast reduction/mastopexy

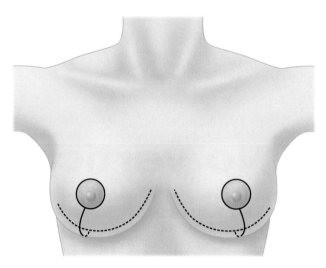

Figure 16.1 The T scar breast reduction has a visible vertical scar in the front of the breast which can distort the areola where the periareolar and vertical scars join at a T junction.

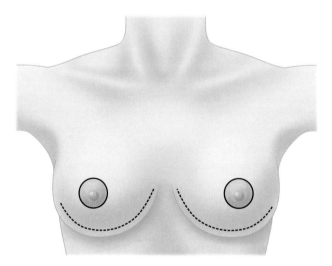

Figure 16.2 The no vertical scar breast reduction has a periareolar scar and a hidden inframammary scar, with no vertical scar coming down the visible front of the breast. The periareolar scar is not touched by any other scars.

regard to obese or overweight patients, most surgeons draw a line somewhere at which point they will not perform the surgery. We calculate normal body weight using standard height/weight tables and give patients the benefit of the doubt using the upper weight deemed appropriate for the largest frames (to account for 'big bones'). We call all weight above this number 'pounds of unhealthy fat', or the patient's POUF number. We draw the line at a POUF number of 10%. If the POUF number is greater than 10% of the patient's healthy upper limit body weight, we provide motivational nutritional weight counseling and do not perform the surgery. However, some authors regularly use the no vertical scar technique with good technical results in severely overweight patients (Nagy et al 2005).

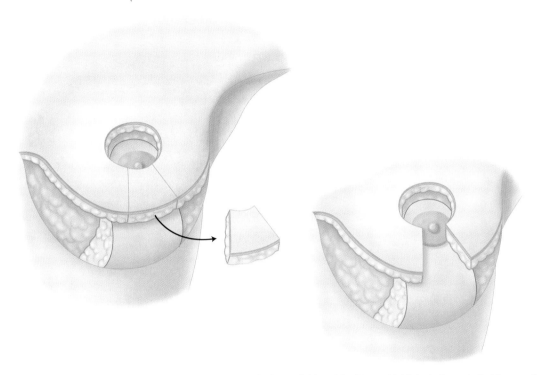

Figure 16.3   The main difference between the no vertical scar (left) and the T scar (right) techniques is that the small quadrilateral piece of skin and fat below the areola is preserved with the no vertical scar technique.

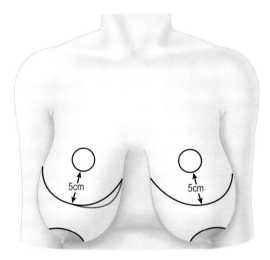

Figure 16.4   The ideal patient has at least 5 cm of normal skin between the new areolar site and the existing areola. Notice the nice smooth curve of the black mark for the proposed inferior border of the skin brassiere flap. The red mark below it on the right medial breast would have given a boxy shape. The medial end of the marked inframammary incision should be hidden under the medial breast mound.

Indications

Consider for a moment how much skin is removed with the skin excision patterns of the three reduction techniques of T scar, vertical scar reduction, and no vertical scar reduction. The vertical scar reduction has the least amount of skin removal of the three techniques. We therefore prefer the Hall-Findlay vertical reduction/mastopexy for the patient who has less skin to excise, and does not have a great deal of ptosis (less than 5 cm of skin between the areola and the new areolar site). This accounts for approximately 25% of the patients in our practice.

If the patient has a lot of ptosis and skin requiring removal as well as breast, then we prefer the no vertical scar reduction. This accounts for approximately 70% of the patients in our practice. Occasionally a patient will present with an excessively wide breast with a lot of horizontal skin needing excision and in this situation we still sometimes use the T scar reduction (≤5% of our cases). However, most of these patients would also do well with the no vertical scar technique because breast tissue can be made smaller with excision, projection can be obtained with breast shaping sutures, and excess lateral horizontal skin can redrape and become part of lateral chest wall skin no longer overlying the breast.

The no vertical scar technique can be used for either reduction or mastopexy. The Hall-Findlay rotation advancement vertical scar operation (rotation of the medial pedicle superiorly and advancement of the lateral pedicle beneath it) may give more projection than the T scar or no vertical scar techniques. However, breast shaping sutures do augment the projection obtained with the no vertical scar and the T scar techniques (Chun et al 2007).

Operative technique

A film with pre-operative markings and intraoperative technique is available for viewing online at https:// www.psvideoworkshop.com/about.htm.

Pre-operative preparation

Markings

The sternal notch is the first place that is marked. It is easily palpable at the top of the midline sternum between both clavicular heads. A line is drawn down the centre of the breast meridian line where the areola will look best (Figure 16.5). If a large part of the lateral breast is to be removed, the nipple/areola axis line can be moved medially as will be appropriate to the final anticipated breast width. The axis of the breast is drawn as a continued straight line below the inframammary fold by keeping it as a straight line seen through two fingers holding up the breast mound. (Figure 16.6)

The new nipple site usually ends up between 19 and 22 cm from the sternal notch, and between 9 and 12 cm from the midline. Larger (22 cm) numbers will apply to larger post-operative breasts, and shorter numbers (19 cm) will apply to smaller post-operative breasts. It is better to err on having a nipple too low than too high, as a very high areola may be visible in a low cut bathing suit. A finger on the breast is used to palpate another finger through the breast at the level of the inframammary fold, and this becomes the new nipple site (Figure 16.5). The areolar recipient site skin excision is marked on the skin brassiere pre-operatively with the patient in the sitting position.

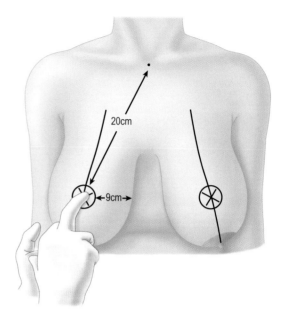

Figure 16.5 A line is drawn down the center of the breast axis. The inframammary fold line is palpated though the breast and the new areolar position is marked at that point on the breast axis line.

It is drawn as a slightly horizontal oval (3.5 cm diameter horizontally, and 3.0 cm diameter vertically) as the oval will stretch to a circle when the skin brassiere flap is pulled down over the breast to the inframammary fold at the time of final closure. The areola is marked as a 4 cm diameter circle also with the patient sitting up. The area of the areolar recipient circle is deliberately marked to be a little smaller than the areola itself in order to achieve a tension free closure in the periareolar scar.

A tension free areolar scar results in a much better areolar scar. This scar is the most visible scar of the reduced breast and the one that the woman will see every day when she is naked (Figure 16.7). It is also the first scar that a significant other will look at when her breast is seen by that person. As it is the showcase scar of the breast it should be treated as we treat the preauricular scar of the facelift; tension free and closed with care (Figure 16.8). The areolar recipient site is deliberately marked a little smaller than the areola itself to get a better tension free periareolar scar when we use the T scar or the vertical scar techniques.

The correct marking of the inframammary fold incision is important. While the vertical reduction has its

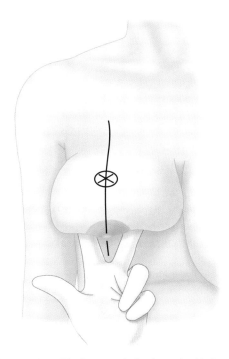

Figure 16.6 The breast axis line is marked below the breast by lifting up on two fingers and seeing both the breast axis line on the breast and the skin below the breast through the fingers.

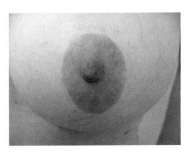

Figure 16.7 Post-operative no vertical scar breast reduction with typical pleasing periareolar scar. There is no distortion of the inferior periareolar scar by a vertical scar, and no vertical scar on the visible breast mound. The inframammary scar is hidden in the inframammary fold below the breast mound.

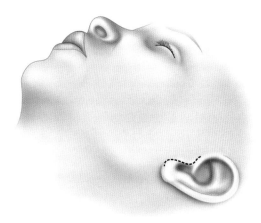

Figure 16.8 The preauricular scar of the facelift is the most visible scar. It is closed tension free and with care. The areolar scar is the most visible scar of the breast reduction/mastopexy. It should also be closed tension free and with care. This is why we measure the areola to be a little larger than the areolar site regardless of which reduction technique we use.

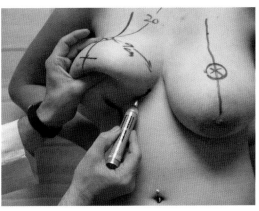

Figure 16.9 The medial end of the inframammary fold incision is marked under the medial fold of the breast so that it will not be visible post operatively.

possible dog ear in the middle of the breast extending to below the inframammary fold, the no vertical scar technique shares the same potential problems of medial and lateral dog-ears and visible scars at the medial and lateral ends of the inframammary fold scars with the T scar technique. To avoid visible medial dog ears in the no vertical and T scar techniques, the medial end of the inframammary fold incision is marked to be hidden under the medial fold of the breast so that it will not be visible post-operatively (Figure 16.9). The medial and central parts of the inframammary incision are drawn in the inframammary fold.

The lateral end of the incision is also marked so that the lateral end of the post-operative inframammary scar will be hidden out of sight in the inframammary fold when the patient is seen from the side in a sitting or standing position. In order to achieve this, the lateral end of the inframammary incision is drawn 1 cm medial to the lateral border of the pre-operative inframammary fold. This is done because the smaller post-operative breast inframammary fold has moved medially. If the patient is overweight and has a lateral chest fat fold, the lateral scar should be kept in this fat fold crease to decrease its visibility. The inferior pedicle with a base of 8–10 cm is marked for de-epithelialization in the same way as for an inferior pedicle T scar reduction.

After the marking of the inframammary fold incision, the lower incision of the skin brassiere flap is marked on the existing breast mound. The center of this incision is marked at 5 cm below the lower border of the areola recipient site. Smooth curves are then drawn from this point medially to reach the medial inframammary fold incision mark (Figure 16.4), and then laterally to reach the lateral inframammary incision mark. To avoid a boxy shape, the medial incision drawing should be a smooth curve upward. The lateral incision drawing will be more horizontal. If there is only 4 cm of unpigmented skin between the new areola site and the existing areola, the technique can still be used by not de-epithelializing the lower 1 cm of the inferior pedicle.

Markings are the same for both reduction and mastopexy patients. In the mastopexy patient, the entire breast is preserved except for the discarded de-epithelialized skin beneath the skin brassiere flap. In mastopexies, all of the skin beneath the skin brassiere flap will be de-epithelialized, unlike in breast reduction patients, where only the inferior pedicle is de-epithelialized.

Positioning and infiltration

The patient is placed in a supine position with the upper extremities on arm boards at approximately 75 degrees from the body to avoid post-operative shoulder pain and traction injuries which sometimes result from the 90 degree position. The area between the arm board and the anesthesiologist is also draped to allow an assistant to easily get above the arm board to provide counter traction to the breast during de-

epithelialization and to assist the surgeon when required. The head area is draped as a 'little tent' between IV poles to permit access to the head by the anesthesia.

A solution containing 160 mL of 0.25% lidocaine and 1:400 000 epinephrine is mixed with 40 mL of 0.5% bupivacaine with 1:100 000 epinephrine; 100 mL (half of the solution) is injected into each breast wherever skin and breast incisions are to be made. The only place where it is not infiltrated is in the intradermal plane where the skin is de-epithelialized in the inferior pedicle region. The reason for this is that the needle itself could possibly damage some of the larger subdermal veins in the pedicle. Epinephrine infiltration decreases intraoperative bleeding to negate the necessity for transfusion. Lidocaine and bupivacaine decrease perioperative narcotic requirements to decrease post-operative nausea and vomiting.

Technique

Tourniquet

A tourniquet is applied around the base of the breast. We use a pack which is tightened with a Kocher clamp. The skin should be checked to make sure that it has not been pinched by the clamp. The tourniquet is palpated at the bases of the breast to see if it is tight enough that it is applying a pressure greater that 120 mmHg, or a number that is higher than the patient's systolic blood pressure. If it is lower than that, arterial blood will get in but venous blood will not be able to get out and the subsequent venous tourniquet will result in more bleeding.

De-epithelialization

De-epithelialization is more a matter of pulling the skin off with the aid of the knife than it is cutting the epithelium off. Pulling hard on the skin to be removed, or avulsing it with the help of the knife, greatly speeds up this part of the operation. This technique allows us to rapidly remove the epidermis in one large sheet as opposed to several time consuming strips. The skin incisions above the tourniquet are all cut before the latter is let down. A knife is used through the epidermis and upper dermis in areas where skin incision healing will be required after the surgery. The coagulation cautery is used to get through the deep dermal and subdermal tissue rich in blood vessels which are cauterized as we cut. The medial and lateral inferior pedicle cuts are made with coagulation cautery as these skin cuts will not be asked to heal to other skin cuts after the surgery. When possible, a 5–10 mm rim of dermis is preserved and de-epithelialized around the areola so that periareolar veins are not cauterized right at the new areolar margin itself. In addition, this preserves a little more of the sensate areolar dermis even though it is buried.

Skin brassiere flap elevation

After skin incisions and inferior pedicle de-epitheliali-zation have been accomplished, a 1.5–2 cm skin bras-siere flap is elevated from the entire breast mound. This skin brassiere flap will be used to cover the reduced or mastopexied breast mound which will be reshaped and repositioned superomedially with breast shaping sutures. The skin brassiere flap is elevated at a thickness of 1.5–2 cm down to the loose areolar tissue of the chest wall (Figure 16.10). The skin flap can be made thinner (1.0 cm thick) laterally to avoid lateral breast bulging. This lateral part of the skin bras-siere flap will no longer be covering the breast after surgery. Instead, it will be covering the lateral chest wall as lateral breast will either be removed in reduc-tions or replaced from this lateral position and tacked to the chest wall medially in mastopexies.

The brassiere skin flap dissection is done with a large #23 blade and carried over the whole breast so that the entire breast mound is skinned (Figure 16.11). This is easy in a younger, glandular breast where pres-sure is maintained on the back of the moving scalpel blade, constantly pressing it against the gland so the sharp edge is cutting between the gland/subdermal fat junction. Large swooping cuts with the blade in this fashion make this a rapid part of the operation.

The skin brassiere flap should not be thinner than 1.5 cm in the bipedicled part below the new areolar hole in order to preserve the blood supply to that skin and fat. The areolar hole in the skin brassiere flap is made with the scalpel aimed obliquely upward (su-periorly) to avoid the fat and blood supply below the areolar hole (Figure 16.12). There are always significant bleeders at about 10 mm in depth which provide a robust blood supply to the skin brassiere flap. We have only lost a little (<2 cm^2) skin below the areolar hole on two occasions in the first year we used

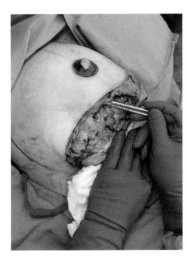

Figure 16.10 The skin brassiere flap is elevated at a thickness of 1.5–2 cm down to the loose areolar tissue of the chest wall. The skin flap can be a made thinner (1 cm thick) laterally to avoid lateral breast bulging. The bipedicled portion of the skin flap below the areola should not be thinned to less than 1.5 cm. To best preserve nerves and blood supply, never expose raw pectoralis major muscle.

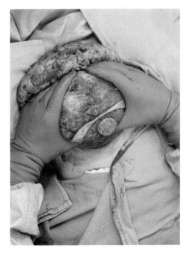

Figure 16.11 The hands are cupping the entire breast mound which has been separated from the skin brassiere flap above. Breast to be removed in this reduction case can be seen above the intact skin which outlines the inferior pedicle.

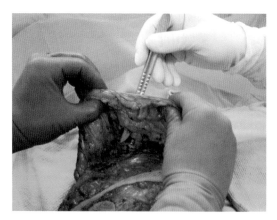

Figure 16.12 A hole is made in the skin brassiere flap to deliver the areola. The hole making blade is aimed superiorly in order to preserve the blood supply to the skin and fat below the areolar hole.

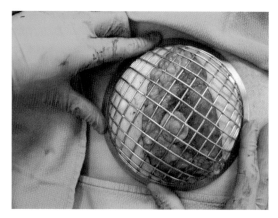

Figure 16.13 The entire breast pedicle and skin flap brassiere are placed in the see through stainless steel breast sizer which has the closest volume to the breast being measured. The same procedure is carried out on both sides to make sure that the two breasts have the same volume before the skin is closed.

this technique because we thinned the bipedicled flap below the areolar hole too aggressively. This skin loss was still less than was sometimes lost in the area of T zone necrosis in the 15 years in which we exclusively used the T scar reduction.

Gland excision

The breast is removed in a horseshoe shaped pattern around the inferior pedicle just as it is in the Tscar reduction. However, an attempt is made to perform most tissue removal laterally. In some of our smaller cases, medial gland excision is not performed at all. Bulging in the armpit is a possible unwanted sequela of no vertical scar breast reduction and this can be avoided by aggressive lateral breast excision and thinning of the lateral skin flap brassiere. It is well known that the nerves and blood vessels travel in the loose areolar tissue over the muscles and in the lateral chest wall. For this reason, a good protective layer of loose areolar tissue over the chest wall and pectoralis muscle is always preserved so that the vascular perforators and the nerves are more likely to be left intact. For this reason, we try to never visualize the pectoralis major muscle.

After the gland excision, intraoperative breast sizers are used to help further resection for final volume adjustment to ensure that the volume of the remaining breast and skin tissue is the same on both sides before the skin is closed (Figure 16.13). We find this technique more accurate than trying to measure breast

volume with our hands. Before the breast shaping sutures are placed, take a few minutes to remove fat from the lateral skin brassiere flap and lateral chest wall so that the lateral skin brassiere flap lies flat and not bulging on the lateral chest wall.

Mastopexy cases

In mastopexy cases, the same 1.5–2 cm skin brassiere flap is elevated from the breast above the de-epithelialized lower half of the breast mound. No breast or dermis is excised. Leave the skin brassiere flap thin laterally so there is no bulge on the chest wall when the breast is tacked down medially. Breast shaping sutures are not essential but give a better result.

Breast shaping sutures

You have dissected a large skin brassiere flap under which you are placing a smaller breast. With both mastopexy and breast reduction, as the patient is lying on her back, the remaining breast will tend to flop laterally and fall into the lateral side of the skin brassiere. The remaining breast also tends to have little projection. With the vertical scar reductions of Lassus, Lejour, and Hall-Findlay, breast shaping sutures are placed in the 'medial and lateral breast pillars' to increase breast projection. This type of breast shaping suture works because white breast tissue scars to white breast tissue in a rigid fashion.

The more white breast tissue there is to suture to itself with breast shaping sutures, the more the scar will hold. The more yellow fat there is, the more the scar will slide. Breast shaping sutures, therefore, are more likely to hold and to be more useful in the younger breast where there is more breast and less fat. The vertical reduction techniques do not have a monopoly on breast 'pillar' or breast shaping sutures. Breast shaping sutures can be used with any kind of breast reduction, including the T scar and the no vertical scar reductions. It only takes approximately 5 minutes to put in two to four breast shaping sutures.

We use breast shaping sutures for both no vertical scar mastopexy and reduction cases. We use 3-0 monocryl (Ethicon, Piscataway, NJ, USA) sutures to suture the breast gland to itself to increase projection and produce a pleasing shape (Figure 16.14), and then we suture the breast to the chest wall superomedially to get it out from under the dependent lateral empty skin brassiere flap pocket until that space heals closed.

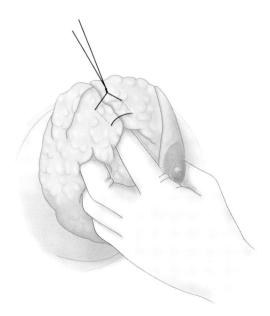

Figure 16.14 Breast shaping sutures: loose big loops (do not kill the tissue inside the loops) with tight knots permit breast to heal to breast in a kissing fashion to increase projection and provide a better shape in a superomedial position while the lateral empty skin brassiere flap heals to the lateral chest wall.

We use our fingers to shape the breast into an attractively shaped projecting breast mound with a lateral concavity, and hold it in that position with two to four sutures of white breast sutured to white breast as much as possible. If only yellow tissue is available, yellow tissue is used. It is very important that breast shaping sutures should not be tied too tightly to strangle the tissue inside the suture loop (Figure 16.14). A suture should be a kiss, not a collision. If the suture loop is strangled tightly, the breast, nerves and blood vessels inside it will suffer ischemic necrosis. We therefore tie solid knots over large loose loops of breast tissue designed to just bring the breast tissue to touch and heal to breast tissue in a kissing fashion. Once the breast mound is attractively shaped and positioned superomedially with breast shaping sutures, it is draped with the skin brassiere flap and the skin is closed.

Closure

Sutures

We use 15–20 deep dermal 3-0 vicryl (Ethicon, Piscataway, NJ, USA) sutures to anchor the inframammary fold incision in each breast. We start with a single suture laterally and then a single suture medially to ensure that there is no lateral or medial dog ear, and the rest of those sutures divide and divide the wound in halves until most of the wound is together. There is more skin on the skin brassiere flap (superior) side of the wound than there is on the inframammary fold (inferior) side of the wound. The skin closure therefore has to be gathered. After the deep dermal interrupted sutures, a running intradermal 3-0 monocryl suture which takes longer bites on the skin brassiere flap side and shorter bites on the inframammary fold side accomplishes this task. It is important that the epidermal edges end up touching each other the entire length of the wound at the time of final closure to avoid dehiscence.

The inframammary closure is one of the more difficult parts of this operation as the skin looks gathered (wrinkled) on the superior part of the inframammary fold incision at the end of the case. We tell our patients that: (1) There will be wrinkles above the inframammary fold incision after the surgery. (2) Most of the wrinkles will be gone most of the time by 3 months after surgery. (3) There will rarely be a left over wrinkle.

(4) These wrinkles are the price they pay to avoid a permanently visible scar down the center of the breast mound. Most patients are not concerned by the wrinkles one way or the other, as they are usually hidden in below the visible mound. We have never been asked to revise any of the rarely leftover wrinkles. The tension free periareolar incision is closed with 8 symmetrically placed buried interrupted 4-0 monocryl sutures followed by small carefully placed bites of a running intradermal 5-0 monocryl suture.

To drain or not to drain

There is plenty of level 1 evidence to show that drains do not reduce the risk of hematoma in breast reduction. However, we still use drains in most cases as they help promote the adherence of the empty lateral skin brassiere flap to the lateral chest wall. We never bring drains through a separate stab incision as this creates an unnecessary scar.

Taping

We do use adhesive strips to cover the wound at the end of the case. However, these tapes are just laid onto the wound, and not pulled across the incision. Pulling on adhesive tapes leads to a shearing force which shears the epidermis off of the dermis and leaves the patient with blisters under the tape. Patients are then improperly labeled 'allergic' to the tapes when they are more appropriately 'allergic' to the person who cranked on the tapes.

Bandages

We use a generous enough supply of gauze bandage to prevent patient concerns which can be generated by seeing a little blood on the bandage. We cover the gauze with a 'one size fits most' type of brassiere that opens to the front and adjusts with adjustable straps.

Operative steps

- Injection of epinephrine containing local anesthesia.
- Tourniquet application, skin incisions, de-epithelialization.
- Elevation of the 1.5–2 cm skin brassiere flap.
- Gland excision.
- Breast shaping sutures.
- Skin closure.

Results

Case 1

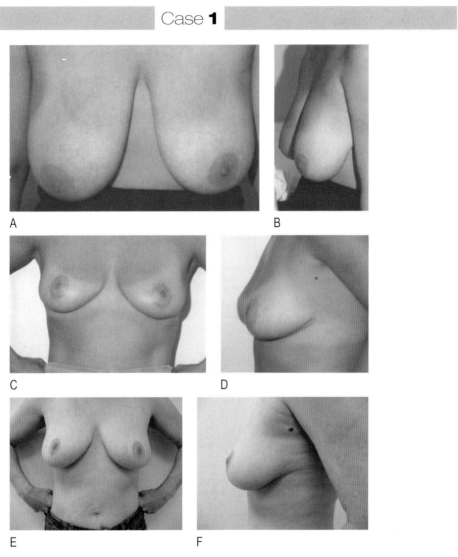

A

B

C

D

E

F

Figure 16.15   A 46-year-old woman with 480 g from (R) breast and 415 g from (L) breast pre-operatively (A,B), 3 months (C,D) and 10 years (E,F) post-operatively. (A,C,E) front and (B,D,F) lateral views.

Case **2**

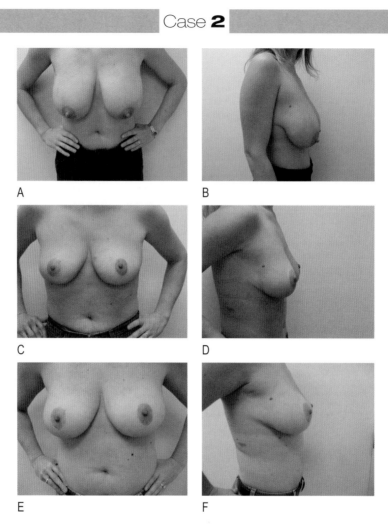

Figure 16.16   A 34-year-old woman with 280 g left and 260 g right reduction anterior and lateral pre-operative views (A,B), 6 months postoperatively (C,D), and 3 years post-operatively (E,F); (A,C,E) front and (B,D,F) lateral views.

Pitfalls and how to correct

Armpit breast deformity (lateral bulge)

The lateral bulge deformity can be avoided by thinning out the skin brassiere flap laterally to 1 cm, by aggressively excising lateral breast tissue, and by suturing the breast mound superomedially until the lateral skin brassiere flap heals to the lateral chest wall. It can be corrected by secondary lateral tissue removal either directly through the inframammary incision or by liposuction under local anesthesia.

Inframammary fold wound dehiscence

This can be avoided by careful closure of the inframammary incision with care to make sure epidermal/dermal contact occurs on both sides of the wound throughout its entire length. If it occurs, the wounds are usually clean and can be resutured secondarily under local anesthesia taking large 1 cm bites of 3-0 nylon (Ethicon, Piscataway, NJ, USA) that will not rip through the skin.

Medial and lateral dog ears/visible incisions

These can be avoided by drawing the incisions so they end up hidden in the inframammary crease when the patient is sitting or standing after wound healing occurs. Visible scars cannot be removed, only revised. Dog ears can be defatted or excised under local anesthesia.

Boxy shape

This can be avoided by drawing the medial inframammary incision as a smooth curve (Figure 16.4). This can be corrected with skin and/or fat excision under local anesthesia as a secondary procedure.

Areola too high

This can be avoided by marking the skin brassiere flap incision line no more than 5 cm below the lower end of the areola recipient site. If it occurs, additional skin below the areola can be excised below the areola at the level of the inframammary fold scar under local anesthesia as you would with the T scar or vertical scar techniques.

Possible skin loss of the bipedicled part of the skin brassiere flap below the areola

This can be avoided by: (1) aiming the scalpel blade obliquely upward (superiorly) when making the areolar recipient site cut in the skin brassiere flap in order to preserve the blood supply to the skin and fat below the areolar hole (Figure 16.12), and (2) by keeping the skin brassiere flap thicker than 1.5 cm below the areolar recipient hole. If skin loss does occur, allow secondary healing as you would with T zone necrosis in the T scar reduction.

Post-operative care

Almost all of our breast reduction/mastopexy patients are outpatients. We see them the morning after surgery in the office and remove the drains if they have any. Our patients are told to take 800 mg of ibuprofen every 4 h if required for the first day or two after surgery. They can augment that with 1 g acetaminophen if required, but this is rarely used. Most patients take two to four doses of ibuprofen before we see them the next day and they are quite comfortable with that.

They are encouraged to stop pain killers as soon as they reach the point of 'it only hurts when I move', which is usually 2–3 days after surgery. They are told that their pain is their body's way of telling them that they are not ready to do what it is they are doing, and that we did not spend 2 billion years evolving pain because it is a bad thing. It is their body's way of helping them get better faster. They are told: 'Don't baby yourself but don't do what hurts. Don't do much if you are on pain killers, because then you don't know what hurts.' With the help of this approach, most of our patients are back to work in 1–4 weeks.

They are allowed to get in the shower the day after surgery. They can wear whatever garment feels best. Many patients feel better with snug fitting sports brassieres. They can wear an underwear liner on the inside of the brassiere if the wound is oozing a little in the first week.

Conclusion

The no vertical scar reduction/mastopexy is another tool which is useful to correct the large or sagging breast with a lot of ptosis. This technique can produce a pleasing breast shape and a nice areola without the distortion or the visibility of a visible vertical scar. We also use the Hall-Findlay and T scar reductions in patients whose result will be better with those techniques.

Further reading

Celebiler O, Sönmez A, Erdim M et al. Patients and surgeons perspectives on the scar components after inferior pedicle breast reduction surgery. Plast Reconstr Surg 2005;116:459; discussion 465.

Chun YS, Lalonde DH, May JW Jr. Internal pedicle shaping to improve aesthetic results in reduction mammaplasty. Plast Reconstr Surg 2007;119:1183.

Hosnuter M, Tosun Z, Kargi E et al. No-vertical-scar technique versus inverted T scar technique in reduction mammoplasty: a two-center comparative study. Aesthet Plast Surg 2005;29:496.

Lalonde DH, French RJ, Lalonde J. The no vertical scar breast reduction: how to delete the vertical scar of the standard T scar breast reduction and produce an excellent breast shape. Perspect Plast Surg 2001;15:103.

Lalonde DH, Lalonde J, French R. The no vertical scar breast reduction: a minor variation that allows you to remove vertical scar portion of the inferior pedicle wise pattern T scar. Aesthet Plast Surg 2003;27:335.

Movassaghi K, Liao E, Morris D et al. Eliminating the vertical scar in breast reduction The Boston modification of the Robertson technique. Aesthet Plast Surg 2006;26:687.

Nagy MW, McCraw JB, Lalonde DH et al. The no vertical scar mammaplasty: a durable approach to a complex problem. Plast Reconstr Surg 2005;116(Suppl):216S.

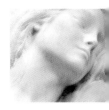

17

Breast shaping in the massive weight loss patient

Dennis J. Hurwitz

Key points

- Spiral flap breast reshaping is indicated with moderately sized ptotic breasts, surrounded by rolls of skin to obtain improved shaped breasts, and an upper body lift.

- Develop an obsessive marking technique for the confidence to commit full inclusion of nearby flaps to the breast and expeditious execution of the operation.

- Suture secure the raised inframammary fold.

- After raising the breast mound, flip up the epigastric flap to the inferior pole and spiral the lateral thoracic flap beneath the superior pole.

- Close the skin over an enlarged round breast mound under some tension, anticipating evolution into a natural breast shape.

Patient selection

After massive weight loss (MWL), breasts lose volume and projection. Both the nipple–areola complexes (NAC) and the mounds descend. Varying with the original size, fat content and shape, cherished feminine contours and softness evolve into flat, pancake shaped, floppy and firm appendages. The empty superior poles extend laterally to unattractive flattening of the anterior axillary folds. Surrounding the breasts are mid torso circumferential rolls of skin that may cascade from scapula to hip. As these patients are concerned about both the mid torso rolls and their breasts, they welcome simultaneous correction.

Excessively large and pendulous breasts are reduced. Due to excess inelastic skin, a Wise reduction pattern with an appropriate nipple pedicle is chosen. Secure suture elevation of the lateral portion of the inframammary fold (IMF) minimizes descent and bottoming out of the breasts. For breasts that may benefit from only moderate degree of augmentation, a superior flap suspension mastopexy with lateral chest wall flap augmentation can be used. When the breasts need considerable augmentation and nearby tissue is sparse, then silicone implants, usually with a mastopexy and suture fixation of the new IMF are offered.

Patients with moderate sized breasts are candidates for autogenous breast reshaping, when the neighboring tissue is full and redundant. In general, MWL patients accept breast implants only if there is no alternative. They are cautioned that recurrent breast ptosis and bottoming out of the implant is common. When autogenous tissue alternative of neighboring mid torso rolls is offered, these patients usually accept the more involved, lengthy and higher risk spiral flap reshaping. The patient must understand and accept the anticipated inverted 'T' mastopexy scars with transverse continuation along the bra line. When there is little back skin laxity and/or the patient objects to a back scar then she is offered a sickle-shaped skin flap excision that extends vertically from the IMF either to the axilla or the hip.

Indications for spiral flap reshaping of the breasts

The spiral flap reshaping of the breasts is best indicated when moderate to severe breast atrophy and ptosis is accompanied by full epigastric and lateral thoracic skin laxity and rolls. Inferior and lateral de-epithelialized axial pattern flaps are elevated in continuity with the Wise pattern mastopexy. These two flaps are based on intercostal perforators. The surgeon needs to understand and respect the dominant blood supply of the breast through a transversely oriented axial pattern blood supply along the third to fifth intercostal vessels. With prior breast reduction surgery the blood supply to the central breast is uncertain.

Breast reshaping is part of an upper body lift, which consists of the transverse removal of mid torso rolls, a reverse abdominoplasty, and suture repositioning of the IMF. The skin laxity and descent of the IMF progressively increases from medial to lateral. There is no redundancy of torso skin where it is broadly adherent over the sternum and spine. Accordingly, my upper body lift (UBL) rarely crosses the midlines. The relatively small amount of excess mid line epigastric skin is taken out by lateral displacement under the medial inframammary incisions. Residual rolls are taken out by secondary skin excisions, or if disturbing to the patient by secondary inverted V midline skin excisions crossing the midline. However, these midline scars are visible in low cut styles and tend to hypertrophy. In unusual cases of considerable mid epigastric skin, and/or symmastia, or mid back rolls, the UBL should continued across the midlines. Contraindications to spiral flap breast reshaping are inadequate redundant

torso soft tissue bulk, unwillingness to accept the wound healing risks and smokers.

Operative technique

Pre-operative preparation

The patient is preferably marked the evening before surgery, avoiding the imperative to rush the markings for the waiting operating room team. The patient has the opportunity to review the markings and ask further questions the next day. Also, the patient is chilled due to the exposure which would leads to pre-operative hypothermia. By using permanent markers, the patient can shower with antibacterial soap the morning of surgery. The UBL and breast reshaping is usually performed after the lower body lift and abdominoplasty. When a single staged total body lift is performed, the UBL and breast reshaping are completed towards the end. Likewise for a multistage plan, the upper lift and breast reshaping along with a brachioplasty constitutes the second stage. As such, one of the objectives of the UBL is to complete treatment of the mid torso laxity not corrected by the first stage. Otherwise the lower abdominoplasty and body lift will have to complete the mid torso correction following the UBL. One indication for that reverse order would be if the patient desires maximum recruitment of limited mid torso tissue for the breast augmentation.

The markings and operation to be described are for a rather typical second stage procedure in a 47-year-old, 5'6" woman, 2 years after losing 220 pounds from an open gastric bypass. Her high weight was 427 pounds and she presented at a stable 205 pounds. She is a full time manufacturing employee and walks several miles daily. Her first stage was a lower body lift, abdominoplasty and bilateral vertical thighplasties with ultrasonic assisted lipoplasty (UAL) (see Figure 17.3) The second stage consisted of an UBL, spiral flaps, brachioplasties and revision of her medial thighplasties (see Figure 17.3).

Marking begins by positioning the breast, NACs and IMFs, followed by the reverse abdominoplasty and back roll excision. Finally, the L brachioplasty is configured; however, the short chest limb of the L is drawn but the actual width of excision cannot be determined until the autogenous breast augmentation is completed (Figure 17.3). The patient sits for the breast and arm, and stands for the upper body markings. The sternal notch and descending anterior midline is marked to the xyphoid. Seven centimeters to either side along the clavicle the mid breast meridians are drawn through the nipple to the chest wall inferior to the IMF. These markings assist in observing for deviations of the NAC or the breast from the ideal breast meridian and to adjust the superior relocation of the NAC. Short transverse lines are drawn along the IMFs and registered on at the same level on the sternum.

Low lying breasts, as confirmed by observation and patient acknowledgment, are pushed several centimeters cephalad until the proper position is attained. The new IMF is registered over the sternum, which tends to be about 3 cm cephalad to the first markings. The new nipple position is marked at or several centimeters higher than the IMF depending a variety of artistic considerations. In general the greater the volume of autogenous augmentation, the less upward positioning of the nipple, because the larger the new breast the greater the tendency towards descending into the lower pole and causing a high riding nipple. The new nipple position is then transposed from the sternal registry to cephalad of the current nipple along the breast meridian line. The differences between the meridians and the two new nipple positions are reconciled. The distances from the sternal notch to the current and future nipples are measured with care taken to avoid excessively long or short distances.

The superior border of each NAC is marked 2 cm cephalad and from that point an inverted V pattern is drawn about 14 cm long and tangential to the medial and lateral edges of each NAC. Again from the superior border of each new NAC a circle roughly 16 cm in diameter is drawn that meets roughly 4.5 cm inferior along the vertical lines. At roughly 75 degree angles transverse lines are drawn towards the sternum and mid axillary line.

Finally, the long inferior line of the Wise pattern includes the excess upper abdominal skin and fat. The surgeon pushes the entire breast mount with the ptotic lower pole cephalad until all the residual laxity of anterior skin is corrected (the umbilicus starts to move cephalad). While holding that tissue upward, a mark is made along the breast meridian that is on line with the new IMF registry over the sternum. Except in extreme cases of midline epigastric skin laxity or near synmastia, the medial inferior incision line rises from that mark along the breast meridian superiorly to meet

the transverse superior medial Wise pattern line at about the sixth rib costal cartilage. The lateral line extension from the breast meridian is made where upward pushing of the skin corrects the anterolateral abdominal skin excess up to the new IMF registered over the sternum. Laterally the inferior and superior Wise pattern lines continue immediately lateral to the breast towards the inferior tip of the scapula, to include all the excess skin of the mid back rolls. The operation starts with the patient prone with the arms roughly at right angles on arms boards. Pre incision infiltration of saline containing 1 mg of epinephrine and 30 mL of 1% lidocaine per liter is customarily done.

Technique

The removal of the back roll by harvest of both lateral thoracic donor flaps (LTF) is begun with de-epithelialization using an electric dermatome set at 32/1000 of an inch. Retained islands of epithelium are removed. The two flaps may be raised simultaneously with the superior and inferior perimeter incisions from the tapered end near the tip of the scapula to the lateral boarder of the latissimus dorsi (LD) muscle. The incisions are made through the skin and subcutaneous tissue to the muscular fascia and then the donor site is undermined for several centimeters. The fasiocutaneous flap is elevated from posterior to lateral over the obliquely oriented coarse fiber LD muscle to just past its lateral border (Figure 17.1A). The laterally based triangular flap lies on the operating room table as the donor site is closed in two layers of a running large braided absorbable suture followed by an intracuticular closure. After the LTFs are wrapped in sterile towels, the patient is turned supine.

The Wise pattern with its inferior epigastric and the LTF extension are de-epithelialized. The precise order of incisions and flap isolation and positioning of this complex operation are not critical, except that the spiral flap positioning occurs after superior mobilization of the breast mound. The medial, superior and lateral Wise pattern skin flaps are incised and elevated from the breast parenchyma for several centimeters. The lateral flap incision is continued as the superior margin incision of the partially elevated lateral thoracic flap. Then the inferior LTF incision is completed to the inferior border of the de-epithelialized Wise pattern. With the perimeter of the LTF completed, the deep surface of the flap is dissected from the serratus muscle

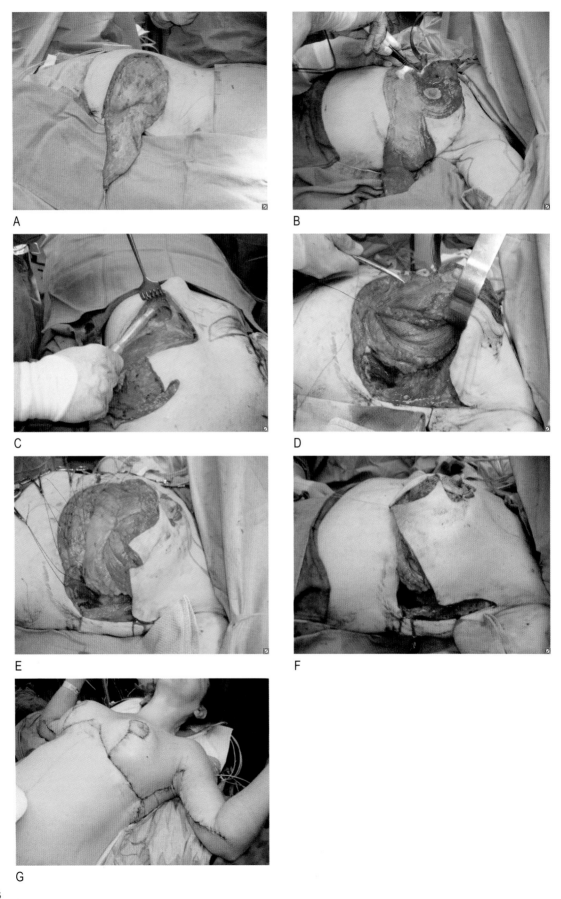

A

B

C

D

E

F

G

Figure 17.1 These are sequential intraoperative views of the upper body lift with spiral flap breast reshaping and brachioplasties. (A) The dissected and de-epithelialized lateral thoracic flap (LTF) lies next to the prone patient with underlying latissimus dorsi muscle exposed. After the donor site is closed, the patient is turned supine and the extended Wise pattern flap is de-epithelialized. (B) With the aid of a Deaver retractor the dissection of the submamammary space for the lateral thoracic flap begins in the parasternal region. The Wise pattern and the extended LTF (on the OR table) are de-epithelialized. (C) Discontinuous undermining of the reverse abdominoplasty flap is being performed with dissector dilators. Prior to that maneuver the border between the Wise pattern and the reverse abdominoplasty was incised and the breast mount advanced several centimeters superiorly. (D) Two Deaver retractors suspend the superior tunnel for the lateral thoracic flap. Parasternal suspension sutures of the new breast mound are in place. (E) The epigastric flap extension of the Wise pattern is flipped up onto the interior breast mound and a series of large braided sutures have been placed between the subcutaneous fascia of the reverse abdominoplasty flap and the sixth rib cartilage and periosteum to advance the reverse abdominoplasty and secure the IMF. (F) The closure starts with approximation of the medial and lateral Wise pattern flaps to each other and the securely advanced reverse abdominoplasty flaps. (G) The appearance on the operating room table at the completion of the upper body lift, breast reshaping with spiral flaps and bilateral brachioplasties.

across the chest to the anterior axillary line where several sizable intercostal perforators can be identified, sounded by Doppler and preserved. The size and vitality of the fully raised flap is assessed. If both qualities are adequate then a crescent shaped submammary superior pole breast space is created for the LTF.

The submammary space for the autogenous augmentation arches from the fifth costochondral cartilage to the third rib at the nipple line and then to the lateral border of the pectoralis muscle about the fourth rib. The dissection may begins at the parasternal sixth rib over the pectoralis major (PM) muscle (Figure 17.1B). Care is taken to avoid injury to the internal mammary perforating vessels from the fifth and superior intercostal spaces. The tunnel is no wider than can be accommodated by the LTF. Exposure of the lateral border of the PM is usually accomplished through the lateral chest vertical extension incision of the L brachioplasties. That incision is carried to the superior margin of the lateral thoracic flap, where it meets it at right angles. Palpation of the lateral border of the PM aids in expeditious identification.

The final incision is now made along the inferior margin of the Wise pattern de-epithelialization. The breast and its inferior extension is then advanced superiorly on the chest wall until the complex reaches the new inframammary fold, saving intercostal perforators at that level. Then either the breast mount reshaping can begin or the reverse abdominoplasty is completed at this time. I generally complete the incision between the upper abdomen and the breast with a scalpel through the subcutaneous fascia. Undermining of the abdominal flap is discontinuous using dissecter

dilators; thereby preserving perforating vasculature (Figure 17.1C). Elevation proceeds to just beyond the costal margin.

The auto augmentation starts with placing an absorbable suture into the distal tip of the LTF to help drag the flap through the superior sub mammary tunnel. The flap should take a crescent like path descending from the midclavicular region to the fifth costchondral junction, where it is secured. Within the tunnel sutures may be use to further suspend or shape the flap. The entire breast still sags laterally. This is corrected by dermal suture suspension of the inferior flap also near the sixth rib costochondral junction (Figure 17.1D). The NAC is then sutured to its new elevated position at 12 o'clock, followed by a three point fixation at 6 o'clock. Then the epigastric extension is flipped up and sutured to the inferior pole to add volume and shape. Now that the breast mound is enlarged, shaped and centralized by the spiral flap, final dermal suture shaping with braided absorbables is done. Then a series of a dozen interrupted braided, permanent sutures are firmly placed from the abdominal advancement flap subcutaneous fascia to the sixth costal cartilage, periosteum and serratus muscle (Figure 17.1E). The waist is flexed and with an upward push on the abdominal skin the sutures are sequentially tied to advance the reverse abdominoplasty and secure the IMF.

Closure

Having secured the NAC position, the distal end of the Wise pattern medial and lateral flaps are joined at the appropriate juncture with the IMF (Figure 17.1F).

These flaps were dissected fairly thin to avoid injury to the transversely oriented breast parenchyma blood supply. The difficult suturing of the inferior margin of the medial and lateral flaps to the newly secured reverse abdominoplasty flap has been eased with the use of Quill™ SRS (Angiotech, Vancouver, British Columbia, Canada). The large tapered needle on a 1 polydioxanone double armed thread facilitates closure with generous horizontal mattress bites. The suturing starts centrally. After placing several throws of the suture in either direction, the ends are pulled to approximate the wound edges. After every two passes the self retaining suture is pulled and cinched to the desired tension. There are no knots to be tied or split. Similarly, the circumareolar closure is facilitated with 2-0 Quill™ SRS sutures with larger bites on the outer circumference and small bites on the areolar. Alignment markings are essential for a speedy and accurate closure.

The patient is then sat up for final adjustments, including trimming for NAC symmetry and roundness. Volume or shape asymmetries are corrected. The combination of volume increase and breast skin removal will make the closure tight and round, which is a good thing, because within a few weeks the breast will become soft and within a year a more natural tear drop shape forms. Finally, an appropriate amount of skin is excised from the chest limb of the L brachioplasty to accommodate the increased anterior chest volume. Closure of the brachioplasty is secure and speedy with running horizontal 0 and 2-0 Quill™ SRS (Figure 17.1G).

Before the completion of the closure a large vacuum drain may be placed through a lateral chest stab wound towards the back donor site. While the drain often removes several hundred milliliters of serum over the next week, I have found no seromas in the cases where no drain was used. I prefer skin glue to seal and protect the wound edges, followed by a light gauze dressing, and non constricting surgical bra and 4 inch Ace® wraps to the arms.

Operative steps

- Bilateral transversely oriented LTFs are de-epithelialized, harvested and the donor sites closed.
- Extended Wise patterns are de-epithelialized to include the epigastric and lateral thoracic extensions.
- Thin medial, superior and lateral Wise pattern flaps are elevated for several centimeters.
- The crescent shaped submammary space for the lateral thoracic flap is dissected under the superior pole of the breast.
- The incision between the reverse abdominoplasty and the extended Wise pattern is made and the low lying breast is raised up the chest from the eight or seventh to the sixth ribs.
- After discontinuously undermining the reverse abdominoplasty flap, it is advanced and sutured to the new IMF about the sixth rib.
- Breast augmentation begins with pulling the de-epithelialized LTF through the submammary tunnel and suturing it to the costal cartilage.
- The laterally sagging breast is centralized with suturing of the inferior de-epithelialized flap to the costal cartilage.
- The epigastric flap is flipped up to fill the inferior pole.
- The Wise pattern flaps and L brachioplasty flaps are appropriately approximated.

Results

Most of our over 80 patients with spiral flap reshaping of the breasts were pleased. One patient required mastectomy for multifocal in situ carcinomas and three patients required needle biopsies for cystic lesions due to dermal cysts. One patient had excisional removal of firm distal flap necrosis and approximately 20% demonstrate distal flap firmness that mostly resolves over a year. Two patients had small saline filled silicone implant augmentation at the time of the spiral flap. Four patients desired larger breasts and had secondary small silicone implant augmentation. Mastopexy and scar revision with further advancement of the lateral IMF were performed in about 20% of the patients. Five further cases are briefly presented.

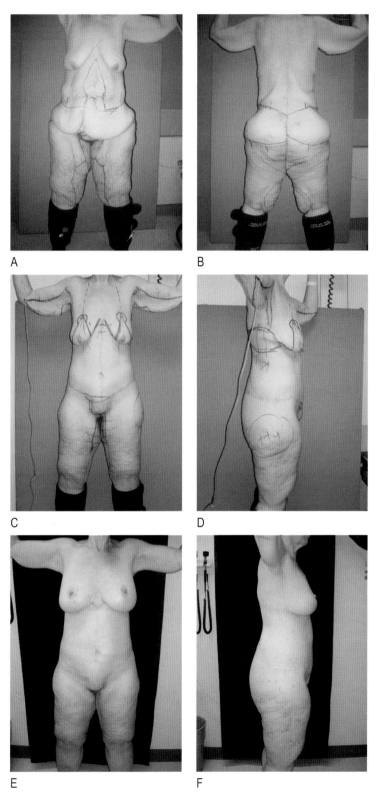

A

B

C

D

E

F

Figure 17.2 These front (A) and back (B) pre-operative views show the surgical markings for first stage of a total body lift that includes an abdominoplasty, lower body lift, bilateral vertical medial thighplasty and UAL of the thighs in a 5' 6", 205 pound, 46-year-old woman who lost 220 pounds after gastric bypass. (C) Front and (D) right lateral views show the surgical markings for the second stage of a total body lift that includes bilateral brachioplasties, upper body lift, and spiral flap reshaping of the breasts. (E) Frontal and (F) right lateral complete 1 year post-operative body views after the second stage completion of her total body lift. She is pleased with her enlarged, raised and better shaped breasts and desires no revision surgery.

Case **2**

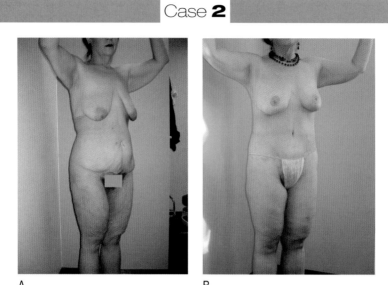

A   B

Figure 17.3 (A) Oblique view of a 5′ 6″, 160 pound, 50-year-old woman who lost 150 pounds after laparoscopic gastric bypass who desires breast reshaping with autogenous tissue and a total body lift. (B) Oblique view 3 years after her abdominoplasty, vertical medial thighplasty, lower body lift, UBL and spiral flap reshaping, followed six months later by bilateral L brachioplasties, facelift and brow lift.

Case **3**

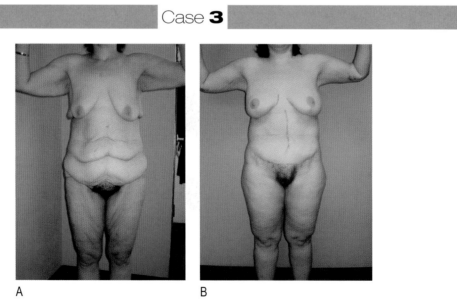

A   B

Figure 17.4 (A) Anterior view of a 5′ 6″, 157 pound, 34-year-old woman who lost 170 pounds after gastric bypass surgery, who requests autogenous breast reshaping with a total body lift. (B) Anterior view nearly three years after her abdominoplasty, lower body lift, upper medial thighplasty, UBL with spiral flap reshaping and bilateral L brachioplasties.

Case **4**

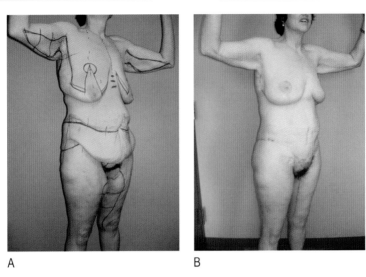

A   B

Figure 17.5   (A) Oblique view of a 5′ 8″, 165 pound, 28-year-old woman who lost 170 pounds through gastric bypass and desires autogenous breast reshaping and a single stage total body lift. (B) Oblique view 2 years after an abdominoplasty, lower body lift, vertical medial thighplasty, bilateral L brachioplasties, UBL with modified spiral flaps. The superior flaps are the sickle version that extends to the axilla. There is no scar along the back bra line.

Case **5**

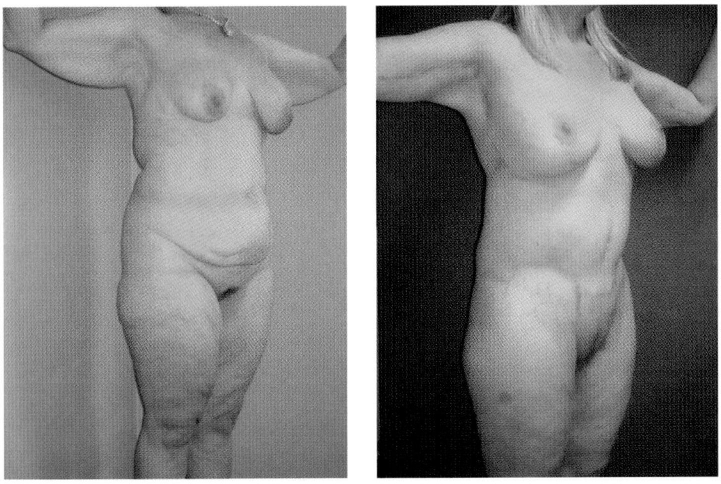

A   B

Figure 17.6   (A) Oblique view of a 5′ 8″, 185 pound, 48-year-old woman who lost 80 pounds through dieting and exercising. She disliked the sagging of her breasts which were augmented with 230 mL silicone gel filled plants 25 years ago. (B) Oblique view of 2 year result of her two stage total body lift. At the second stage her implants were removed and she had spiral flap reshaping with an UBL and bilateral L brachioplasties. At a third stage revision the lateral edge of the right breast was advanced.

Pitfalls and how to correct

The most common problem is that the breasts may be broad and boxy (Figure 17.5). This is due to the lateral position of the pedicle of the lateral thoracic flap. This appearance is more likely in the heavier breast. This problem is avoided by dissecting the pedicle as far medially as necessary; however, significant trans-serratus muscle perforators may be damaged. The safest way to approach this problem is to treat it secondarily by advancing the lateral IMF without resection of the lateral bulge. The lateral breast needs to be independently secured to serratus fascia at a medial and higher level. A wedge resection of skin between the NAC and IMF can be helpful in coning the breast.

The lateral IMF may drift inferiorly (Figure 17.6). The problem is due to slippage of the suture approximation of the reverse abdominoplasty to the serratus fascia, and recurrent laxity of the tissues. At the primary operation adequately mobilize the reverse abdominoplasty and suture with braided sutures taking large bites of the subcutaneous fascia and the serratus fascia and muscles. Tie all sutures while pulling the tissues together. Revision corrections are done the same way and tend to be a great improvement.

Post-operative care

The patient is admitted for three days of general care, and management of pain and fluids. The patient wears a support bra except for bathing for six weeks. The color of the NAC and Wise pattern flaps is checked periodically and, if congested and there is tension, sutures maybe removed. Patients at high risk for deep vein thrombosis receive chemoprophylaxis. The patient resumes her high protein diet with ProCare supplement as soon as possible, Vigorous physical activity is resumed between 4 and 6 weeks.

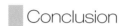 Conclusion

In properly selected massive weight loss patients, the breasts can be reliably augmented and better shaped with neighboring excess tissue called the spiral flap. The technique which includes an upper body lift is described herein for plastic surgeons versed in autogenous breast reconstruction.

Further reading

Holstrom H, Lossing C. The lateral thoracodorsal flap in breast reconstruction. Plast Reconstr Surg 1986;577:933–941.

Hurwitz D J. Single stage total body lift after massive weight loss. Ann Plast Surg 2004;52:435–441.

Hurwitz D. Breast reduction and mastopexy after massive weight loss. In: Spear SL (Ed). Surgery of the Breast. Philadelphia: Lippincott Williams & Wilkins; 2006: 1193–1209.

Hurwitz DJ, Agha-Mohammadi S. Post bariatric surgery breast reshaping: The Spiral Flap. Ann Plast Surg 2006;56;481–486.

Hurwitz DJ, Golla D. Breast reshaping after massive weight loss. In: Spear SL, Davidson S (Eds). New Trends in Breast Reduction and Mastopexy. Seminars in Plastic Surgery 18. New York: Thieme; 2004: 179–187.

Hurwitz DJ, Holland SW. The L Brachioplasty: An innovative approach to correct excess tissue of the upper arm, axilla and lateral chest Plast Reconstr Surg 2006;117:403–411.

Kwei S, Borud LJ, Lee BT. Mastopexy with autologous augmentation after MWL: The intercostal artery Perforator (ICAP) Flap. Ann Plast Surg 2006;57:361.

Levine JI, Soucid NE, Allen RJ. Algorithm for autologous breast reconstruction for partial mastectomy defects. Plast Reconstr Surg 2005;116:762.

Rubin JP, O'Toole J, Agha-Mohammadi S, Approach to the breast after weight loss. In: Matarasso RJP (Ed). Aesthetic Surgery after Massive Weight Loss. Philadelphia: Saunders Elsevier; 2006: 37.

Van Landuyt K, Hamdi M, Blondeel P, Monstrey S, Autologous augmentation of pedicled perforator flaps: Ann Plast Surg 2004;53:322–327.

Wuringer E, Mader N, Posch E, et al. Nerve and vessel supplying ligamentous suspension of the mammary gland. Plast Reconstr Surg 1998;101:1486.

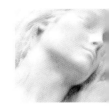

18

Complications in breast augmentation: maximizing patient outcomes with some surgical solutions to common problems

Bradley P. Bengtson

Key points

- We learn most from complications and our difficult revision patients.

- The key to maximizing patient outcomes and developing best practices is through refining the process of breast augmentation and minimizing complications.

- Common major complications of breast augmentations will be presented, along with some techniques for surgical revision.

- Specific techniques are discussed for capsular contracture, fold malposition, symmastia.

- Extrusion/potential infection will be presented.

- Capsular flap and neopocket techniques will be described in augmentation revision patients for malposition including the inframammary fold and symmastia.

Introduction

Learn from the mistakes of others.
You will never live long enough to make them all yourself

Sam Levenson

It has been said, 'If you do not have any complications, then you are not performing enough surgery.' Complications and revsion surgery are inevitable. Although our goal for surgical revisions should be zero and 'perfection', every plastic surgeon even a month into practice understands this goal is unattainable. One of my surgical mottos is: Pursue perfection, but accept excellence. Breast augmentation by its nature is elective and, because implants will not last forever, every patient we augment will require a breast revision surgery. The key to minimizing patient complications, maximizing patient outcomes and enhancing our surgical lives is to constantly pursue and improve the process of breast augmentation, determine which complications we can actually impact and lower, and then choose to make the necessary changes in our practices to achieve these goals. I am the first to recognize that changing the way we practice is difficult. Many studies have shown that once a physcian develops a routine for more than 5–7 years, few will change. Hopefully, after reviewing this brief chapter you will be challenged to look specifically how you are performing breast augmentation and as necessary adapt and change your approach to avoid the complication versus just viewing this chapter as correcting or enhancing a complication once it occurs.

As surgeons, unless we document, follow, photograph, are self-critical and objectively measure our patients and outcomes, we will underestimate our complications and overestimate the number of procedures we perform, and quite frankly the quality of our results. The turning point for me was beginning the Style 410 cohesive gel implant study. Being involved in an FDA, CRO reviewed, highly scrutinized new implant study brings with it immediate accountability. I would encourage each surgeon reading this text to make a conscious commitment to begin today to start a patient database (sample format included) tracking all of their breast augmentation patients and their outcomes. Once you make this choice and begin following your patients in this way, then can begin the positve patient cycle shown in Tables 18.1 and 18.2. So where

Table 18.1 Reporting outcomes data

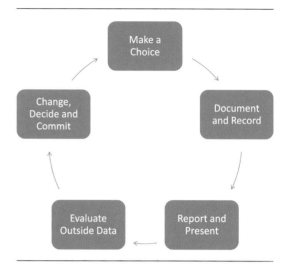

Table 18.2 So where is this going?

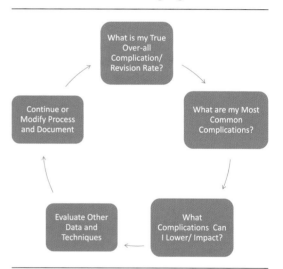

is this all going? We need to understand that breast augmentation is a process and that equally important as a refined meticulous surgical technique is preoperative patient assessment and education, implant selection and tissue based planning, and defined postoperative follow-up. We should constantly review our ever-advancing science and technique, evaluate data and documented experiences and constantly move toward 'excellence'. It is with this background and approach that I have prepared this chapter.

Complications may be presented in many different formats and ways. By their nature, they are difficult to

Table 18.3

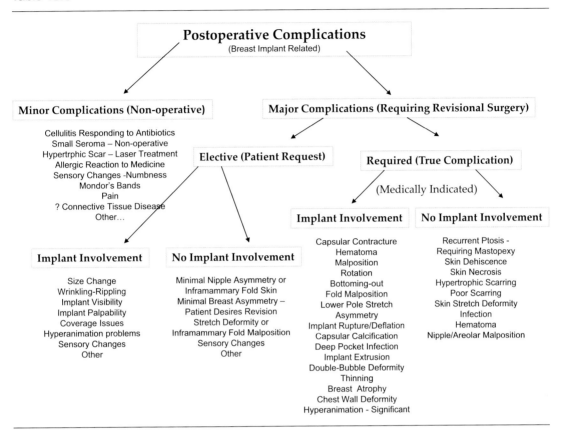

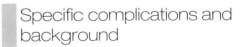

categorize with many patients having multiple problems such as malposition, thinning of overlying tissues, palpable and visible wrinkling and rippling simultaneously. We must also be careful not to create a new problem while we are correcting another, such as creating a fold malposition while correcting a capsular contracture. Shown here in Table 18.3 is one method. It has been modified since its initial publication (Bengtson 2005) and is not perfect but helps to show the most common complications in breast implant surgery. It also is not an excuse or an attempt to minimize a complication. All complications are not however equal in significance, and stratification is helpful in sorting both importance and frequency.

By adopting a standardized approach to the process of breast augmentation, complications may not be eliminated but untoward events and revisions can be minimized. We should also improve over time. I will be presenting a few of the most common complications in breast augmentation revsion, suggest ways to

minimize or prevent their occurrence, and describe some current approaches and techniques to correct, improve or enhance a specific complication and include specific patient case studies and outcomes.

Specific complications and background

Capsular contracture

Actual techniques in treating patients with capsular contracture depend upon multiple factors. Some of these include: the style and generation of the device, the position of the current implant pocket, if any complications occurred at the primary operation, the degree of glandular atrophy and coverage over the implant, any calcification of the capsule, prior size, manufacturer and surface of the implant, to name a few. If you did not perform the prior operation(s), obtaining the prior operative note and medical record is important along with weighing and assessing the implant intraoperatively. Saline implants not only have greater projection and radial diameter when inflated, they also weigh more. The shell of the implant has weight and adds 7–15% to the final weight of the device. Saline devices are filled at surgery, the shell has weight, and saline is more dense than gel. Silicone gel devices are pre-filled and their mL or weight includes the shell.

Options for revision in a patient with a capsular contraction have been well delineated. BASPI and additional options include: capsulotomy only, capsulectomy–partial or complete, capsular flap or neo-pocket with collapse of the capsule placing the new implant on top of the prior capsule, changing pocket planes, usually subglandular to partial subpectoral or dual-plane, and more recently adding a soft tissue matrix such as Alloderm or Strattice. It should also be mentioned that implant removal with or without capsulectomy may be performed without replacement. This is always an outpoint. The true etiology of capsular contracture is unknown; however the most common theories include a low-grade bacteria: bacterial theory and the hypertrophic scar theory secondary to blood, fluid or tissue trauma. It is likely that one or both play a role in each individual patient. Because the exact etiology is unknown, similar to deep vein thrombosis, I recommend doing everything possible to lower the incidence of capsular contracture or prevent it. In addition, technical points to maximize success and limit recurrence include: meticulous hemostasis and atraumatic technique, use of surgical drains with any capsulectomy, antibiotic irrigation such as the Adam's solution, perioperative antibiotics, and the use of op-site or tegaderm over the nipple. If implant rupture is suspected placement of a protective barrier drape over the entire incision area and chest/breast region will limit contamination and silicone skin contact (Figure 18.1).

Further background

The most common patient presentations include a subglandular capsular contraction where a position change is performed following capsulectomy and implant removal or a patient with a prior partial sub-muscular implant that has developed a capsular con-

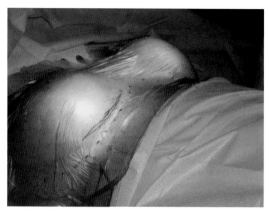

Figure 18.1 In cases of suspected implant rupture, a large op site dressing may be placed over the operative field including well below the incision to prevent contamination and skin–silicone contact. It also has the added benefit of decreasing contamination with coverage of the nipple.

tracture. Patient examples of each of these scenarios will be presented.

Capsular contraction

- Baker IV capsular contracture and an early generation silicone device placed in the subglandular position with visible distortion and asymmetry.
- Proper pre-operative informed consent including management of patient expectations and implant range and patient asymmetry information documented.
- Patient goals and desires are discussed and factored.
- Tissue based planning is performed and documented taking into consideration the measurements including the base width of the breast (BW), skin stretch (SS) or breast elasticity, sternal notch to nipple distances (SN-N), nipple to inframammary fold distances (N-IMF), contribution of the breast parenchyma. Assessment of the patient's chest wall and any breast ptosis and breast asymmetry are recorded.
- Surgical marking of the midline, IMF and pre-operative measurements are performed.
- Implant selection is confirmed.
- The new IMF incision is preferred and has been found to have the lowest complication rate and recurrent capsular contracture rate, although

periareolar may be used. The incision can be very accurately positioned directly in the IMF based on 'High Five', a selector device or other planning methods.

Operative technique for correction capsular contraction

- Large op-site dressing is applied to the entire field if implant rupture is suspected (Figure 18.1).
- A minimum of a 5 cm incision is made directly in the predetermined IMF.
- Pocket position is determined with partial submuscular prioritized for both soft tissue coverage and reduction of recurrent capsular contracture.
- New virgin pocket with heavily textured implant.
- Short acting anesthetics and muscle paralysis are used with multiple anti-nausea agents.

- In the case of a prior subglandular implant, if an older generation, thick or calcified, the entire capsule is removed including the implant preferably without capsulotomy (Figure 18.2). If a newer generation device is encountered, and thinning is present, the capsule against the muscle may be removed and anterior capsule left intact. This is dramatically facilitated with a double handle retractor, spatula retractor, lighted retractor, suction and consideration for tumescent fluid (Figure 18.3).
- In the case of a prior submuscular implant, a neopocket with capsular flap is made or a capsulectomy, complete or partial, may be performed (Figure 18.4).
- Atraumatic and bloodless precise pocket dissection is performed with prospective hemostasis either with creation of a new submuscular pocket or a

Case **1**

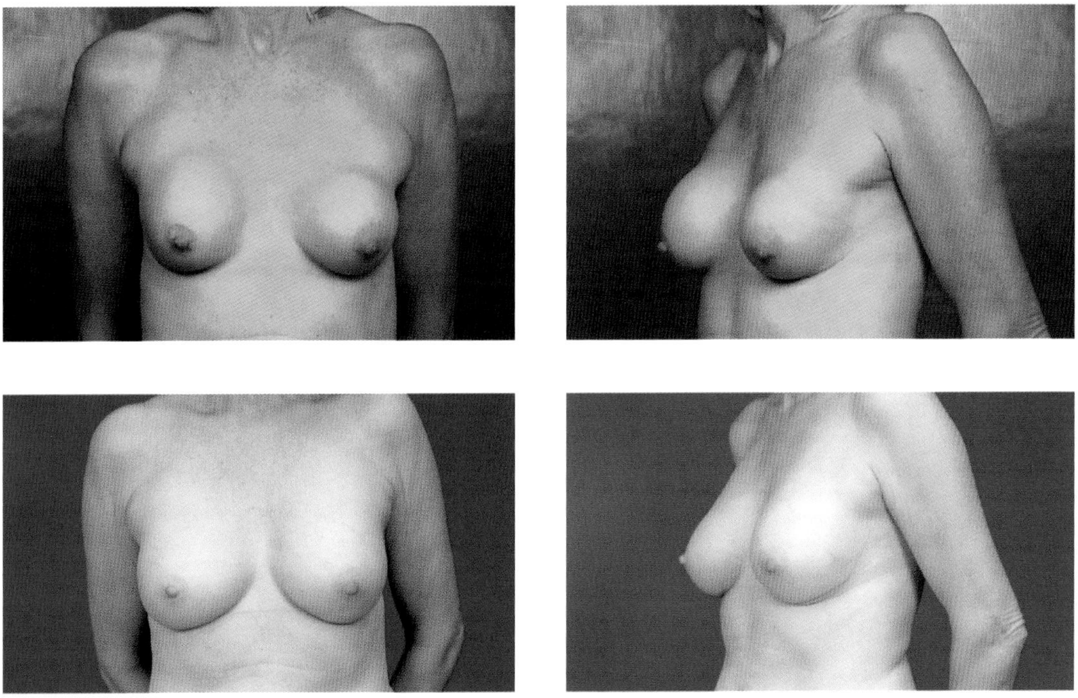

Figure 18.2   This patient had bilateral Baker IV capsules following a subglandular implant with 240 mL smooth silicone implants 16 years prior to surgery. Her tissue-based planning measurements included a 13 cm breast base width, 3 cm of skin stretch, 22 cm SN-N distance, and 8.5 cm N-IMF distances. Style 410 FM 350 g implants were placed in the partial submuscular, dual-plane placement position with her result shown at 5 years with no recurrence of capsular contraction and implants in good position.

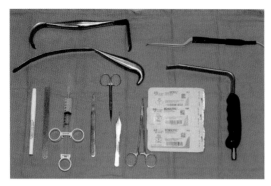

Figure 18.3 Instrumentation for breast augmentation revision cases is similar to primary cases. Spatula, retractor along with the double handle, lighted retractors and smoke evacuators are extremely helpful. 2-0 vicryl is used to set the IMF, 3-0 vicryl for a deep running closure and 4-0 monocryl for the subcuticular layer.

neopocket with a capsular flap method or capsulectomy.

● I prefer to begin the pocket dissection centrally proceeding laterally being careful not to over-dissect the lateral pocket, then defining the fold maintaining a fascial shelf when possible with prospective hemostatsis with monopolar cautery coagulating the perforating vessels as they come in above the muscle insertions, then medial and high in the pocket.

● The muscle fibers, including false insertions on the ribs are dissected free with preservation of the sternal insertions.

● Hand-in-glove pocket dissection is performed for form stable implants. Lateral pocket dissection is implant independent but for smooth devices the superior or cranial pocket is developed to the second rib.

Case 2

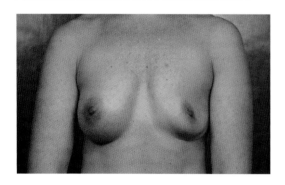
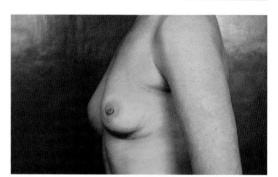
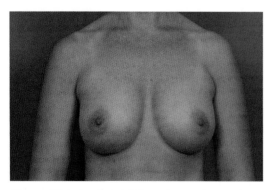
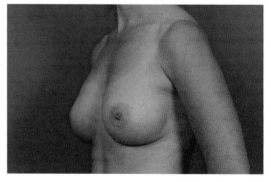

Figure 18.4 Implant deflation submuscular to submuscular with neopocket. This patient had a prior partial submuscular placement of 350 mL smooth saline implants 6 years prior to surgery. Her tissue based planning measurements included a 13.5 cm breast base width, 2 cm of skin stretch, 21 cm SN-N distance, and 9 cm N-IMF distances. Style 410 FM 440 g implants were placed back into a new partial submuscular, dual-plane placement position following a capsular flap, Neopocket procedure with her results shown at 30 months.

- Triple antibiotic irrigation using the Adam's solution (50 K units of bacitracin, 1 g of cefazolin and 80 mg of gentamicin in 250–500 mL physiological saline).
- No touch handling and placement of the implant is used with the surgeon touching the implant only and dipping his/her finger in antibiotic solution if pocket is re-entered including a glove change just prior to implant placement. Consideration for an insertion sleeve, particularly with textured devices (Figure 18.5).
- I like to put the implant in the first web-space of my left hand with constant pressure against the incision and spin the implant in with alternating index and thumb pressure versus a rocking back and forth from side to side motion.
- The patient is sat up at 90 degrees and symmetry checked. No blunt dissection with all additional pocket manipulation under direct vision with cautery and retractors.

- Closure is performed in multiple layers. I use a 2-0 vicryl to set or redefine the fold (Figure 18.6) followed by a 3-0 vicryl running suture to approximate the fascia and deep dermis followed by 4-0 monocryl running subcuticular closure.
- Particular attention is paid to the subcuticular closure medially and laterally to avoid a dehiscence and revision and the running suture approximates the incision completely.
- Steristrips, Dermabond® or a silicone sheet bandage is applied.
- Drains should be considered mandatory for any patient having a capsulectomy.
- No straps or bands are used and bras are optional. The surgeon should not rely on any external forces to try to correct a pocket malposition but may be used for support. If used, the bra should be loose at the fold and not pulling the breast up with push up bras.

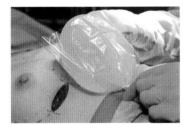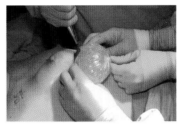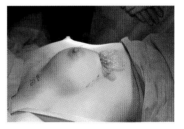

Figure 18.5 Insertion sleeve. A temporary plastic insertion sleeve is particularly useful when inserting heavily textured implants. I cut the sleeve in half and place antibiotic pocket irrigation fluid inside the pocket and sleeve. The assistant retracts and holds the twisted sleeve at the 6 o'clock position. After the inplant is in position, fingers are inserted inside the sleeve lifting up the implant off the chest and the posterior or deep side of the sleeve is removed first followed by the anterior sleeve.

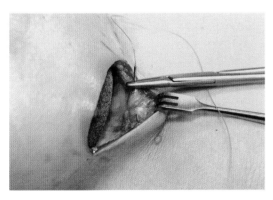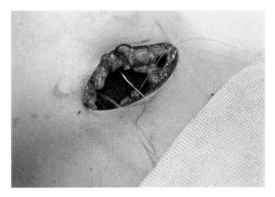

Figure 18.6 Fold reset. Securing of the inframammary fold position may be helpful in preventing malposition postoperatively. Keeping a fascial bridge medially, using a heavily textured implant facilitates maintaining position but even when using smooth devices the IMF may be further secured by placing a 2-0 vicryl suture in the chest wall and triangulating it to the superficial breast fascia. One or two sutures may be placed.

- Fast track recovery program: full arm ROM beginning in recovery and immediate return to full normal routine activity, and dinner the night of surgery okay.

Operative steps reviewed

- Opsite™ if implant rupture suspected.
- Minimum 5 cm incision.
- Pocket position determined.
- Short acting anesthetics and muscle paralysis.
- Atraumatic, bloodless and precise pocket dissection.
- Intra-operative antibiotics and antibiotic pocket irrigation.
- No touch implant techniques–implant placement spun in.
- Confirm pocket and IMF symmetry–sitting position in OR.
- Multiple layer–complete closure.
- Bra optional but no push-up.
- Immediate range of motion (ROM).
- Fast track recovery program.

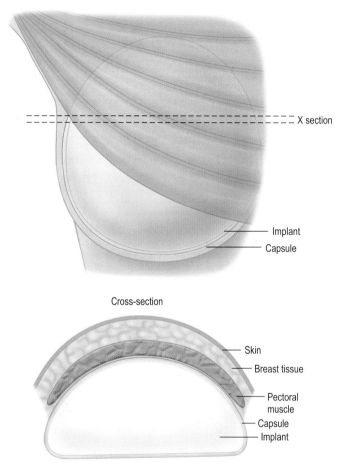

Figure 18.7 Capsular flap/neopocket procedure. The first description of the capsular flap is from Silver, presented at ASPS in Montreal in 1971. Its main application is where a prior implant already in the submuscular position is replaced back into the submuscular position, and it is particularly useful with heavily textured devices although it also works with smooth surface implants. Dissection is facilitated keeping the old implant in position and developing the plane between the anterior capsule and the pectoralis major. The old implant is then removed, capsule collapsed, trimmed and closed and the new implant is placed on top of the collapsed surface and back into the sub-pectoral space. The prior capsular space is shown where the previous smooth implant was present..

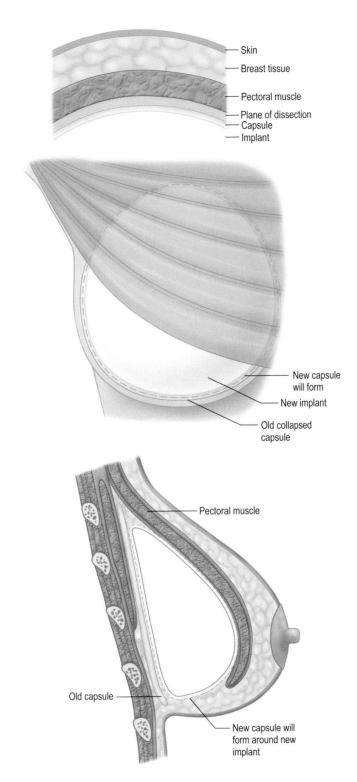

- Skin
- Breast tissue
- Pectoral muscle
- Plane of dissection
- Capsule
- Implant

- New capsule will form
- New implant
- Old collapsed capsule

- Pectoral muscle

- Old capsule
- New capsule will form around new implant

Figure 18.7 *Continued.*

Special technique: capsular flap neopocket procedure description

Utilization of capsular tissue in breast revision surgery is not a new concept. Both Silver in 1971 and Snyder in 1975 have described using the posterior capsule as an additional layer for breast augmentation revision. Per Heden in *Clinics of Plastic Surgery* in 2001 brought this technique back to the forefront noting that the new Style 410 cohesive gel implants require a brand new virgin pocket. Interestingly, in 1992 in a pig model we experimentally showed the rich vascularity of capsular tissue and showed it could support a skin graft. Clinically, we now have used this technique in over 200 patients for a variety of clinical situations including its original description for exposure of an implant and capsular contraction, as well as symmastia repair, malposition and areas of thinning and tissue weakness. I have found the posterior capsule useful but more unreliable centrally and more difficult to dissect. I prefer to use the anterior capsule layer if the patient's soft tissues are 2 cm thick, or at least 1 cm using the 410 device.

Capsular flap procedure

- The typical patient benefiting from this procedure has an implant in the partial subpectoral position and has a capsular contraction.
- It is useful with smooth devices and really mandatory when replacing with a heavily textured implant.
- A minimum 6 cm incision facilitates the dissection as does local infiltration or tumescent technique.
- Proper instrumentation is also critical with a double handled retractor, spatula retractor, Bovie extender, and smoke evacuator (Figure 18.3).
- The implant is left in place and a new plane is dissected on top of the anterior capsular surface and below the pectoralis.
- Care is taken not to over-dissect the pocket particularly when repairing a synmastia or malposition and placing a textured anatomical implant.
- Following dissection superiorly the medial and lateral pocket dimensions are defined.
- Capsulotomy at the base of the implant is performed and additional capsule trimmed and capsule closed on tension with a 3-0 vicryl to avoid sliding
- New implant is positioned with no touch technique following antibiotic pocket irrigation.

- A surgical drain is placed and closure performed in layers as previously described including a 2-0 vicryl setting of the inframammary fold.
- Still photographic images are shown (Figure 18.7).

Malposition

Implant malposition is the second most commonly reported complication in breast augmentation and thus revisional breast surgery. Malposition may be subdivided into:

1. Lateral malposition.
2. Fold malposition.
3. Lower pole stretch deformity / fold remaining intact.
4. Double bubble deformity/fold malposition or implant breast diameter mismatch.
5. Symmastia /loss of sternal muscle attachments.
6. A combination of these deformities.

Although not all, the vast majority of implant malpositions are preventable and may result from ignoring tissue based planning principles or not basing the implant selection on breast tissue assessment such as choosing an implant with too wide a base diameter, or over-projecting device based on the patient's soft tissue stretch. Malpositions may also result from a technical error with over-dissection of the lateral breast pocket or inframammary fold, or excessive release of the pectoralis muscles off of the sternum (symmastia). Patients should be informed that creating cleavage is not surgically recommended and informed about the consequences of symmastia with release of pectoralis major off of the sternum. Cleavage definition should be accomplished with bras or clothing. Additionally, malposition may occur when any device overpowers the breast soft tissues and their weight exceeds the internal support of the breast and soft tissues. This is extremely variable patient to patient, but the surgeon and the patient should accept that the larger and heavier the implant, the greater the likelihood of malposition. Other factors that affect malposition include genetics with poor skin tone, and degree of ptosis, and whether a concurrent mastopexy is performed; prior weight loss and pregnancies may all affect stretch deformities; however, many cases are preventable.

Another factor resulting in lower pole stretch and the degree of force being applied to the lower pole of the breast is implant style. Saline implants result in a greater degree of lower pole stretch than gel devices. In addition, there is much less stretch to the lower pole with Style 410 highly cohesive gel implants. In my first 300 primary augmentation patients the average stretch with up to 6 year follow-up is 2 cm on stretch and 1 cm at rest. Likely, the main reason for this is the heavily textured devices' interface with the submuscular pocket capsule helping to hold the device up, resulting in less pressure on the base of the breast.

Further background

Malposition of the inframammary fold is one of the more common complications and may occur as an isolated event or with a myriad of other deformities including lateral malposition. Fold malposition in my experience and corroborated by the literature is more common when a breast augmentation is performed from a distant site such as a non-endoscopically controlled transaxillary approach. The incidence of fold malposition in my previous practice through the transaxillary route was 17%, which is one reason why I have converted to the new inframammary incision.

It is critical to distinguish between a patient with IMF malposition versus lower pole stretch, because the treatment and surgical correction is different, recognizing some patients may have both. If I performed the primary operation, I record the measurements from the nipple to the fold on stretch, set the IMF and place the incision directly in the fold. Thus, if the incision is consistent in position, but the N-IMF has increased in length then lower pole stretch has occurred. If however there is an increase in the N-IMF distance and the incision is riding up on the breast, resulting in implant show below the incision, fold malposition has occurred. One method of fold malposition correction is shown. If lower pole stretch has occurred I resect a quarter-moon shape in the lower pole in an attempt to standardize the nipple to fold distance bilaterally. If there is both a fold malposition and stretch component, I perform both simultaneously.

Operative technique for correction of IMF malposition

- Symmetric markings of the midline and IMF are performed in the sitting or standing position. This may be facilitated with a level.
- I prefer a minimum of a 6 cm incision in the inframammary fold. If a skin resection is planned secondary to stretch this is included in the design.
- Senn retractors are placed below the incision and the plane between the capsule and subcutaneous space is dissected with Bovie cautery to just below the capsular space that has displaced.
- All surgery performed with precise, defined prospective hemostasis with no blunt dissection.
- With the implant still in position, dissection is then carried out cranially or superiorly 2 cm if no tissue matrix support is planned or to the lower border of muscle if acellular dermis or other material is planned.
- Capsulotomy at the inferiormost portion of the capsule is performed along the entire IMF so all capsule has been removed from beneath the skin in the area of fold malposition.
- Permanent sutures, I prefer 2-0 Ethibond™, are then placed securing the skin to the chest wall leaving a 6–8 mm ridge everted to have an edge to suture to.
- Two additional 4-0 polypropylene sutures are placed in a horizontal mattress fashion through skin, then chest wall or rectus fascia and out again and tied at the end of the procedure without a bolster. These are removed at 1 week.
- Any additional implant exchange or other pocket procedures are performed.
- The pocket is then irrigated with Adam's solution with intraoperative antibiotics administered in surgery and antibiotics initiated 2 days pre-operatively.
- No touch technique is used as described previously and implant placed back into the pocket with symmetry confirmed in the sitting position.
- The inferior leading edge of the capsule is then trimmed as necessary or imbricated upon itself as an additional layer of support further holding the implant up in position.
- If an acellular dermal matrix or other support is utilized, it is sutured to the leading edge of the pectoralis muscle as an extension and then into the IMF moving from lateral to medial after being tacked into position.
- Drains are used with any soft tissue matrix or for any bleeding whatsoever.
- Closure is then performed in multiple layers with 3-0 vicryl in the deep fascia, 4-0 monocryl in the deep dermis followed by a 4-0 monocryl subcuticular suture.
- A loose bra is applied along with a single panel from an abdominal binder for support beneath the breast.

- No bouncing motion or impact aerobics for 6 weeks and no downward pressure on the breast.
- I have had no recurrences with this technique in over 20 patients with up to a 7 year follow-up.

Operative steps reviewed

- Minimum 6 cm incision in IMF.
- Atraumatic, bloodless and precise pocket dissection.
- Antibiotics 2 days preoperatively intra-operative antibiotics and pocket irrigation.
- No touch implant techniques.

- Capsulectomy beneath skin below IM fold.
- Skin sutured with permanent suture back down to chest wall.
- Horizontal mattress reinforcing sutures.
- Confirm pocket and IMF symmetry, sitting position in operating room.
- Capsular closure for further support at fold.
- Multiple layer–complete closure.
- Minimal to no overcorrection on the table.
- Supportive bra and single panel binder below breast.
- No stress to IMF for minimum of 6 weeks.

Case **3**

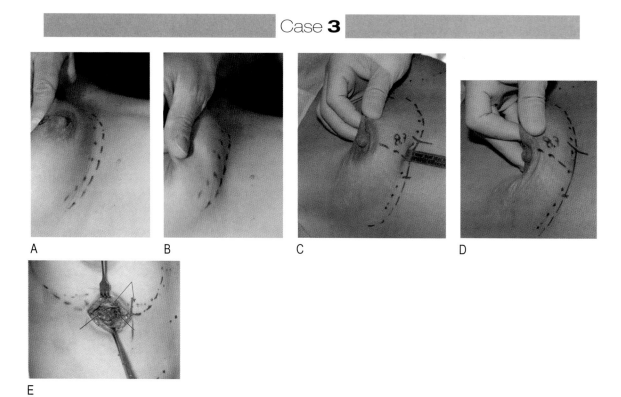

A   B   C   D

E

Figure 18.8 (A-D) Malpositioned IMF. There is a difference in the inframammary fold in the sitting/standing position and the actual fold anatomically as it inserts on the chest. Because of this anatomic difference, a breast implant may be lower than the pre-operative fold as transmitted to the skin. This is also the reason why the transverse inframammary scar rides up in a tight breast reduction closure when present. Muntan and Nava and Acland's group have nice histologic descriptions that give insight as to how this may occur clinically. (E) The red arrow denotes superficial fascia of the breast that transmits to the sitting fold location additional red arrow. The blue arrows show the true inframammary fold and location of the base of the implant.

Case **4**

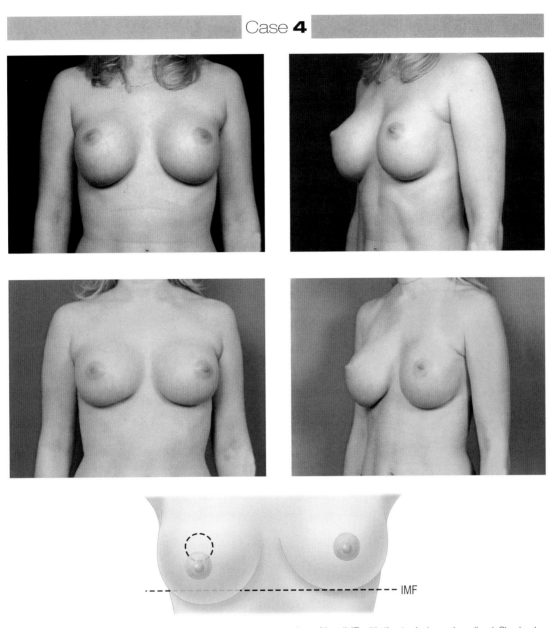

Figure 18.9 Malpositioned IMF. This patient had reconstruction of her IMF with the technique described. She had 390 mL smooth saline implants filled to 420 mL and when explanted secondary to the saline fill and shell weight equalled 450 g. Capsular flap was performed along with resection of the redundant capsule in the region below the fold with replacement and replacement utilizing a 397 mL Style 15 smooth silicone device. The fold was secured with 2-0 Ethibond® deep back down to the chest wall and further by horizontal mattress 4-0 polypropylene removed at 1 week. Her result is shown at 24 months.

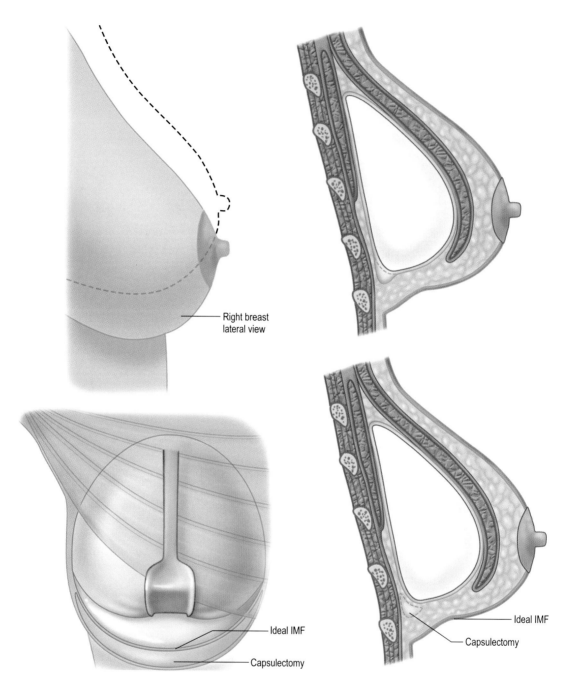

Right breast
lateral view

Ideal IMF

Capsulectomy

Ideal IMF

Capsulectomy

Figure 18.9 *Continued.*

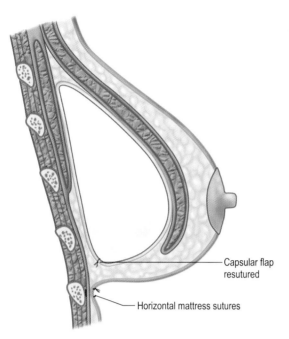

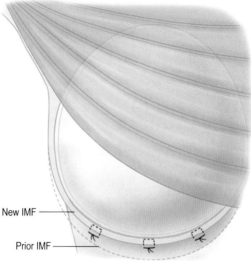

Capsular flap
resutured

Horizontal mattress sutures

New IMF

Prior IMF

Figure 18.9   *Continued.*

Malposition symmastia

Synmastia fortunately occurs more infrequently than IMF or lateral malposition. This complex problem is a result of pectoralis muscle fibers being dissected off their sternal attachments. Although multiple stage reconstructions have been described, single stage revisions can be very effective. Correction is similar to IMF correction with suturing of the underlying capsule back down to the sternum, creation of a neopocket with a capsular flap and consideration for the reinforcement with a acellular dermal matrix.

Operative technique for symmastia correction

- General anesthesia is required.
- Pre-operative, intra-operative and post-operative antibiotics are utilized along with antibiotic pocket irrigation as previously described.
- A minimum of a 6 cm IMF incision is made or periareolar approach used.
- Capsular flap with a neopocket is made either elevating posterior capsule off the chest wall beginning 4–5 cm lateral to the desired medial implant position or if adequate anterior soft tissue coverage is indeed available (rare) a complete

neopocket as described above may be used. This is the desired approach and important (or total capsulectomy) if a textured shaped implant is used to avoid rotation.
- This also is an ideal indication for Strattice or other acellular dermal matrix to further reinforce the medial pocket and adding additional soft tissue coverage medially over the implant where visible wrinkling and rippling is a common concurrent problem.
- Suturing of the pre-sternal soft tissues back down to the chest wall may be performed for further reinforcement similar to a IMF repair if exposed.
- Drains are used and a multilayer closure is performed as described previously.

Operative steps reviewed

- Minimum 6 cm incision in IMF.
- Atraumatic, bloodless and precise pocket dissection.
- Antibiotics 2 days pre-operative, intra-operative antibiotics and antibiotic pocket irrigation.
- No touch implant techniques.
- Suturing of the soft tissues overlying the sternum may be helpful depending on capsular flap technique used.

- Skin may be sutured with permanent suture back down to chest wall but is not required.
- Consider additional soft tissue matrix support internally.

- Confirm pocket and IMF symmetry, sitting position in operating room.
- Final result achieved on the table. No over correction required.

Case **5**

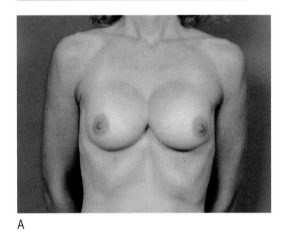
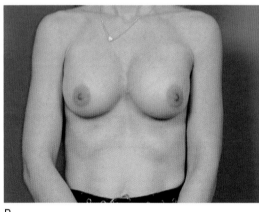

A   B

Figure 18.10   Malposition symmastia. This patient 3 years prior underwent submuscular placement of 300 mL smooth saline implants filled to 320 mL bilaterally and developed symmastia. Bilateral capsular flaps with neopockets were made and Style 410 FM 350 g implants were placed using the technique described with her post-operative result shown at 3 years.

Extrusion - infection

Background

Treatment of infections around a breast implant remains a controversial topic, although some recent studies have suggested retention of the implant except in the face of extensive purulence. Some articles included in the Further Reading section address this issue including BASPI. My surgical approach to this rare occurrence is similar to potential or near extrusion. If caught early with no Gram stain appearance of bacteria, debridement, irrigation, capsular flaps and or local muscle flaps may be effective without an interval time of explantation. With evidence of true bacterial contamination or frank purulence, I recommend an interval of explantation of a minimum of 3 months and preferably 6 months or longer.

Operative technique for near extrusion

- Patients are likely already on antibiotics. If they are not however a course is begun. In addition to peri-operative, and post-operative specific antibiotics, pocket irrigation is performed.
- Debridement of thinned damaged tissue preferably prior to actual exposure of the implant as soon as possible.
- Capsular flap elevation either the posterior capsule off of the chest wall, anterior turn down capsular flap, or both. Local muscle or fascial flaps particularly rectus abdominus muscle or fascia may also be utilized.
- Drains, implant placement with no touch techniques, and multiple layer closure as previously described is performed.

- Again, a soft tissue matrix for further support should be considered.

Operative steps reviewed

- Minimum 6 cm incision in IMF.
- Atraumatic, bloodless and precise pocket dissection.

- Antibiotics 2 days pre-operative, intra-operative antibiotics and antibiotic pocket irrigation.
- No touch implant techniques.
- Consider additional soft tissue matrix support.
- Confirm pocket and IMF symmetry–sitting position in operating room.

Case **6**

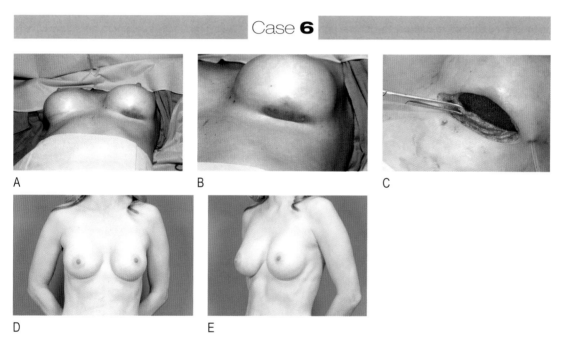

A   B   C

D   E

Figure 18.11 (A-C) Extrusion/infection. This patient had near extrusion following secondary augmentation revision with a Style 410 cohesive gel, 290 gm FF implant. She was immediately returned to surgery and the pocket was debrided and irrigated with antibiotic solution. The thin skin was resected and a posterior wall capsular flap was raised, a new implant placed and skin reapproximated over the capsular closure. She was kept on antibiotics for 2 weeks post-operatively and went on to heal primarily with no further skin breakdown, thinning, infection or capsular contracture. (D,E) Additional clinical photographs are shown at 1 year following revision.

Post-operative care

My post-operative care following revisional breast surgery is similar to primary augmentation except for activity instructions. I have patients resume normal routine activities within 48 hours, and provide detailed instructions for the first 6 weeks. It is vital that the post-operative instructions are seamlessly integrated into the pre-operative planning. In revision breast surgery, I limit vigorous physical activity for 6 weeks. Additionally, I have patients take an antibiotic for 1

week post-operatively and they typically are managing surgical drains. Because the etiology of capsular contracture is likely multifactorial and uncertain, I do everything I know of that may lower its incidence: electrocautery dissection, meticulous hemostasis and use of drains to minimize and limit blood and fluid collection, along with pocket antibiotic irrigation to decrease any bacterial load. In capsular contraction revision patients with smooth devices, I instruct on vertical implant displacement exercises twice daily for

30 s each compressing the breast up in the pocket and pushing medially. For highly cohesive implant patients, no implant massage is performed. For IMF and symmastia revisions and prior extrusion patients, I do not have them stress their repairs with any pressure.

The future of surgery

The future for breast augmentation is exciting. There is an initiative underway to improve the process of breast augmentation at all levels from pre-operative patient evaluation, education and informed consent to tissue based planning and implant selection to refining of surgical techniques and defined post-operative care. Advancing through this process, complications will decrease, patient experiences, results and satisfaction will increase and most importantly patients will benefit. In addition, breast implant technology continues to evolve and improve, and new materials such as acellular dermal matrices, techniques, procedures, and instrumentation continue to progress. The future is bright, but our main focus should remain on reducing complications versus developing new technology and procedures to treat them.

Conclusion

Breast augmentation complications and revision breast surgery continue to be a challenge in plastic surgery with revision and reoperation rates remaining 15–30%. Change can indeed occur and rates dramatically decreased by advancing the entire process of breast augmentation, naming, claiming, recording and tracking our results and choosing to alter our approaches based on accurate outcomes data. Patients and surgeon will benefit directly. The best way to deal with a complication is to do what we can to completely avoid them in the first place. In the meantime, presented are some surgical solutions and methodology for correction of some very difficult problems. I hope they add to your armamentarium.

. . . .

Further reading

Adams WP. The process of breast augmentation: four sequential steps to optimizing outcomes for patients. Plast Reconstr Surg 2008; in press.

Adams WP, Bengtson BP, Glicksman C et al. Decision and management algorithms to address patient and food and drug administration concerns regarding breast augmentation and implants. Plast Reconstr Surg 2004;114:1252–1257.

Adams WP, Rios JL, Smith SJ. Enhancing patient outcomes in aesthetic and reconstructive breast surgery using triple antibiotic breast irrigation: six-year prospective clinical study. Advances in breast augmentation. Plast Reconstr Surg 2006;118(7Suppl):46S–52S.

Adams WP, Teitelbaum S, Bengtson BP, et al. Breast Augmentation Roundtable. Advances in breast augmentation. Plast Reconstr Surg 2006; 118(7Suppl):175S–187S.

Bengtson BP. Four Year Experience with style 410 highly cohesive gel implant. Presented at the American Association of Aesthetic Plastic Surgery Meeting, New Orleans, 2005.

Brown MH, Shenker R, Silver S. Cohesive silicone gel breast implants in aesthetic and reconstructive breast surgery. Plast Reconstr Surg 2005;116:768–779.

Burkhardt BR, Dempsey PD, Schnur PL et al. Capsular contracture: A prospective study of the effect of local antibacterial agents. Plast Reconstr Surg 1986;77:919.

Handel N, Cordray T, Guitierrez J. Long-term study of outcomes, complications, and patient satisfaction with breast implants. Plast Reconstr Surg 2006;117: 757–767.

Inamed directions for use and Inamed Corp. Silicone gel and saline implant PMA clinical trials. Available at: http://www.fda.gov/cdrh/breastimplants/index.html.

Nava M, Quattrone P, Riggio E. Focus on the breast fascial system: a new approach for inframammary fold reconstruction. Plast Reconstr Surg 1998;102: 1034-1045.

Mentor directions for use and mentor corp. Silicone gel and saline implant PMA clinical trials. http://www.fda.gov/cdrh/breastimplants/index.html.

Muntan CD, Sundine MJ, Rink RD, Acland RD. Inframammary fold: a histologic reappraisal. Plast Reconstr Surg 2000;105:549–556.

Rempel JH. Treatment of an exposed breast implant by a muscle flap and by fascia graft. Ann Plast Surg 1978;1:229.

Spear SL, Bogue DP, Thomassen JM. Synmastia after breast augmentation. Advances in breast augmentation. Plast Reconstr Surg 2006;118(7Suppl):168S–171S,

Spear SL, Bulan EJ, Venturi ML. Breast augmentation. Advances in breast augmentation. Plast Reconstr Surg 2006;118(7Suppl):188S–196S.

Spear SL, Carter ME, Ganz JC. The correction of capsular contracture by conversion to 'dual-plane' positioning: technique and outcomes. Advances in breast augmentation. Plast Reconstr Surg 2006; 118(7Suppl):103S–113S.

Spear S, Cunningham B. The breast implant safety supplement. Plast Reconstr Surg 2007; Dec.

Spear SL, Howard MA, Boehmler JH et al. The infected or exposed breast implant: management and treatment strategies. Plast Reconstr Surg 2004;113:1634–1644.

Tebbetts JB. Dual plane breast augmentation: optimizing implant soft tissue relationships in a wide range of breast types. Plast Reconstr Surg 2001;107:1255–1272.

Tebbetts JB. A system for breast implant selection based on patient tissue characteristics and implant-soft tissue dynamics. Plast Reconstr Surg 2002;109:1396–1409.

Tebbetts JB. 'Out points' criteria for breast implant removal without replacement and criteria to minimize reoperations following breast augmentation. Plast Reconstr Surg 2004;114:1258–1262.

Tebbetts JB, Adams WP. Five critical decisions in breast augmentation using five measurements in 5 minutes: the high five decision support process. Advances in breast augmentation. Plast Reconstr Surg 2006;118(7Suppl):35S–45S.

Wong CH, Samuel MM, Tan BK, et al. Capsular contracture in subglandular breast augmentation with textured versus smooth breast implants: a systematic review. Plast Reconstr Surg 2006;118:1224–1236.

Wood S, Spear SL. What do women need to know and when do they need to know it? Silicone Breast Implants: Outcomes and Safety Supplement, Plast Reconstr Surg 2007;118(7Suppl):135S–139S.

Index

Index

moderate, 155, 156, *158*, *160*
no vertical breast reduction/mastoplexy, 231–2
periareolar incision, 20
pre-operative evaluation, 2
recurrent, mastopexy complications, 165
semi-cohesive gel implant indications, *76*, *78*, *79*
severe, 155, 156, *159*
silicone implants, 49
breast reconstruction
autologous fat transplantation, *139*, 141, *142*
saline implant patient selection, 41
breast size
decrease, secondary augmentation, 114–15, *118*
discussion *see* pre-operative evaluation
increase, secondary augmentation, 114
preference evaluation, circumvertical breast reduction
technique, 188
breast tissue
amount, saline implant patient selection, 39–40
thinning/atrophy, patient selection for semi-cohesive
gel implants, 64
breast upper pole
breast fat distribution, secondary augmentation, 96
thickness, pre-operative physical examination, 4, *5*
vertical mammaplasty, 219
breast width (BW) measurement, mastopexy, 154
broad/boxy breasts, massive weight loss (MWL) patient
complications, *251*, 252

C
caliper pinch thickness, secondary augmentation, 101
capsular contracture, 83, 105, 107–9, *117*, 255–62
antibiotics, 109–10
bacterial infection, 256
causes, 40
correction techniques, 107–8, *119*, 257–8, *259*
antibiotics, 259
aseptic techniques, 259
capsular flap/neopocket procedure, 262
closure, 259
drains, 259
dressing, *256*, *257*
instruments, *257*, *258*
pre-operative preparation *see below*
prior subglandular implants, 257, *257*, 260–1
prior submuscular implant, 257, *258*
device role, 109–10
drains, 110
hypertrophic scar theory, 256
implant rupture, 256, *256*
incision choice, 109
pharmacologic agents, 109
pre-operative preparation, 256–7
prior operative notes, 256
revision options, 256
risk of, informed consent, 13
saline implants, 40
secondary augmentation, 98

sterility, 110
subglandular, *119*
capsular flap/neopocket procedure, capsular contracture
correction, 262
capsulectomy, 108
skin envelope problems, with mastopexy, 106–7
submammary, 108–9
capsulorrhaphy, superior malposition correction,
111–12
central pedicle, mastopexy, *162*
centrifugation, fat processing, 130, *130*
chest wall flap, vertical mammaplasty, 219
circumvertical breast reduction technique, 187–99
closure, *190*, 190–1, *191*
complications/pitfalls, 198
hematomas, 192
skin slough, 192
indications, 188
inverted T technique, 188
marking, 188
operative steps, 191
patient selection, 188
pre-operative preparation, 188
results, 187, 191–2, *194–7*
technique, *188*, 188–90, *189*, *193*
anesthesia, 188, 191
cone suture, 188–9, 191, *192*
de-epithelialization, 188, 191, *191*
parenchyma removal, 188, 191, *192*
sutures, 189–90, *190*, 191
wound division, 191, *193*
w-pattern parenchyma removal, 187
circumvertical incision, mastopexy, *161*, *163*
cleavage, pre-operative physical examination, 2
clinical studies
cohesive gel implants, 254
complication avoidance, 254
closure
Benelli periareolar technique, 170, *172*, *174*
capsular contracture correction, 259
circumvertical breast reduction technique *see*
circumvertical breast reduction technique
concentric mastopexy without parenchymal
reshaping, 169
Góes periareolar technique with mesh support, 173,
177, *178*
incision selection, 25
inframammary fold malposition correction, 263
inframammary incision, 18–19, *19*
massive weight loss patient *see* massive weight loss
(MWL) patient
no vertical breast reduction/mastoplexy *see* no
vertical breast reduction/mastoplexy
periareolar approach complications, 175
periareolar incision, 21–2, *22*
semi-cohesive gel implants, 80
subfascial transaxillary breast augmentation, 88, *88*
subpectoral approach, 31, *31*

Index

Index

Index

Index

Index